Parenting from Womb to Adolescent

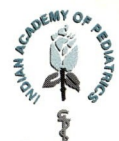

IAP GDBP Academy

Parenting from Womb to Adolescent

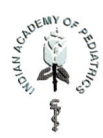

IAP GDBP Academy

Chief Editor

Suchit Tamboli
MBBS DCH PGDMLS PGDAP

National Chairperson, IAP GDBP Chapter 2014–15
Consultant Pediatrician
Chiranjiv Child Development and Research Institute
Ahmednagar, Maharashtra

Associate Editor

Santosh Nimbalkar
MBBS DCH PGDDN

Consultant Pediatrician
Morya Multispeciality Hospital
Kolhapur, Maharashtra

CBS Publishers & Distributors Pvt Ltd

New Delhi • Bengaluru • Chennai • Kochi • Mumbai • Pune
Hyderabad • Kolkata • Nagpur • Patna • Vijayawada

Disclaimer

Science and technology are constantly changing fields. New research and experience broaden the scope of information and knowledge. The editors, contributors have tried their best in giving information available to them while preparing the material for this book. Although, all efforts have been made to ensure optimum accuracy of the material, yet it is quite possible that some errors might have been left uncorrected. The publisher, the printer, editors and contributors will not be held responsible for any inadvertent errors or inaccuracies.

Parenting from **Womb** to **Adolescent**

ISBN: 978-81-239-2587-5

Copyright © Indian Academy of Pediatrics and Publisher

First Edition: 2015

Published by Satish Kumar Jain and produced by Varun Jain for

CBS Publishers & Distributors Pvt Ltd

4819/XI Prahlad Street, 24 Ansari Road, Daryaganj, New Delhi 110 002, India.

Ph: 23289259, 23266861, 23266867   Website: www.cbspd.com
Fax: 011-23243014   e-mail: delhi@cbspd.com; cbspubs@airtelmail.in.

Corporate Office: 204 FIE, Industrial Area, Patparganj, Delhi 110 092

Ph: 4934 4934   Fax: 4934 4935   e-mail: publishing@cbspd.com; publicity@cbspd.com

Branches

- **Bengaluru:** Seema House 2975, 17th Cross, K.R. Road, Banasankari 2nd Stage, Bengaluru 560 070, Karnataka
  Ph: +91-80-26771678/79   Fax: +91-80-26771680   e-mail: bangalore@cbspd.com
- **Chennai:** 7, Subbaraya Street, Shenoy Nagar, Chennai 600 030, Tamil Nadu
  Ph: +91-44-42032115   Fax: +91-44-42032115   e-mail: chennai@cbspd.com
- **Kochi:** 36/14 Kalluvilakam, Lissie Hospital Road, Kochi 682 018, Kerala
  Ph: +91-484-4059061/65   Fax: +91-484-4059065   e-mail: kochi@cbspd.com
- **Mumbai:** 83-C, Dr E Moses Road, Worli, Mumbai-400018, Maharashtra
  Ph: +91-22-24902340/41   Fax: +91-22-24902342   e-mail: mumbai@cbspd.com
- **Pune:** Bhuruk Prestige, Sr. No. 52/12/2 + 1 + 3/2 Narhe, Haveli (Near Katraj-Dehu Road Bypass), Pune 411 041, Maharashtra
  Ph: +91-20-64704058/59, 32392277 Fax: +91-20-24300160   e-mail: pune@cbspd.com

Representatives

- **Hyderabad** 0-9885175004   • **Kolkata** 0-9831437309, 0-9051152362
- **Nagpur** 0-9021734563   • **Patna** 0-9334159340   • **Vijayawada** 0-9000660880

Printed at: India Binding House, Noida, UP

To

my sons: Kshitij and Anvesh

Dr Santosh's sons: Shantanu and Indraneel

without them the word parenting may not have been understood by us.

For all parents who always try to bring best out of their children.

Foreword

I read "Parenting from Womb to Adolescent" with interest. This is one of the most important areas of information for a country like ours. We are a "young nation" committed to develop a large pool of skilled workers in every subject. Our beloved Prime Minister has emphasized this again and again.

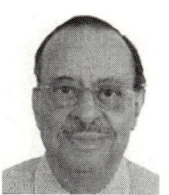

How could we develop this pool? By creating a secure bond between parents, caregivers and growing children, besides emotional attachment (which does not need any training!) right direction in every aspect of growth and development needs to be used as reinforcement.

I am happy to note that the contributors of this book are not only medicos but also psychologists, sociologists, teachers, administrators and other health caregivers. Dr Suchit Tamboli was trained in developmental medicine at KEM Hospital, Pune. Pioneering work on this subject was done at this institute since the eighties. Dr Tamboli has taken this subject to further heights.

I am confident that this book will have wide readership cutting across all specialties. This will act as a reference book for families who want to know more about "parenting".

I congratulate IAP GDBP for taking this initiative. My best wishes for its success.

Dr Anand Pandit
MD FRCPCH (UK)
Honorary Professor and Director
Department of Pediatrics, Neonatology
TDH Rehabilitation Centre
Morris Child Development Centre

Foreword

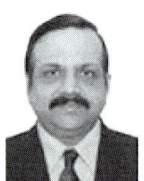

It is both a pleasure and a privilege to write the foreword to this book *Parenting from Womb to Adolescent*. Parenting our children is one of the most weighty responsibilities we have in our whole lives. Yet a few of us receive any formal training in how to be good parents. This book aims to enable parents with an essential tool to improve the quality of our parenting.

This book has emphasized the importance of an early start by preparing 'to be parents' to be physically and emotionally strong with proper premarital counseling. This book also includes vital information on the importance of monitoring growth, balanced diet, exercise, pre-school education, as well a full session on common discipline mistakes and the solutions. I am sure this will be a great book for pediatricians, students as well as parents.

I am sure that the pediatricians and parents will appreciate the magnanimous and magnificent effort taken by the Dr Suchit Tamboli, Dr Santosh Nimbalkar and all the contributors in bringing out this wonderful book.

Dr SS Kamath
President—Elect 2014
Indian Academy of Pediatrics (IAP)

Foreword

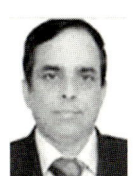

It gives me immense pleasure to present this book *Parenting from Womb to Adolescent* published under the banner of Indian Academy of Pediatrics, Growth, Development and Behavioral Pediatrics Chapter.

At times it gets very difficult for a busy practicing doctor to find the right information about problems related to growth, development and behavioral pediatrics. They do not know how to answer the parents in OPD. This book provides scientific way to answer them. Parents will also find this book of great help in upbringing their children.

I congratulate the chief editor and present chairperson of Chapter Dr Suchit Tamboli and associate editor Dr Santosh Nimbalkar and the team for their efforts to bring this wonderful book on parenting.

My sincere thanks also goes to the authors who have taken their valuable time to contribute to this book. I hope this book will be useful to the practitioners and parents for whom it is published and will become their desk companion.

Dr Vijay N Yewale
President, IAP 2014

Contributors

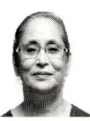
Shabina Ahmed MD
Consultant Paediatrician
(Developmental) and
Director
Assam Autism Foundation
Guwahati

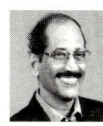
Chandrashekhar Dabhadkar
MD DCH PGD-DN FIAP
Consultant Pediatrician at
Mahad (Raigad)
Maharashtra

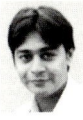
Amol Annadate MD DCH
Pediatric and Neonatal
intensivist, Anand Hospital
and Postgraduate
Teaching Institute. Vaijapur
Aurangabad, Maharashtra

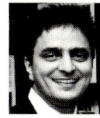
Samir Dalwai
MD DCH DNB FCPS LLB
Developmental and
Behavioral Pediatrician,
New Horizon Child
Development Centre
Mumbai, Maharashtra

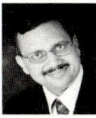
Anurag Bajpai MD FRACP
Pediatric and Adolescent
Endocrinologist, Fortis
Memorial Research Institute
Gurgaon

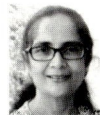
Sushma Desai MD DCH
Practicing Pediatrician and
Adolescent Counselor
Surat, Gujarat

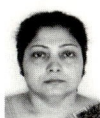
Monideepa Banerjee MD
Clinical Director of
Paediatrics Peerless
Hospital, Kolkata
West Bengal

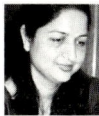
Preeti Deshpande
MBBS DGO
Consultant Gynecologist
Deshpande Maternity and
Surgical and IVF Centre
Ahmednagar, Maharashtra

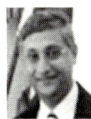
Anjan Bhattacharya
MBBS DCH MRCP MRCPCH
Developmental
Pedictrician, Child
Development Centre
(CRC) Apollo Gleneagles Hospital
Kolkata, West Bengal

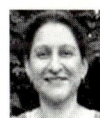
Preeti Galgali
MD PGDAP
Adolescent Medicine
Specialist and Director
Bangalore Adolescent
Care and Counseling Centre
Bengaluru Karnataka

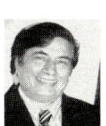
Shrikant Chorghade
MBBS DCH
Consultant Paediatrician
and Behavioral Consultant
Nagpur, Maharashtra

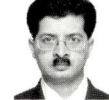
Sunil Godbole MD
Consultant Paediatrician
Deenanath Mangeshkar
Hospital and Research
Centre, Pune
Maharashtra

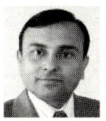
Jaydeep Choudhari
MD DC
Associate Professor
Department of Pediatrics
Institute of Child Health
Kolkata

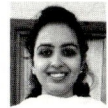
Supriya Phanse Gupte
MD ΓICMCH
Consultant Pediatric
Endocrinologist, Columbia
Asia Hospital, Pune
Maharashtra

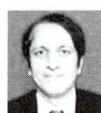

Pramod Jog
MD DNB FIAP FICMCH

Professor, Department of
Pediatrics, Padma Shri
Dr DY Patil Medical College
and Research Centre, IAP President—
Elect 2016 Pune, Maharashtra

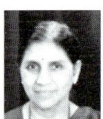

Archana Joshi MD DCH
Joshi Children Hospital and
Neonatal Intensive Care
Unit, Virar, Mumbai
Maharashtra

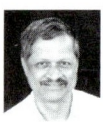

Hemant Joshi MD DCH
Joshi Children Hospital and
Neonatal Intensive Care
Unit, Virar, Mumbai
Maharashtra

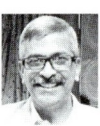

Atul Kanikar MD DCH
Adolescent Care
Pediatrician
Nasik, Maharashtra

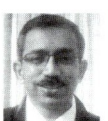

Sandip Kelkar MD DCH
Consultant Pediatrician
Prathamesh Hospital
Jupiter Hospital and
Kaushalya Hospital
Thane, Maharashtra

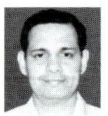

Vaman Khadilkar MD DCH
MRCP

Consultant Pediatric and
Adolescent Endocrinologist
Jehangir Hospital, Pune
Maharashtra

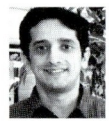

Upendra Kinjawadekar
MD DCH

Consultant Pediatrician
Navi Mumbai, Maharashtra

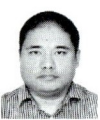

**Chingthang
Kshetrimayum** MD
Resident Fellow
Department of
Neonatology, MSRMH Bengaluru,
Karnataka

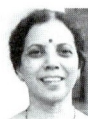

Sandhya Kulkarni
MSc (Biophysic), DMRIT

Associate Director and
Chairperson
New Horizons Institute of
Education and Research
Mumbai, Maharashtra

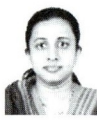

Shailaja Mane
MD PGDPC PGDMLS PGDAP FRIPH

Professor, Department of
Pediatrics, Padma Shri
Dr D.Y. Patil Medical
College and Research
Centre, Pune. Maharashtra

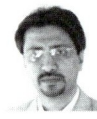

Zafar Meenai MBBS DCH
Consultant Developmental
Pediatrician, Coordinator
Child Development Cell
People's College of
Medical Sciences and
Research Center, Bhopal
(MP)

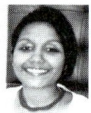

Nita Mehta
MA (Clinical Psychology) DHRM

Clinical Psychologist and
In-Charge, New Horizons
Health and Research Foundation,
Mumbai, Maharashtra

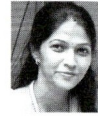

Deepti Kanade Modak
MA (Clinical Psychology), DHRM
Clinical Psychologist and
In-Charge, New Horizons
Health and Research
Foundation, Mumbai, Maharashtra

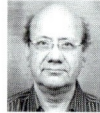

Anil Mokashi MD DCH PhD
Consultant Paediatrician
and PG Teacher
Dr. Anil Mokashi Hospital
Newase Road, Baramati
Maharashtra

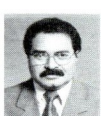

MKC Nair MD DCH
Director Professor
Child Development
Centre,Government
Medical College Campus
Thiruvananthapuram-11; Kerala

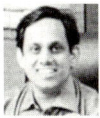

Santosh Nimbalkar
MBBS DCH PGDDN

Consultant Paediatrician
Morya Multispeciality
Hospital, Kolhapur
Maharashtra

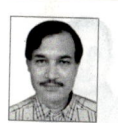

Sailaja Nandan Parida
MD FIAP FNNF
Consultant Paediatrician
Asian Institute of Public
Health, Bhubaneswar
Odisha

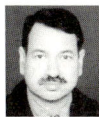

Ashok Rai
MD PhD FIAP FIAMS

Consultant Pediatrician
Apollo Hospital, Varanasi
and Kilkari Institute of Child
Health, Varanasi

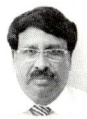

Jaydeb Ray MD DNB DCH
Professor of Pediatrics
ICH, Kolkata
West Bengal

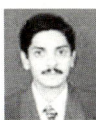

Chandrakant Sanklecha
MD

Consultant Gynecologist
and Obstetrician
Nasik, Maharashtra

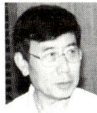

Ksh Chourjit Singh
MD DCH

Professor and Head
Department of Pediatrics
Jawaharlal Nehru Institute
of Medical Sciences,
Imphal, Manipur

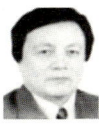

N Heramani Singh MD
Professor and Head
Department of Psychiatry
Regional Institute of
Medical Sciences Imphal
Manipur

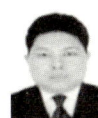

S. Gojendra Singh MD
Assistant Professor
Department of Psychiatry
Regional Institute of
Medical Sciences, Imphal,
Manipur

Suchit Tamboli
MBBS DCH PGDMLS PGDAP

National Chairperson, IAP
GDBP Chapter 2014–15
Consultant Pediatrician
Chiranjiv Child Development and
Research Institute, Ahmednagar
Maharashtra

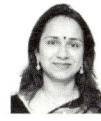

Anjana Thadani
MBBS DNB DCH FCPS

Consultant Developmental
Pediatrician and Director
Niramaya Hospitals
Navi Mumbai, Maharashtra

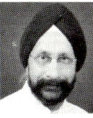

JS Tuteja MD DCH
Consultant Pediatrician
Indore (MP)

Preface

Parenting is the key word of 21st century. Every parent wants his child to be the best in this competitive world.

While bringing best out of their child they must remember that the children require love, security and mental satisfaction. If you know your child well by proper scientific methods you can make your child successful in his life. You must identify the qualities in your child. Parents should perform the role of Krishna as in Mahabharat war. They should know how to stimulate and when to counsel their child. They must understand the potential of their children.

Parenting starts before marriage and you must know that adolescent girl's wt 45 kg and ht 145 cm is essential for the marriage. She should increase wt by 9–11 kg in pregnancy to get healthy baby of 2.5 to 3 kg.

After delivery the child should have 5 important milestones to be observed till one year of age as follows:

1. Social smile—2 months
2. Neck holding—4 months
3. Sitting—8 months
4. Standing—12 months
5. Understand meaningful words and utter baba, mama, dada—12 months

Parents must not label the child but they should label his bad behavior. They should stimulate, encourage and reinforce the child positively by giving age-appropriate toys and conducive environment according to their mental age.

In pre-school age group the curriculum must enrich the child in gross motor, fine motor, personal social, mental, expressive and receptive language. They must put their child in first standard after completion of 6 years only. Completing 6 years is important for their skills to develop. Emotional literacy can be taught since 4 years of age. IQ, EQ & SQ will help the child to develop up to their maximum potential. Emotional intelligence is essential to become successful in their life.

In the school age group study skills and behavioral problems like anxiety, depression, phobias affect the performance of the child.

In adolescent age group social media, drugs, sexual abuse, peer pressure plays important role in molding the character of the adolescent.

Life skills help them to become a mature person in their life.

This book will help students of medicine, general practitioners, pediatrician, teachers, parents to understand the child from **Womb to Adolescent.**

Suchit Tamboli
Chief Editor
Santosh Nimbalkar
Associate Editor

Acknowledgments

We are grateful to our executive committee of growth, development and behavioral chapter who always have encouraging words.

Our sincere thanks to the various contributors from all over the country for their tireless efforts to submit the articles.

We are also thankful to Dr Vijay Yewale (President, IAP 2014), Dr Pravin Mehta (Secretary, IAP 2014), Dr SS Kamath (President, IAP 2015), Dr Pramod Jog (President, IAP 2016) for their active help.

We are really very grateful to Dr Anand Pandit, who is pioneer of this field in India and my teacher for always being there without whom we are no where.

Thanks to CBS Publishers & Distributors, Mumbai, for publishing this book. We must thanks specially to Mr Ramesh Krishnamachari for his commitment and follow-up without whom this book may not have reach in time to you all.

We are also grateful to Mrs Neha Tamboli and Mrs Sangeeta Nimbalkar for their active help and encouragement. We are thankful to Miss Shraddha for her tireless efforts on computers to make this book successful.

We are grateful to all those who have given their valuable contributions.

Suchit Tamboli
Chief Editor
Santosh Nimbalkar
Associate Editor

Contents

Section 3: Growth and Nutrition of Child

Section 4: Toddler

Section 5: School Age

Section 6: Special Child

Section 7: Adolescent

Section

1

Parenting—before and after Marriage

1

Importance of Parenting Classes before Marriage

MKC Nair

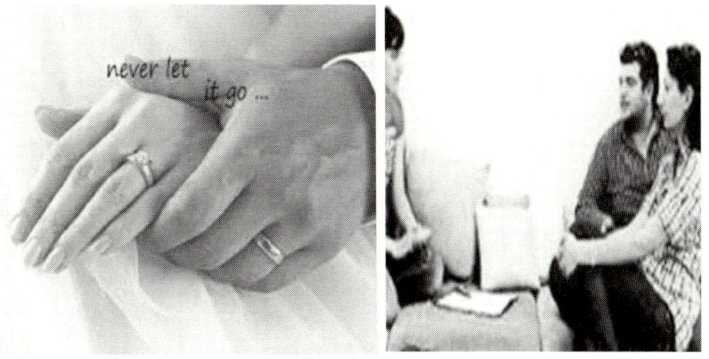

Parenting is an art and science at the same time. There are definite scientific principles for appropriate parenting, though the art of parenting is often learned from our own parents. Some of us are blessed with an offspring early on after marriage, some a little later and quite a few who never. Whether early or late, most of us go through this stage of the life cycle totally unprepared. For many, it is just another natural phenomenon in life to welcome the new one and it is, in essence the fulfillment of life itself. We never ask ourselves whether we are prepared for parenthood—mentally, emotionally, physically and financially. And it is not uncommon that we wonder why all these preparations are needed for receiving the "God given gift". Like in any other matter, planning for a family is also essential as it helps us to understand what pregnancy and parenthood is all about. And to really grasp the complicated dimension of parenting one must start right from when life begins.

Premarital Counseling Services

Although parenting classes/premarital counseling should be given after legal age for marriage is achieved, in the Indian context, because of early marriage age, the same could be offered more effectively to any adolescent over 15 years of age. But for this we need total support and commitment of parents that is not often forthcoming. The finding of a CDC Kerala study, supported by Indian council of medical research (ICMR), done to assess parents' and teachers' attitude towards adolescent reproductive sexual health education showed; (i) 65.2% of parents and 40.9% teachers have not discussed growth and development issues with their adolescents; (ii) more than 50% of parents were not sure whether information on topics like masturbation, dating, safe sex, contraceptives, pregnancy, abortion and childcare should be provided to adolescents. (iii) 44% of parents agreed that information on HIV/AIDS/STD should be provided; and (iv) only 5.2% teachers and 1.1% parents discussed sexual aspects with adolescents. It is huge task to reach out to millions of above 15 boys and girls and hence we should use services of all community health care providers, including trained nursing students, anganwadi workers of Integrated Child Development Services and ASHA workers of National Rural Health Mission, India. The key messages in the community premarital counseling module should be as follows:

- The ideal time to have a baby is between the ages of 20–35 years of age, when girls are physically and psychologically grown up to conceive a baby.
- A pre-pregnant weight of at least 40 kg and a height of at least 140 cm is ideal, as it reduces the chances of giving birth to a low birth weight baby (<2.5 kg)
- To those mothers at risk for giving birth to a child with chromosomal abnormalities like Downs syndrome, chromo-somal studies and prenatal diagnosis is a must, though not always feasible.
- Intra uterine infections like toxoplasmosis can cause irreversible damage to the growing fetus and hence the pregnant lady should avoid contact with domestic animals, as they are the carriers of many infections.

- All adolescent girls should be vaccinated against rubella as infection occurring during pregnancy will cause problems in the fetus like low birth weight, small head, deafness, cataract, various birth defects, etc.
- Vaccination against human papillomavirus (HPV) is advisable for girls to prevent cervical cancer after many years, though high cost of the vaccine is a barrier.
- A medical checkup is important to rule out common sexually transmitted infections (STIs) like gonorrhoea, syphilis, chancroid, herpes and HIV/AIDS.
- A gynecological check-up before marriage is important to detect menstrual abnormalities, vaginal infections and polycystic ovary syndrome (PCOS) all with increasing chances of producing infertility.
- 5 mg of folic acid daily soon after marriage till pregnancy could prevent neural tube defects (large head, split spinal cord) up to 75% in the baby.
- Avoid drugs during 2nd half of menstrual cycle as fertilization occurs around 14th day.

Content of Counseling Sessions

Thus, the counseling session should include:
  i. Family life and life skill education
 ii. Enhancing coping strategies
iii. Improving communication strategies
 iv. Guidance on morality/spirituality issues
  v. Self-empowerment both economic and social
 vi. Vaccination for prevention of rubella, hepatitis B, human papillomavirus infections
vii. Screening for STIs/ HIV, lifestyle disease markers, mental health, reproductive health
viii. Medical examination including breast and external genitalia
 ix. Transabdominal ultrasound examination if indicated
  x. Sex and sexuality skills needed in family life including understanding needs of self as well as the partner.

While examining any adolescent and particularly a female adolescent, it is a must (a) to have presence of her mother, (b) explain what specific examination you are going to do and why and (c) get her permission at every stage of examination in a reassuring way.

Points to remember

1. Parenting is an art and science
2. Planning   to become parent is important
3. Premarital counseling should be given from 15 years of age
4. Counseling session should prepare them physically and emotionally strong to become good parents.

1

I Want a Healthy Baby— Counseling for just Married Couple

MKC Nair

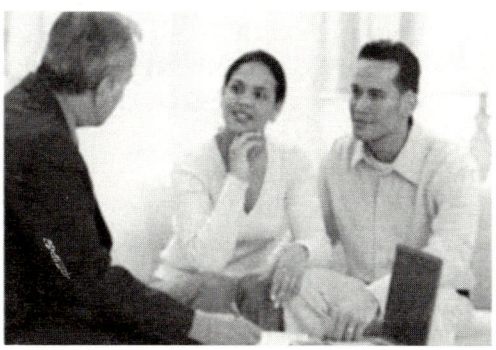

When life begins with the union of the sperm and the ovum to form the zygote, there starts the role of parents. Many enter into this phase of life without any planning or preparations and for most it may not be by choice but sudden or random. As in all aspects of life one must make preparations for parenting too. Both the husband and wife need to equip themselves— financially, emotionally, and socially. What are the different aspects that have to be looked into? How to be equipped for this?

1. Both partners must educate themselves with all necessary information on pregnancy and childcare. Maintaining birth spacing of at least 3 yrs is recommended for the mothers' and the baby's health.

2. During pregnancy, women should have more number of feeds, of small quantities. A balanced diet rich in iron and protein should be taken during pregnancy. Hence, a mother to be should have plenty of greens, grams and grains.

3. Extra folic acid intake three months before and after conception could significantly reduce the risk of having a baby with birth defects such as neural tube defects—spina bifida and anencephaly.

4. Avoid medication without prescription in the second half of menstrual cycle, if you are planning to be pregnant.

5. Health checkup is a must for parents to be to rule out reproductive health problems, mental health problems and for adjusting dose of medication for medical problems like epilepsy, asthma, diabetes or hypertension.

6. Before getting pregnant, make sure to take vaccination against rubella to avoid a baby born with congenital heart defects, low birth weight, developmental delay, visual and/ or hearing impairment.

7. Taking drugs, tobacco and alcohol during pregnancy carry risk especially on the fetus and hence it is advisable to avoid them including passive smoking through the husband.

8. Remember that fetal harm can result from prior parental exposure to toxicants either directly affecting the maternal or paternal reproductive organs or getting stored in the body and later mobilized during pregnancy.

9. During pregnancy mother has to eat enough to meet the nutritional needs of the baby, to have the strength and vitality for labor and also breastfeeding after delivery.

10. In the second trimester, a pregnant woman needs 300 kcal more than in the pre pregnancy stage. Hence, proper intake of food both in terms of quantity and quality is important. Pregnant woman should have a balanced diet of greens, grams and grains. The diet should consist in addition to the principal food at least half liter of milk, 1 egg or equivalent, plenty of green vegetables and fruits.

Tips for Care during Pregnancy

Each day of pregnancy may be eventful for the mother to be. Hence it is natural to have many doubts and apprehensions in all the trimesters of pregnancy-right from confirming pregnancy to delivery, especially so for the first timers.

During the first trimester, which is the extremely crucial period of fetal development

    i. Antenatal visits should be carried out once in a month

   ii. Avoid unaccustomed exertion and long distance travel by bad road

  iii. Avoid sexual intercourse during the first trimester as this might cause miscarriage in some one who has a tendency for it.

   iv. Consult your doctor if you contract any viral infections or other illness.

    v. Consult your doctor before taking any drugs to confirm its safety

   vi. Eat nutritious food, home made, with lots of green leafy vegetables.

  vii. Throughout pregnancy period maintain good personal hygiene especially of the genital area so as to avoid infections.

In the Second Trimester

    i. The movement (life) of the baby can be felt at about the 18th week of conception. If not doctor should be consulted.

   ii. 2 doses of TT vaccinations at an interval of 6 weeks should be taken.

  iii. Do your antenatal exercises as per the doctor's advice.

   iv. Do not strain yourself physically.

    v. Skin changes especially pigmentation of the face is common during this period. Don't worry, as this is likely to disappear after delivery.

In the Third Trimester

    i. Make regular antenatal visits. More frequent visits are needed as term approaches.

   ii. If the nipples are retracted, correction should be done in the later months of pregnancy by finger manipulation or by using nipple shields.

  iii. Discuss with the doctor, labour and delivery, especially if there is any risk factor like hypertension, diabetes, etc.

Make sure that a hospital selected for delivery has resuscitation facilities for the baby and emergency cesarean section or at least vehicle facility for emergency referral.

iv. Prepare the older child to welcome the younger one. Make necessary preparations clothes, money, vehicles and human resource for the approaching delivery.

v. Consult the doctor if there is any swelling of the feet and hands, excessive tiredness and pallor, white discharge, itching in the genital area.

vi. If a lowered fetal movement, bleeding or sudden gush of water leakage from the vagina is noticed report to the doctor immediately.

vii. Avoid sexual intercourse during the last 6 weeks as this may lead to premature delivery.

viii. Painful uterine contractions at an interval of 10 minutes or earlier and continuing for at least an hour, may be suggestive of labor pain. Seek medical attention as early as possible.

ix. During pregnancy mother has to eat enough to meet the nutritional needs of the baby, to have the strength and vitality for labor and also breastfeeding after delivery.

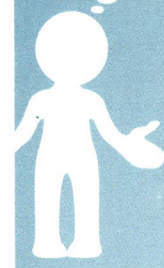

Points to remember

1. Both the husband and wife need to equip themselves—financially, emotionally, socially to become good parents.
2. Mother should take proper care with medical guidance to deliver physically and mentally healthy baby.

Home Sweet Home

Shrikant Chorghade

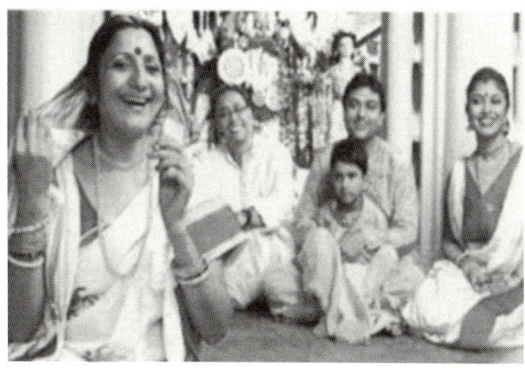

Personality development of a child since birth onwards is determined by many variables. The most important amongst them is the relationship with the family members. Home is the primary environment for every child. The home doesn't only provide food, shelter and education but it is responsible for the shaping of the child's personality.

Scientific study about influence of home on an individual has been done in various cultural settings. The conclusion reveals four major reasons of prime importance of home, and its effect on development of child's personality.

a. **Time spent in the home:** The home environment is responsible for shaping up of child's personality. Home provides this environment where the growing child spends most of its time. This prolonged association with home environment and relationship sows the seeds of personality.

b. **Control on behavior:** Family members exert control on the behavior of a child. Parents have undoubtedly the greatest influence but in a joint family set up, grandparents, uncles and aunts, older siblings, baby sitters, other paid servants play the role of surrogate parents who also have influence on the child. Amongst parent, a mother has more control than father as she spends much more time with the child. In a nuclear family, usually child's behavior is controlled by the mother while father has control of money matters. Permanency on the control is determined by the time spent with the child by the caretakers; hence a mother has maximum control over behavior of a child.

c. **Emotionally determined relations:** Persistence of family relationship reinforces the effect on the emotional life of a child. Emotional bonding with the members of the family is so strong that it is likely to persist in the child even after the death of the member concerned. It is not uncommon that father or mother are respected and worshiped even after their death.

d. **Early experiences:** Child's early social experiences take place in home settings. Mr. Glasner has rightly said "personalities are formed in the first instance within the womb of family relationship". Child's attitudes, values and patterns of social behavior are determined by early social experiences in home settings. During early years of a child, the parents exert maximum social influence. The parenting style which parents deploy, serves as formative force on child's social behavior. The frustrations parents impose, the rewards and incentives which are offered, the methods of discipline to control the behavior of a child are all responsible for social development of a child.

e. **Security in home:** With an anchorage of family relationship the child develops a feeling of security in home. The child can maximally enjoy his triumphs and glory in home settings. His sorrows and defeats are also smoothened in home. A child feels inadequate and unhappy without this heaven called 'home'.

In home settings the family members influence the shaping of child's personality in two ways.

    I. Directly   II. Indirectly

i. **Direct influence of family:** Every member in a family loves a child and gives a feeling of security which motivates a child to learn by trial and error. At the same time every member in the family tries to teach the child as and when in varied fields. A child is disciplined, and is taught social and moral values. The child is made aware about the right and wrong thing, socially acceptable and unacceptable behaviors. This helps the child to build up its personality. Whatever may the parenting style, parenting does affect a child's development. In a nuclear family mother and father are the only people in home available for offering love and feeling of security and teaching social and moral values and skills. While in a joint family, there may be grandparents, uncles, aunts, and cousins in addition to parents and older siblings. All of them have their share to contribute child's development. In a nuclear family in addition to parents there may be older siblings, babysitters, paid servants who try to teach mannerism, values and skills. The same thing will happen in a joint family.

ii. **Indirect influence:** A child may or may not listen to what the parents or grant parents try to teach or inculcate. At the same time the child silently observes and tries to imitate speech, mannerism expressions, skills and hobbies of members in the family. This happens naturally with child's own initiative and choice and desire. In a joint family a child has wide variety of personality patterns and mannerism to imitate.

The children are silent observers and imitators of the family members regarding the ways they handle their emotions and stress. A child living with parents who are nervous, anxious and lacking in sense of humor, makes the child anxious, nervous and subject to outburst of anger. On the other hand a child who is brought up by warm affectionate, happy and interesting parents becomes gregarious, showing interest and affection while dealing with the family members or outsiders.

Nagging parents or family members may beget a team of nagging people. Happy and cheerful parents or family members can set a pattern of happy and contented children. The more

3

significant a family member is to the child; greater will be the effect and impact of his and her expressions, mannerisms and behavior on the growing child.

Other indirect effect occurs as due "mirror image" of the child. This effect is the result of the way child is looked at, labeled, and treated by the family members and significant people around. A child, who is constantly criticized and demeaned, develops poor self-concept and inferiority complex. While a child who is praised, encouraged and rewarded has a positive self-image and a higher self-respect resulting into a self-confident personality.

Another indirect effect can be due to the attitude of family members towards other siblings. If the parents or other family members show favoritism to other siblings in the family the child may develop jealousy towards the favored child sibling and attitude of jealousy and resentment toward people of authority outside the home set up.

Friction and conflicts in a family also have indirect impact on a child. Friction between parents in a nuclear family or any two members in a joint family affects the emotional climate in home, causing stress in the child. If other family members start taking sides in this conflict there may occur increase in severity of turbulence making the child anxious and stressful.

Any major event in the family has indirect impact on the emotional state of the child. Death in the family, long-term illness in a family, a child may feel neglected imbibing a feeling of insecurity in a child resulting into behavioral aberrations. Even celebrations can imbibe a similar feeling if child is not a participant in the celebrations. Success of other siblings, favoritism to other siblings also affects a child's emotional balance negatively.

Points to remember

1. Home is the primary environment for every child.
2. Relationship with the family members is important factor for personality development of child.

Section

2

Parenting—Pregnancy and Neonatal Period

As soon as
Pregnancy is Diagnosed

Preeti Deshpande

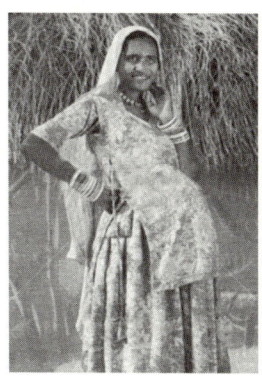

Congratulations, you are pregnant!

Behind every wish, there is hidden responsibility. You are thinking of getting pregnant then you are responsible for one new life. Pregnancy is a dream and a way to ultimate fulfillment—the achievement of motherhood. It begins with conception and the beginning of life and culminates in the arrival of a lovely new human being.

To understand this awe-inspiring process which converts a single cell into small baby kicking away with life, you should know a few things.

Points to keep in mind if you want to be a mother

- The best age for having baby is between 20 to 30 years of age
- You should be physically fit and free from undue anxieties and on healthy nutritious diet at least 3 months before conception.

- Avoid medication, X-ray, smoking, alcohol consumption before and after pregnancy.
- If working in a hazardous department (risk of exposure to X-ray/chemicals), move to safer department or take adequate precautions.
- In case you are suffering from any medical disorder like high BP, diabetes, heart disease then consult your doctor and bring them under control before you go in for pregnancy.
- Any hereditary disorder in the family should be discussed with your doctor.

4

Once you have decided and taken care of these things, to succeed, you must be aware of fertile period in your cycle. The best chance of conception is around the period of ovulation so medication (like for postponement of menstrual cycle for religious occasions, etc.) should be avoided.

We obstetrician think that pregnancy should not be by chance but it should be by plan. It is to be planned when you are physically, mentally, socially and economically fit.

These are a few points which you should know about pregnancy

- Duration of pregnancy is 40 weeks
- First day of LMP (Last Menstrual Period) is to be taken into consideration. From LMP, we can calculate EDD (Expected Date of Delivery) 7 days and 9 months to be added to LMP.
- From LMP we can calculate exact gestational age of that particular date so that you can compare growth of the baby.
- 9 months are divided into 3 trimesters (each of 3 months). Each trimester has its own event, preparation and minor problems to be coped with, as the baby grows within.
- When a period is missed, one should go to the doctor and confirm the pregnancy.
- Once the pregnancy has been confirmed, you now choose your obstetrician. You have to decide which hospital or under which doctor you want treatment. Do consider the

distance between your home and the hospital. Firstly enquire about that hospital (it should be well-equipped, a pediatrician should be available), doctor, their degree, their experience. Once you are convinced, keep faith in the doctor.

- *Sex of the baby*—there are certain specific cells which decide the sex of the baby. Ordinary body cells contain 46 chromosomes but reproductive cells—eggs and sperm have only half the number. A chromosome contains coded information regarding hereditary traits of the individual. Information regarding sex of the baby is stored in sex chromosomes labelled as X chromosome and Y chromosome. All eggs carry a single X chromosome, although some sperms carry the X chromosome and others the Y chromosome. When a sperm carrying the X chromosome unites with the ovum, a girl child is born (XX). And when sperm carrying Y chromosome unites with the ovum, a boy is born (XY). **The male sperm determines the sex of your baby. It is decided at the time of fertilization and no subsequent efforts will change it.**

- In 1st trimester, many patients will complaint of nausea and vomiting. It is called as morning sickness. It will remain till the end of the 1st trimester. It is worse in the morning and may continue throughout the day. The cause is hormonal changes which are taking place in the body. There are medications which doctor will prescribe to you. Diet should also be modified accordingly. Frequent small feeds should be taken throughout the day. Smell of certain food will aggravate or precipitate the symptoms. They should be avoided.

On your first visit, your few necessary investigations are to be done.

- Haemoglobin
- Blood group
- Blood sugar
- Hepatitis B antigen
- HIV testing
- VDRL

- Thyroid function
- Urine exam

These are the basic lab investigations

- Ultrasound in first trimester is to be done to confirm pregnancy
- To see single or multiple pregnancy
- To know exact gestational age
- This is very important
- Ultrasound is very safe in pregnancy. It doesn't harm baby and if possible it is to be done every two monthly
- At around 22nd to 24th week anomaly scan is to be done. This scan is to rule out any congenital anomaly, each organ is checked for that.
- At around 32 week one more scan is advised. At this stage growth of the baby, status of the liquor, growth retardation is noted.
- At the 35 36th weeks ultrasound is done for positions of the baby

Nowadays few special investigations recommended

The *triple marker screen test* analyzes how likely an unborn baby is to have certain genetic disorders. It is also known as a multiple marker test. The exam measures the levels of three important substances in the placenta: alpha-fetoprotein (AFP), human chorionic gonadotropin (HCG), and estriol.

Triple marker screening is administered as a blood test for women who are between 17 and 18 weeks pregnant. An alternative to this test is the quadruple marker screen test, which also looks at inhibin A.

Down syndrome

Edwards syndrome neural tube defects (such as spina bifida and anencephaly).

NST (Non Stress Test) this investigation is done for fetal wellbeing. After 32 week onwards.

Diet for a Healthy Pregnancy

Now that you're a mum-to-be, it is important to eat well. This will make sure you get all the nutrients you and your developing baby need.

If your diet is poor to begin with, it is even more important to make sure you have a healthy diet now. You need more vitamins and minerals, especially folic acid and iron.

You need a few more calories during your pregnancy as well. Getting your diet right for pregnancy is more about what you eat than about how much. Limit junk food, as it has lots of calories with few or no nutrients.

Eat a variety of foods from these different food groups each day:

Milk and dairy products: Skimmed milk, yogurt/curd, buttermilk (chhaach), cottage cheese (paneer). These foods are high in calcium, protein and vitamin B_{12}. Talk to your doctor about what to eat if you are lactose intolerant.

4

Cereals, whole grains, dals, pulses and nuts: These are good sources of protein if you do not eat meat. Vegetarians need about 45 grams of nuts and 2/3 of a cup of legumes for protein each day. One egg, 14 grams of nuts, or ¼ cup of legumes is considered equivalent to roughly 28 grams of meat, poultry, or fish.

Vegetables and fruits: These provide vitamins, minerals and fibre.

Meat, fish and poultry: These provide concentrated proteins.

Fluids: Drink lots of fluids, especially water and fresh fruit juices. Make sure you drink clean boiled or filtered water. Carry your own water when out of the house, or buy bottled water from a reputed brand. Most diseases are caused by waterborne viruses. Go easy on packaged juices as they have very high sugar content.

Fats and oils: Ghee, butter, coconut milk and oil are high in saturated fats, which are not very healthy. Vanaspati oil is high in trans fats, which are as bad for you as saturated fats. A better source of fat is vegetable oils because these contain more unsaturated fat.

Dairy products, along with sea fish and sea salt or iodised salt are all good sources of iodine. You need plenty of iodine in your diet to help your baby's development.

Even though everyone will advise you to eat for two, the average woman does not need any extra calories during the first six months of pregnancy. Your body actually becomes more efficient at extracting the required energy and nutrients from your diet when you're expecting a baby.

Although latest research suggests that a pregnant mum only needs 200 extra calories a day in her last trimester, most doctors recommend 300 extra calories a day in the second and third trimesters.

But, you may need more or less calories if you were underweight or overweight before getting pregnant or if you are pregnant with more than one baby. Your doctor will be able to recommend what calorie count best suits you during your pregnancy.

You can add 200 additional calories to your daily diet with: 2 rotis without ghee one plain dosa with a dollop of coconut chutney, 2 bananas, 2 scrambled eggs.

Your own appetite is the best indication of how much food you need to eat and you may find it fluctuating during the course of your pregnancy:

In the first few weeks you may not feel like eating proper meals, especially if you suffer from nausea or sickness. Try then to eat smaller but more frequent meals throughout the day. During the middle part of your pregnancy your appetite may come back. You may be hungry and feel like eating more than usual.

Towards the end of your pregnancy your appetite will probably increase. If you suffer from acidity, heartburn or a full feeling after eating you may find it helpful to have small frequent meals.

The best rule is to eat when you are hungry and to choose healthy food rather than calorie-rich dishes with little nutritive value.

Morning sickness or food aversions may make it hard to eat well during pregnancy. A vitamin and mineral supplement may be a good idea to help you get all the vitamins and minerals you need.

Folic acid is particularly important. Your doctor will recommend you take 5mg of folic acid in a supplement until at least the 12th week of pregnancy. A lack of this B vitamin has been linked with neural tube birth defects such as spina bifida. You may also need to take iron supplements. Your doctor will check your iron levels regularly and advise you on how much to take.

Talk with your doctor about your diet if:
You are a strict vegetarian
You have gestational diabetes
You have anaemia
You have a history of low-birth weight babies.

In these cases you may need extra vitamins and minerals, or you might have to eat a special diet.

Remember, though, that more is not always better. Very high doses of vitamins and minerals could be harmful to your baby. Always check with your doctor before taking any medicines or tablets, even if they are herbal.

Dieting during pregnancy could harm you and your baby. Some diets can leave you low on iron, folic acid or other important vitamins and minerals.

Weight gain is one of the most positive signs of a healthy pregnancy. Women who eat well and gain the appropriate amount of weight are more likely to have healthy babies.

So if you're eating fresh, wholesome foods and gaining weight, relax. You're supposed to be getting bigger!

The average weight gain during pregnancy is between 8 kg and 15 kg.

Bear in mind that weight gain varies among women, and how much weight you put on during your pregnancy depends on many factors.

So concentrate on eating a healthy diet of plenty of starchy carbohydrates, fruits and vegetables, reasonable amounts of protein, milk and dairy foods, and just a little in the way of fats and sugars.

When you put on weight may be as important as the amount you put on. You may gain the least weight during the first trimester. Your weight should then steadily increase throughout the second trimester, and you may put on the most weight over the third trimester, when your baby is growing the most.

If you are over 90 kg or under 50 kg, your doctor may advise a special diet.

Even if you're not hungry, chances are your baby is, so try to eat every four hours.

Sometimes morning (or all-day) sickness, food aversions, acidity, or indigestion make eating difficult.

Try eating five or six small meals each day, instead of three large ones. Your baby needs regular sustenance, and you need to keep up your energy levels, so try not to miss meals.

Eating high-fibre and wholegrain foods will help to keep you feeling full, and will be more nutritious, too.

The Best Exercises in Pregnancy

There are lots of good reasons to keep active when you're pregnant.

Exercise improves your muscle tone, strength and endurance, which may make it easier for you to adapt to the changes that pregnancy brings.

Regular exercise will

- Help you to carry the weight you gain in pregnancy.
- Prepare you for the physical challenge of labour and birth.
- Improve your mood, and give you energy.
- Help you to sleep better.
- Make getting back into shape after your baby is born easier.
- Give you the chance to meet other mums-to-be, if you opt for a class.

The ideal exercise in pregnancy will get your heart pumping and keep you supple, without causing physical stress. Many activities, such as running and weight training, are fine in the beginning, but you may need to modify your workout as you grow bigger.

You'll really feel the benefit if you do a combination of: Aerobic exercise, which works your heart and lungs. Muscle-strengthening exercise, which improves your strength, flexibility and posture.

To get the full benefits, you'll need to exercise at least three times a week, ideally more. Try to find something that you enjoy, as you'll be more likely to stick to it in the longer term.

Build activity into your daily life, too. For example, taking the stairs instead of the lift, and doing housework or gardening, counts as exercise.

The following types of exercise are safe in pregnancy, though some may not be suitable for the last few months, and you may need to lessen the activity as your pregnancy progresses. Talk to your doctor before starting any exercise that's new to you.

Walking

4

Brisk walking keeps you fit without jarring your knees and ankles, and gives your heart a workout. It is safe throughout pregnancy, and can be built into your daily routine. Aim to walk for at least 30 minutes a day, five times a week. So walk to the shops rather than drive, take the bus only part of the way, or do a brisk a few laps of the park or pavements in your lunch hour.

Running

Running is one of the quickest and most efficient ways to work your heart and body, and you can vary the distance as your energy levels allow.

However, if running is new to you, pregnancy is probably not the time to start. It's best to stick to more gentle exercise, such as walking or swimming.

Swimming

Swimming is an ideal, and safe, form of exercise in pregnancy. It exercises your arms and legs, and works your heart and lungs. The bigger your bump gets, the more you'll enjoy feeling weightless in the water.

If you enjoy group activity, you could join an aquanatal class or aqua aerobics class. Exercising while standing in water is gentle on your joints and supports your bump. It can help to ease back pain and swelling in your legs in late pregnancy.

Yoga

Pregnancy yoga helps to maintain muscle tone and flexibility and improve your posture. It's kinder to your joints than more vigorous types of exercise. However, you should also do some aerobic activity, such as brisk walking, a few times a week, to give your heart a workout.

Stretching helps to keep you supple, though don't overdo it. Think about gently opening and extending your body, rather than pushing yourself. Your yoga teacher will show you how to relax your body and mind.

Make sure that your yoga teacher is experienced in providing advice for pregnant women. It's best to go along to a pregnancy yoga class, rather than start with a DVD.

The exercises you learn may help you with relaxation and breathing in labour, too.

Aerobics

Going along to a weekly aerobics class gives you a regular time to exercise. It's safe, as long as you keep the exercises low impact, to protect your joints. If you sign up for an antenatal class, you can feel reassured that each movement is safe for you and your baby.

Mental Health

Physical as well as mental wellbeing of mother is important during pregnancy. Hence be positive. Think positive, try to keep away from anything which will induce stress, depression, tension.

- Read good books.
- Hygiene and cleanliness are very important.
- Breastfeeding is another important aspect. Get proper guidance and information about it.
- Travelling should be avoided. If possible, prefer trains.
- At around term, keep your delivery bag ready and packed in case you have to leave for the hospital in a hurry. Don't forget to include your antenatal card and reports.

Pregnancy is a beautiful journey which you should enjoy with certain responsibility under the guidance of your obstetrician.

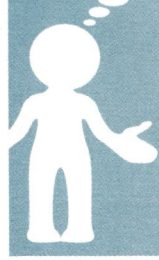

Points to remember

1. The best age for having baby is between 20 and 30 years of age
2. Proper investigations and medical advice is necessary.
3. Balanced diet and exercise is important to deliver healthy baby

4

Garbh Sanskar:
Is it Really Helpful

Chandrakant Sankalecha

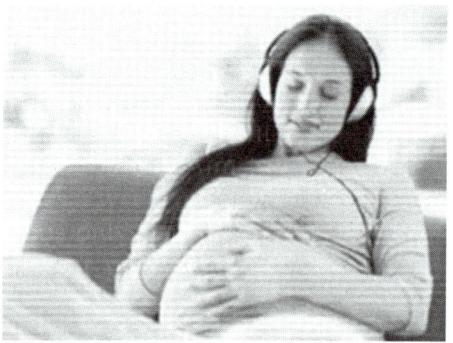 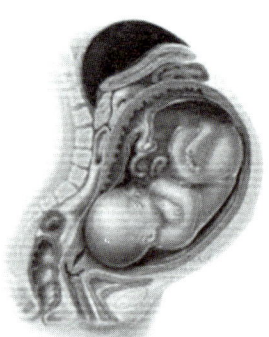

INTRODUCTION

In today's world of everything instant, garbh sanskar (GS) is becoming an important part of antenatal care. With rapid improvement in technology and access to it, the pace of life has noticeably increased. As a result, a person is always short of time for any activity and wants to make up for this *less* or *no* time with something instantly rewarding.

With increased pace of life, competition has increased at all levels. A perception has been created in the minds of people that one has to be *superior* to others even to survive let alone progress. Everybody wants their children to be more competitive, to have an edge over others. For this they are ready to participate in any activity without verifying its usefulness. The already ruthless market forces become even more aggressive at such times and try to trap the potential takers. What better vulnerable group than the anxious and ignorant 'would be parent' wanting desperately to go up the socioeconomic ladder? Many classes and workshops of GS are being conducted. It is difficult to critically evaluate the usefulness of this ritual, if we can call it so. Those advocating GS give examples mainly from ancient scriptures and holy books. There is no way to verify the claims. Outcome of GS is also ill-defined, to say the least.

GARBH SANSKAR

There is no universally accepted definition.

It is about keeping oneself in a good state emotionally, mentally and physically for the sake of growing baby. Modern antenatal care has the same aim. What GS claims to achieve is grooming the child in mother's womb to make it *better* and actually shaping its future.

Most of the books, websites and self proclaimed masters of G-S quote Ayurveda as its basis. 'Sharirsthan' chapter in Ayurveda contains references of GS (Ashtang Hruday by Vagbhat; 3rd–6th century AD). The references are non-specific and open to different interpretations. It is a masterly treatise but some things mentioned in it have been proven incorrect.

- An embryo is formed first and 'life' enters in it after a month.
- Couples doing intercourse on even days after menses will get male child and those doing it on odd days will get a female child.

As there is no single standard reference book, 7 books that are available in the market were studied. Several internet sites were also visited. Though there are differences in the actual methods of performing GS, basic components remain common to all:

- Listening to music
- Thinking positive and being stress-free
- Eating healthy food
- Yoga, meditation and prayer
- Being creative
- Communicating (talking) with the unborn child

CLAIMS

If we perform GS properly, the next generation will be *supraja*. (Supraja: su-good in quality; praja-people). The child that is born will be *tejasvi* (having an aura, though implied meaning varies). It will have an ideal personality. We can decide what kind of person it should be. We can shape its future, improve its intelligence. We can teach many things while it is still in the womb so as to have an edge over others. The child will have very good bonding with the parents.

ABHIMANYU VERSUS SHIVAJI

5

The most commonly cited example of garbh sanskar is from the epic Mahabharat, that of Abhimanyu. He listened to the war strategy while in the mother's womb. He remembered it at the age of 16 and actually implemented it.

When Jijabai was pregnant, she had to literally run from one place to another for safety. Her father and brother were killed during that period and she herself thought of committing suicide. Still Shivaji was born to her who established first independent kingdom in Western India. What garbh sanskar did Jijabai perform?

UNDISPUTED FACTS

1. *Diet:* Pregnant women should have healthy and nutritious diet. It will prevent anaemia, nutritional deficiencies, IUGR and preterm labor.

2. *Exercise:* Both GS and modern medicine advocate regular exercise for the pregnant woman. It helps the mother during labour and postpartum period. Though maternal exercise does not have direct beneficial effect on the fetus, it does so indirectly by keeping the mother in a positive frame of mind.

3. *Pranayam, Yoga, Meditation:* Pranayam or breathing exercises help mother during labour. They make her confident and better prepared to face the challenges of delivery. Yoga and meditation have a calming effect and are proven stress busters.

4. *Thinking positive:* Having a positive attitude helps a person to overcome any illness. Pregnancy creates a lot of anxiety and fear in the mind of the woman. There are many

associated minor ailments like nausea, vomiting, backache, abdominal pain, etc. There may be additional risk factors like PIH, previous bad obstetric history and anemia. Positive attitude would certainly help pregnant women to cope with these.

CONTROVERSIES

1. *Listening to music*: Main purpose of this is to make the woman happy and peaceful. Any music—folk/classical/Western/disco—that makes the mother happy should do. But GS advocates specific shlokas and particular music only. Some studies were conducted wherein certain music was played to a group of pregnant women. After the child was born, the same music when played had calming effect on the baby. There are no trials to test if this music had same calming effect on other children whose mothers did not listen to it during pregnancy. There are no trials to show whether different styles of music had the same effect. There are no ways to see if it has direct effect on the *baby*.

   There are many examples of deaf and dumb people who contributed to the welfare of mankind in a big way. Some of the world's greatest artists have been deaf and dumb.
   What kind of sanskars they might have received in utero?

2. *Talking to the child:* GS gives lot of importance to this. The mother is supposed to talk to the child in her womb at a particular time of the day. She should say good things about her family and can narrate stories from religious books.
   Theoretically, the fetus can *listen* from 5th month onwards as auditory apparatus and brain start developing. But as auditory pathway is not fully myelinated, there is partial connection between ear and brain. Pregnant uterus is in close contact with maternal aorta and vena cava. The loud rustling noise of blood flowing through these great vessels must be deafening to the child. How can it listen to the mother's *talk*? Even if it listens, can it understand the words, the language? What about other people in the house talking to the mother?

5

Many characteristics are genetically determined and cannot be modified or altered with external influences.

Twins born to a woman have everything common. They have same mother with same thoughts in her mind, same sanskars, and same environment. Still there may be profound differences in the intelligence and abilities of two siblings.

IS THERE ANY HARM?

Insisting on a particular kind of music has no proven benefit. Similarly talking to the child in the womb does not make any sense. It may help mother in her bonding to the child but it won't help the child in any way. Then why are these included in the GS?

Reasons may be many. It makes the package attractive. It gives the therapy a personal and emotional touch. Its benefit can neither be proved nor disproved. As the pregnant woman is emotionally labile, she is unlikely to question it.

Many people opt for GS fully knowing that there is no proven benefit. The argument is—*what is the harm*? But this is flawed logic. It can cause adverse effect.

THE HARM

When couples perform GS religiously, they are convinced that their child will be extraordinary, intelligent and smart. They become demanding. They do not accept anything less than first rank in the studies and winner's trophy in the competitions. If these expectations are not fulfilled, the child is harassed, pressurised and bullied. There is tension in the house. Pressure of performance may make child's life miserable and lead to depression and psychological problems.

Some centres charge heavily for GS workshops and classes. They sell products like cassettes, books, charts and Ayurvedic preparations to the participants at a heavy premium.

Hoping that GS will take care of the unborn child, many couples do away with the basic tests like ultrasound and haemogram. Some even stop taking iron supplements.

5

CONCLUSION

GS as advocated by books, websites and self proclaimed masters is a mix of proven and unproven practices which may have potentially harmful effects in the long run.

Exercise, good diet, meditation and positive attitude are beneficial to the mother and child. These should form an integral part of any antenatal care. Other practices like talking to the child may not be of any use to the fetus.

No ritual whatsoever will guarantee a birth of a smarter, brighter and more intelligent child. Raised expectations of parents may cause more harm than good to the children.

One needs to be aware that GS workshops may have the motif of selling unreasonable dreams just to earn money.

5

WHAT IS SANSKAR?

There is no English word for *sanskar*. Broadly speaking it is to purify, refine the inner conscience. To inculcate human values into the subconscious of a person such that they become a part of his/her nature and guide him/her throughout life. Character building is the main purpose of this process which continues well into the late childhood and shapes the psychological, emotional and social makeup of a person. Parents, teachers and peers play a major role in this.

An example often given is that of a diamond. Raw diamond looks like an ordinary stone. It is cleaned, impurities removed (purification), polished, cut (removing deficiency) and then made into an ornament (value enrichment). These three processes constitute *sanskar*.

What we have to keep in mind is that it has to be a *diamond stone* in the beginning.

We cannot make *any* stone into diamond by mere purification, making up the deficiency and value enrichment.

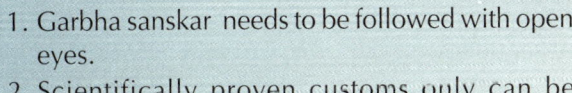

Points to remember

1. Garbha sanskar needs to be followed with open eyes.
2. Scientifically proven customs only can be followed.
3. Limitations of garbh sanskar needs to be understood by parents.

6 Neonatal Behavior: Behavioral Competence of Newborns

Sailaja Nandan Parida

IMPORTANCE OF NEONATAL BEHAVIOR

Each and every baby is unique and has powerful influence in shaping the way through which he develops his relationship with the parents or other caregivers and the environment around him. In short newborn behavior relates to his personality and aimed at drawing the attention of the parents or others persons toward solving his simple physical needs and problems. Many parents do not know what normal newborn behavior is. But they can be assured that though their babies develop at different rates still most of them would display many of the same behavior, when compared with babies of same age.

Neurobehavioral Perspective

The systematic examination and evaluation of a baby at birth and thereafter was attempted by Apgar 1960, Prichtel and Beintema 1964, Parmeeli in 1973, where one could identify gross abnormality in function but not milder dysfunctions of the CNS.[1] Much less attention was given to elicit neonate's ability to orient and organize his responses to positive social stimuli, because of the idea that the newborn operates only at subcortical level. Subsequently few landmark research by Pritchel, Rosenblith and others could find out the difference between state behaviors and reflex activity, newborn's capacity to habituate, the responses to positive social stimuli which were proposed as indicators of intact CNS of the baby.[2]

The principle of ontogenetic adaptation

It has been observed that the neonate seen at any stage of development has developed competency for that particular age, rather than an imperfect precursor model of later stages. As per Dr. Brazelton, human newborn at any gestational age is to be seen as a biological and social partner in a highly organized feedback system to interact with the caregivers, constantly eliciting and seeking attention to be nurtured well.

The principle of continuous organism

Environmental interaction applies to the CNS differentiation and development. This also corroborates to the concept of Fetal Origin of Neonatal Behavior. The continuity of fetal behavior to the postnatal life and beyond is an indicator of intact neurobehavioral development. The integrity of the fetal nervous system can be assessed antenatal. The intactness of fetal CNS is determined by observing the gross movements, spontaneous motility and even observing the unstimulated and resting fetus for spontaneous behavior. All these recording are influenced by maternal anxiety, mood and illness through 4D ultrasound. Stanjevic and Kurjack in their review[3] suggested that all those movements those were present in fetal life has to be present in the neonatal life of the same baby, these movements could be eye blinking, mouth and eye opening, smiling, hand movements directed towards other parts of the face like, mouth, eye and ears. It is possible to identify babies with emerging neurological impairment by looking for abnormal movements *in utero*. These abnormal patterns indicate disruption of continuity of the maturative process of the CNS.

ASSESSMENT OF THE NEWBORN

It is important to evaluate the newborn behavior in the early days of life to understand the interaction and bonding between the parents and the baby. Though genetic endowment has a major contribution for development of human behavior, many other factors like maternal nutrition, drugs and infections during antenatal and postnatal period do exert their influence on health and behavior of the newborn. Subtle differences in behavior is also seen in between boys and girls., where girls show higher level of functioning than boys.[4] The early care professionals may have to devote more time to the boys by talking to them to improve their auditory and alertness abilities which in turn helps them to regulate their state.

The process of birth is a very stressful event for both, the mother and her baby. Each neonate passes through a phase of transition from fully dependent intrauterine environment to an independent existence to grow as a human being though the neonate already has nine months of intrauterine experience when born; he enters this world with what is akin to a survival checklist. The neonate after birth spends enormous energy in establishing homeostasis of various organ systems. The most immediate and basic challenges are to regulate breathing, maintain thermal stability and regulate autonomic and motor functions, before concentrating on areas like development and growth. The next level of development is the ability to process and response to various stimuli around him. A baby's response and ability to process it appropriately provides key information on care giving. Most babies are social from birth, bonding between the parents and the baby is enhanced if the newborn responds to the voices of parents and others and focuses on their faces, until and unless the baby is too premature or sick, when the parents and infant relation ship is likely to be compromised.[5] Which can be evident as cognitive deficit and other behavioral disorders during follow-up visits (Fig. 6.1).

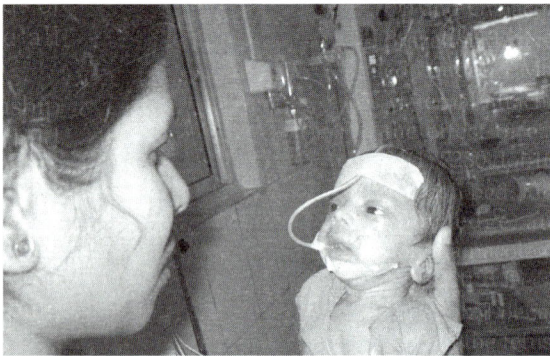

Fig. 6.1: An eye fixing with caregiver

The fetus is minimally conscious by 24 weeks of gestation, after which the level of consciousness steadily increases, unless disrupted by adverse intrauterine conditions. Consciousness otherwise described as the state is the most important aspect in assessing the response of the baby. It is important to note that a conscious baby only can elicit responses from the caregivers. When the baby is conscious he is awake and aware of the body and self, can process tactile, olfactory, auditory stimuli at cortical level, can show emotions, imitates facial expressions and has the power to habituate. Sensory experience and pain elicit specific hemodynamic responses in the somato sensory cortex. Pain thresh hold is lower in premature infants and higher in awake infants.[6] Pain can be minimized by giving sweet substances like sucrose to the baby, Cuddling and even by Kangaroo Mother Care.

6

Usually the baby passes between two sleep and three awake states. The sleep states are defined as

1. Deep sleep where there are no spontaneous body movements, with closed eyes and regular breathing.
2. Light sleep otherwise also known as REM sleep, with irregular respiration and random body and limb movements.
3. Four awake states are: (1) drowsy or semi dozing, (2) alert, (3) alert and active, (4) alert and crying.
4. Neonates usually sleep 30 minutes to 4 hours at a time, up to 20 hours a day. By 3 months most babies sleep 6 to 8 hours during the night.
5. Abnormal sleep wake pattern in a neonate is a predictor of aberrant neurobehavioral outcome in later life.

The fetus can hear in utero by 26 weeks of gestation, which has been depicted in Mahabharat. Abhimanyu in his mother's womb was able to listen the techniques of only entering the Chakravyuh from his father Arjun, as long as his mother was awake. Soon after birth the baby can distinguish between different sounds and recognize familiar voices, indirectly encouraging parents to talk to him often. It has also been documented that the fetus can responds to touch of the mothers abdomen and gets agitated during the procedures like amniocentesis.[7]

6

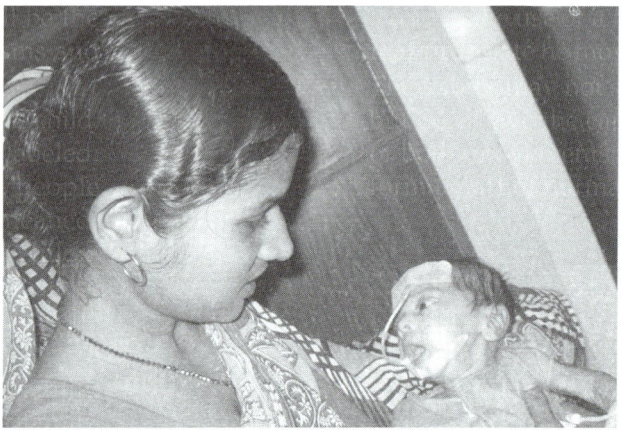

Fig. 6.2: Recognising and listening to mother

Habituation to a stimulus is learned in utero, which empowers the baby to seek comfort by ignoring unpleasant environmental stimuli after birth, and thus conserving energy for growth and development. If a baby has trouble in blocking out the unwanted stimulus the parents should know that they have to support their baby by providing him comfort in a quiet and dimly lighted room. The recent practice of nursing the babies in quiet NICUs with diffuse lights, with soft pleasing music will not only help babies grow better, but develop a healthy behavioral competence in future.

Within minutes after birth a neonate can follows a face like pattern, can taste the difference and shows preference for breast milk over cows milk and can even express boredom when shown an abstract picture for a long time by shifting his gaze to a different one even though he has poor visual acuity.[8–10]

The newborns can smile, and premature smile more often than mature ones. Smile is mediated at subcortical level, though smile is not indicative of happiness in a neonate but has got a powerful impact on the mind of the parents.

The infant always strives for a balance between two opposing physiological responses that is exploratory or reaching out and avoiding and withdrawing response. If stimulation is appropriate the infant actively move towards those stimuli takes it and make use of it for his own development. If the stimulus is inappropriate he moves away from it and try to defend himself. The babies may not speak a word till they are about a year old but they have the capacity to communicate through a plethora of body movements. Intense visual response and cries. Which form a part of normal behavior?

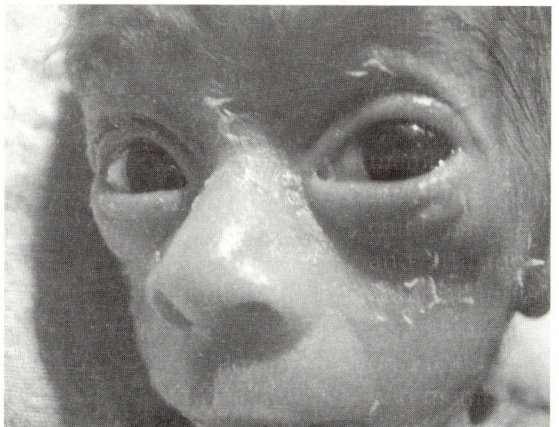

Fig. 6.3: Intense eye contact speaks a thousand words

Excessive crying, sleeping or feeding problems when found in a baby can be predictor of behavioral problems in child hood.[11]

NEONATAL BEHAVIORAL ASSESSMENT SCALE

The complexity of the newborn behavior has led to the develop ment of the Brazeltons Neonatal Behavioral Assessment Scale (BNBAS) by Dr T. Berry Brazelton and his colleagues in the year 1973. When Dr Brazelton started working on the project he had two things in his mind (1) To assess the functional integrity of the baby and (2) as a clinician to understand the newborn baby's contribution to the parent infant biological system? He felt that unless one understood the neonate well, lacked the skill to communicate with the eager parents about the individuality of their baby. After eight decades of the original publication and many more research on the subject the basic objective of the scale is still maintained.[12]

The scale looks at a wide range of neonatal behavior and can be used up to two months of age. The baby is seen as an active participant in a dynamic situation. The scale also demands that the observer become reliably sensitive to the dynamics of the newborn. The, babies state or consciousness is the single most important element in behavioral examination, The NBAS examiner looks at how the infant controls his states and manages the transition from one state to another. The basic score sheet includes 28 behavioral items to be scored on a nine-point scale. There are also 18 elicited responses to be scored on a three-point scale. The NABS observers are trained to get the best performance from the baby by doing everything possible to support the baby to succeed the assessment procedure. At the end of the examination, the examiner has got a complete picture of the newborns personality, that can be used for better care giving by providing specific physical needs of the baby. It has also been observed that recovery curves on repeat examination were due to transient influences on neurodevelopment while the items those were below average remained low in spite of a nurturing environment indicates a more permanent insult to the neuronal axis. The NABS items those were below average but began to recover on repeat examination could help us in planning an early interventional programme for the affected baby.

Increasing worldwide survival rate of high-risk babies is an emerging public health problem for both developed and developing countries. Clinical examination of such babies still plays an important role in identifying and tailoring the specific care giving strategies for them and NABS is a step forward in achieving this goal. As proposed by Dr Brazelton, the babies are to be respected as social partners and as individuals with their own unique qualities who can effectively engage and some extent guide caregivers to support their growth and development.

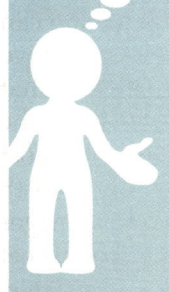

Points to remember

1. Genetic endowment has a major contribution for development of human behavior; many other factors like maternal nutrition, drugs and infections during antenatal and postnatal period do exert their influence on health and behavior of the newborn.

2. Babies have the capacity to communicate through a plethora of body movements. Intense visual response and cries which form a part of normal behavior.

3. The babies are to be respected as social partners and as individuals with their own unique qualities who can effectively engage and some extent guide caregivers to support their growth and development.

6

FURTHER READING

1. Apgar V.A. A proposal for new method of evaluation of the newborn infant. Current research in anesthesia and analgesia: 1960, 32:260.

2. Heidelise Als, Tronic E,Lester BM,Brazelton T B, BNBAS, journal of abnormal child Psychology: 1977; 5(3), 215

3. Continuty from fetal to neonatal behavior: lesson leaned and future challenges, STANOJEVIC, Kurjik Asim, Donald School Journal in Ob and Gynacol: April–June 2011;5(2): 107–118.

4. Brazelton TB,Nugent JK. Neonatal behavioral assessment scale 3rd ed.London 7 Mac Keith Press ; 1995.

5. Maternal attachment representations after very preterm birth and the effect of early intervention, Infant Behavior Dev. 2011Feb; 34(1):7280.doi:10.1016/j.infant beh.2010.09.009.Epub2010 Nov9

6. Turkish ped. Efe E, Dickman S, Atlas N, Boneval C: Surgical nurses knowledge and attitude regarding pain assessment and nonphamacological methods in newborn' pain relief, Pain Manag Nurs. 2013 Dec;14(4):343-50.doi:10.1016/j.pmn.2011. 08.003.E Pub.

7. Brimholz J,Benacerraf B. Fetal hearing. Scince.1983; 222:516(5)Drifc JO,Can the fetus listen and learn Br J Obstet Gynaeccol 1985;92:777

8. Carpenter G.Mothers face and the new born, New Scientist, 1974; 61:742.

9. Lozoff B, Britenham GM, Trause MA, Kennell JH, Klaus MH. The mother newborn relationship: limits of adaptability, J Peditr. 1977; 91:1

10. Brazelton TB. Behavioral competence of the newborn infant Sem Perinatol 1979;3:3.

11. Hemi MH,Wolke D, Schneider S, Association between problems with cryingsleeping,or feeding in infancy and long term behavioral outcomes in childhood: a meta analysis, Arch Dis Child. 2011 July;96(7):622 9.doi:10.1136 adc.2010.191312.Epub2011April20

12. Brazelton TB. Neonatal Behavioral Assessment Scale 2nd Ed, Spastics Int Med Publication,Black Well Scientific Publication, London, JB Lippincott Co, Pheladelphia 1984.

6

NICU Baby's Parents Worry—Time to Get Best of Your Child

MKC Nair

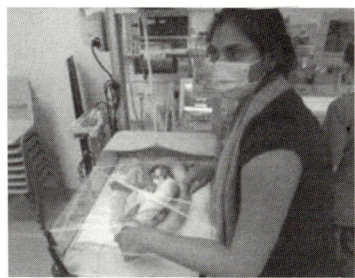 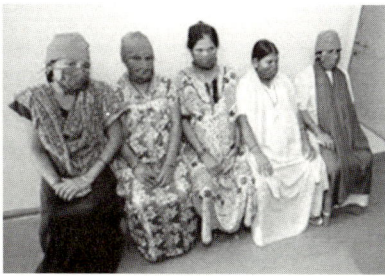

Effective communication with parents of critically ill NICU babies is of utmost importance. Family members who had been accurately informed about expected events were often found to experience less anxiety and expend less effort in trying to cope with their loss. Frequent, accurate and truthful discussions with parents alleviates the sense of uncertainty and fosters confidence in the team's capability. The strategies to enhance communication with parents include: (i) introduce NICU team to the parents, (ii) use only simple explanations with parents, (iii) explain each procedure/therapy in detail, (iv) encourage suggestions from parents; and (v) see them through entire crisis calmly. Waiting related stress add on to the stress of parents and hence every effort should be taken to provide a comfortable waiting area, fixed time updates by resident doctor, provision for communicating emergencies and access to NICU chief (if absolutely essential). It is equally important to take steps to reduce the work pressure/burn-out among NICU staff by providing effective leadership, giving guidelines on work responsibilities, avoiding work overload, providing adequate holidays, encouraging group activities and organizing stress management training. The indicators of difficulty to accept severity of illness in newborn include; (a) anger against the NICU team, (b) resistance in compliance with therapy, (c) insistence on futile therapeutic ventures, (d) emotional withdrawal from the baby, and (e) sudden increase in religious fervor.

The parents also have to be made to understand some details of the present morbidity, possible brain damage and strategies for reducing poor outcome. A risk factor is something that increases the likelihood of getting a disease or condition, but the division of risk as mild, moderate and high is often arbitrary. Which 'high risk' newborns require periodic screening, ideally needs to be determined locally. It must also be remembered that many babies not considered "at-risk" may also manifest developmental problems as they grow.

In simple words we need to tell them that neonatal brain damage primarily occurs due to:

  i. Lack of oxygen

  i. Lack of glucose, and

 iii. Adequate blood perfusion to the developing brain.

Newborn encephalopathy represents the neurological manifestations of central nervous system injury due to any cause obvious or not so obvious, that occurs in the first few hours or days of life. The importance of intrauterine asphyxia in the genesis of hypoxic-ischemic brain injury is well known. A seizure by far the most frightening event for the parents, mostly secondary to hypoxia or hypoglycemia or seizure by itself can disrupt the development of maturing nervous system. A cascade of biochemical/molecular pathways is normally responsible for brain plasticity or activity-dependent development of the maturing nervous system. Depending on the degree of brain immaturity, seizures may disrupt the processes of cell division, migration, myelination, sequential expression, receptor formation, and stabilization of synapses, each of which contributes to brain damage and degrees of neurological sequel. Most neurodevelopmental impairments among very preterm babies are likely to be the consequence of brain damage of perinatal origin. Majority of these lesions can be identified in the neonatal period with the use of cranial ultrasound. Intraventricular hemorrhage (IVH) – peri ventricular hemorrhage (PVH) and white matter damage (WMD) are the best-recognized preterm brain injuries associated with adverse neuro developmental outcomes.

Apart from known risk factors the **early warning signals** would be history of infertility, abortion, and hyperemesis in the prenatal period; low birth weight, convulsions requiring more than one drug in the natal period; difficulty in handling, difficulty in feeding and difficulty in putting to sleep in postnatal period. History of unexplained excessive crying suggests early hypertonia that may lead on to spasticity later. There are also babies presenting with developmental delay and spasticity, who do not have identifiable risk factors and hence development-friendly well-baby clinic offers the best opportunity to detect them routinely and it is a feasible strategy, as shown in the Trivandrum experience. Ultimately, in order to reduce neuro-developmental disabilities and their social impact, we need a comprehensive strategy

7

i. To reduce or ameliorate neurological impairments by pre-natal and natal interventions;

ii. To reduce disability by early stimulation and developmental therapy;

iii. To reduce handicap by specific age appropriate social interventions, thus optimally intervening in the disability process.

Neurodevelopmental follow-up assessment: At the time of discharge appointment for follow-up visits have to be given at 2 weeks, 2 months, 4 months, 6 months, 8 months, 12 months and 2 years corrected age. The selection of the developmental tests depends on many factors and is to be judiciously undertaken. The following new scales developed and validated at Child Development Centre, Kerala and published have made it possible to screen and assess these babies without any fees to be paid for the test material. The simple screening tools include:

1. CDC, Kerala, Grading for motor milestones (0–1 year) for the three important motor milestones in the first year—Head holding, Sitting and Standing.
2. Trivandrum Developmental Screening Chart (TDSC: 0–6 years) for developmental screening by physician in office practice and health workers in the community.
3. Language Evaluation Scale Trivandrum (LEST: 0–3 years) to identify young children with early speech, language and communication delay.
4. Developmental Assessment Tool for Anganwadis (DATA: 2–6 years) to identify developmental problems in the community by Anganwadi workers.
5. Trivandrum Autism Behavioral Checklist (TABC) to screen for autism spectrum disorders.

The busy pediatrician can seek the assistance of trained transdisciplinary paramedical personnel like the PG diploma in clinical child development degree holders of child development centre, Kerala, who are optimally trained paramedical professionals to undertake developmental screening, formal developmental assessment and developmental therapy.

Points to remember

1. Effective communication with parents of critically ill NICU babies is of utmost importance
2. Neonatal brain damage primarily occurs due to lack of oxygen, lack of glucose and adequate blood perfusion to the developing brain.
3. Reduce or ameliorate neurological impairments by prenatal and natal interventions and reducing disability by early stimulation and developmental therapy is very important part of treatment of NICU babies.

FURTHER READING

1. The High Risk Newborn. Nair MKC, Jain N, Murkhi S, Parthasarathy A (Eds.) Jaypee Brothers Medical Publishers, New Delhi, First edition 2007.
2. MKC Nair. Child Development (Special Supplement). Indian Pediatrics 2009; 46: S7–S90.
3. MKC Nair, Russell PS (Eds). Supplement issue on Adolescent Care Counseling: Part-I. Indian Journal of Pediatrics—An International Journal. 2012; 79: S1–S91.
4. MKC Nair, Russell PS (Eds). Supplement issue on Adolescent Care Counseling: Part-II. Indian Journal of Pediatrics—An International Journal 2013; 79: S129–S255.

7

Breastfeeding and Complementary Feeding

Anil Mokashi, Santosh Nimbalkar

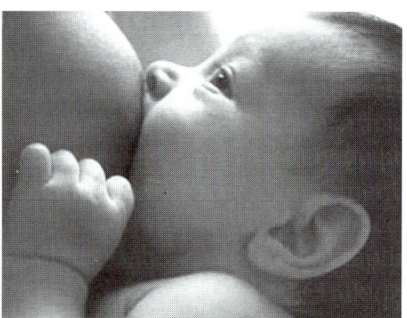

INTRODUCTION

Babies need adequate nutrition, affection and protection. Breastfeeding meets all these needs and gives babies the best start in life. Breastfeeding is natural. Like mother's love, there is no substitute for mother's milk. For successful breastfeeding, you need correct information and support of the family and the community.

This article has been designed to help women during pregnancy and after child birth to make breastfeeding much easier. This article can be used by parents and all those who care for the mothers and babies and also by those who want to encourage, support and promote breastfeeding.

- It deals with the natural course of breastfeeding and complementary feeding for the baby up to 2 years of age.
- It also deals with how to breastfeed a baby with ease and how to prevent and manage problems during breastfeeding.

- It guides about how working women can continue to breastfeed and how to express breast milk.
- It helps dispel myths/age old beliefs related to breastfeeding.
- It aims to provide answers to frequently asked questions by mothers.

It is recommended that all infants should be fed exclusively on breast milk until they are six months of age and continued to be breastfed till 2 years or beyond. Breastfeeding is advantageous for all—you, your baby and the society.

Before your baby is born he is protected within your womb from all infections and after birth breastfeeding takes over the protection process. The milk which you secrete for the first few days known as **colostrum** should be given to your baby as it provides resistance to your baby against various diseases and infections.

Your milk is made especially for your own baby. It is the right nutrition for the growth of your baby. It is easy to digest and it contains protective substances which help prevent infection especially loose stools. You can give it even when you are ill, pregnant or menstruating.

Benefits Your Baby Enjoys

Breastfeeding provides numerous benefits to your babies which are as follows:

- Breast milk contains adequate calories and provides the right kind of proteins, fats, lactose, vitamins, iron, minerals, water and enzymes in the amounts necessary for your baby.
- Breast milk contains iron, water soluble Vitamins D, A, C and E more than cow's milk.
- Breast milk is clean, free from bacteria and has anti-infective properties.
- It also contains substances which prevent harmful bacteria from growing in intestines and causing loose stools.
- It is ready to serve when the baby wants it, needs no preparation and it has the right temperature.
- It is economical and free from contamination.

- Breastfeeding enhances the emotional bond between the child and the mother and provides warmth, love and affection and is more than food.
- Breastfeeding protects the child against several infections including respiratory infections.
- Breastfed babies are less prone to have diabetes, heart diseases, eczema, asthma and other allergic disorders later in life.
- Breastfed babies have been shown to have a **higher IQ (Intelligence Quotient)** and develop better mathematical abilities than infants who are not breastfed.
- Breastfeeding **enhances brain development.** There is better visual development and visual acuity leading to learning readiness.

Benefits You Enjoy as a Mother

Breastfeeding has many advantages to the mother, which include the following:

- It reduces post-delivery bleeding and chances of anemia.
- Obesity is less common among breastfeeding mothers as it helps the mother regain her normal figure.
- It has a contraceptive effect.
- It has a protective effect against breast and ovarian cancers.
- If you exclusively breastfeed your baby, you will have better adjustment with your baby.

Benefits the Society Enjoys

Breastfeeding lowers health care costs by reducing illness and deaths of children under five years of age and thus reduces the strain on the family budget.

Exclusive breastfeeding: Exclusive breastfeeding means giving a baby no other food or drink including water, in addition to breastfeeding with the exception of syrup or drops of vitamins, minerals and medicines.

Complementary feeding: The infant receives breast milk along with solid and semi-solid foods.

Antenatal Counseling and Breastfeeding

Antenatal counseling is the job of lactation management counsellor. It gives you an opportunity to get introduced to the expecting mother so that she knows whom to approach in case she has many problems.

With mothers in groups

- Explain the benefits of breastfeeding.
- Give simple relevant information on how to breastfeed.
- Explain what happens after delivery.
- Discuss mothers' questions.

8

With each mother individually

- Ask about previous breastfeeding experience.
- Ask if she has any questions or worries.
- Examine her breasts only if she is worried about them.
- Build her confidence and explain that you will help her.

Dangers of prelacteal feeds

Prelacteal feeds are artificial feeds or drinks given to a baby before breastfeeding is initiated.

They are dangerous because:

- They replace colostrum as the baby's earliest feeds.
- The baby is more likely to develop infections, such as diarrhea, septicemia and meningitis.
- He is more likely to develop intolerance to the proteins in the artificial feed, and allergies, such as eczema.
- They interfere with suckling.
- The baby's hunger is satisfied, and hence breastfeeds less.
- If she/he is fed from a bottle with an artificial teat, she/he may have more difficulty at the breast (nipple confusion).
- The baby suckles and stimulates the breast less.
- Breast milk takes longer to "come in" and it is more difficult to establish breastfeeding if a baby has even a few prelacteal feeds; mother is more likely to have difficulties, such as engorgement. Breastfeeding is more likely to stop early when a baby is exclusively breastfed from birth.

Advantages of Rooming-in and Demand Feeding

Rooming is (ideally bedding-in) and demand feeding help bonding and breastfeeding.

Advantages of rooming-in
- Mother can respond to baby, which helps bonding.
- Babies cry less, so less temptation to give bottle feeds.

Advantages of Demand Feeding

- Breast milk "comes in " sooner.
- Baby gains weight faster.
- Fewer difficulties such as engorgement.

How to help a mother with an early breastfeed?

Avoid hurry and noise

Take quietly and be unhurried, even if you have only a few minutes to ask the mother how she feels and how breastfeeding is going. Let her tell you how she feels, before you give any information or suggestions.

Observe a breastfeed

Try to see the mother when she is feeding her baby and quietly watch what is happening. If the baby's position and attachment are good, tell her how well she and the baby are doing. You do not need to show her what to do.

Help with positioning if necessary

If the mother is having difficulty, or if her baby is not well attached, give her appropriate help.

Give her relevant information

Make sure that she understands about demand feeding, about the signs that a baby gives that show that he is ready to feed, and explain how her milk will "come in".

Answer the mother's questions

She may have some questions that she wants to ask. Explain simply and clearly what she needs to know.

How does the mother hold her baby while breastfeeding?

Correct position: Baby's body close, facing breast. Face to face and attention from mother.

Incorrect position: Baby's body away from mother. Baby's neck twisted. No mother–baby eye contact.

How does the mother hold her breast?

Correct holding: Resting her fingers on her chest wall. Her first finger forms a support at the base of the breast.

Incorrect holding: Holding her breast to close to the nipple.

8

Body Position

Signs that breastfeeding is going well
- Mother relaxed and comfortable.
- Baby's head and body in straight line.
- Baby's face facing the breast.
- Baby's nose opposite the nipple.
- Baby's body close to mother's (baby's bottom supported).
- Baby reaches breast from below.
- Breast well supported (optional).

Signs of Possible Difficulty

- Shoulder tense, leans over baby.
- Baby's head and body is not in a straight line.
- Baby's face not facing breast.
- Baby's nose away from nipple.
- Baby's body not close to mother.
- Baby reached breast from above.
- Breast supported in scissors hold or nipple being pushed in babies mouth.

Positioning a Baby at the Breast

Introduction: Always observe mother breastfeeding before you help her. See what she is doing. Try to understand her situation clearly. Do not rush to make her do something different. Some mothers breastfeed to their babies satisfactorily. There is no point in disturbing and teaching something new.

How to help a mother who is sitting?

- Make sure that she is sitting in a comfortable position.
- Sit down yourself so that you also are comfortable and relaxed and at a same level.
- Explain to the mother how to hold her baby.

Make these four key points clear

- The baby's head and body should be in a straight line.
- Baby face should face the breast, with nose opposite the nipple.
- Mother should hold the baby close to her with skin to skin contact.
- She should support his bottom, and not just his head and shoulders.
- Show her how to support her breast with her 'C' shaped cupped hand.
- She should rest her fingers on her chest wall under her breast so that her first finger forms a support at the base of the breast. She can use her thumb to press the top of her breast slightly. This can improve the shape of the breast so that it is for her baby to attach well. She could not hold her breast too near to the nipple.
- Explain how she should touch her baby's lips with her nipple so that she/he open his/her mouth.
- Explain that she/he should wait until her/his baby's mouth is wide open before she moves him/her onto her/his breast. His/her mouth needs to be open to take a large mouthful of breast.
- Explain or show her how to quickly move her baby to her breast when she/he are opening his/her mouth wide. She should bring her baby to her breast and not herself or her breast to the baby. She should arm her baby's lip below her nipple so that his/her tongue will touch her breast.
- Last she/he should have an eye to eye contact with the baby while the baby is enjoying feeds.

How to help a mother who is lying down?

Help the mother to lie down in a comfortable, relaxed position. It is better she is not "propped up" on her elbow. This can make it difficult for the baby to attach to the breast. Show her how to hold her baby. Exactly the same four key points are important, as for a mother is sitting, she can support her baby with her lower arm. She can support her breast if necessary with her upper arm. If she does not support her breast, she can hold her baby with her upper arm.

Then Advice to the Mother

Advice her not to wash her breasts more than once a day, and to use soap, or rub hard with a towel. Breasts do not need to be washed before or after feeds. Normal washing as for the rest of the body is all that is necessary. Washing removes natural oils from the skin, and makes soreness more likely. Advice her not to use medicated lotions and ointments because these can irritate the skin, and there is no evidence that they are useful.

Not Accepting Breastfeed and Crying

Introduction

Many families start top milk because child refuses to feed. That leads to complete stopping of breastfeeding. If baby is "crying too much", mother and relatives think that the breast milk may be inadequate. She starts animal milk. We have to tell her about her baby's crying and refusal to feed.

Kinds of Refusal

There are different kinds of refusal:

- Sometimes baby attaches to the breast, but then does not suckle or swallow, or suckles very weakly.
- Sometimes a baby suckles for a minute and then comes off the breast crying. She/he may do this several times during a single feed.
- Sometimes a baby takes one breast, but refuses the other.

8

- A baby who cries a lot can upset the relationship between him / her and his / her mother and can cause tension among other family members.

You need to know how to decide why a baby is refusing to breastfeed, and how to help the mother and baby enjoy breastfeeding again.

Why a baby may refuse to breastfeed?

Is the baby ill, in pain or sedated?

- *Illness:* The baby may attach to the breast, but suckles less than before.
- *Blocked nose:* Sore mouth [Candida infection (thrush)], an older baby teething. The baby suckles a few times, and then stops and cries.
- *Pain:* Pressure on a bruise from forceps or vacuum extraction. The baby cries and fights as his/her mother tries to breastfeed him.
- *Sedation:* A baby may be sleepy because:
  a. Drugs that his/her mother was given during delivery
  b. Drugs that she is taking for psychiatric treatment
  c. Drugs given to the baby.

Is there a difficulty with the breastfeeding technique?

Sometimes breastfeeding has become unpleasant or frustrating for a baby.

Possible causes

- Feeding from a bottle, or sucking on a pacifier (dummy)
- Not getting much milk, because of poor attachment or engagement
- Pressure on the back of the baby's head, by his mother or a helper positioning him roughly, with poor technique. The pressure makes him/her want to "fight"
- His/her mother holding or shaking the breast, which interferes with attachment
- Restriction of breastfeeds; for example, breastfeeding only at certain times.

Has a change upset the baby?

Babies have strong feeling, and if they are upset they may refuse to breastfeed. They may not cry but simply refuse to suckle. This is most common when a baby is aged 3–12 months. She/he suddenly refuse several breastfeeds. This behaviour is sometimes called a "nursing strike".

Possible causes

- A new caretaker, or too many caretakers
- A change in the family routine, for example, moving house, visiting relatives
- Illness of his/her mother, or a breast infection
- His/her mother menstruating
- A change in his/her mother's smell, for example, different soap, or different food, different scent.

8

Is it "Apparent" and Not "Real" Refusal?

Sometimes a baby behaves in a way which makes his/her mother think that she/he is refusing to breastfeed. However, she/he is not really refusing. When a newborn baby "roots" for the breast, she/he moves his/her head from side to side as if she/he is saying "no". However, this is normal behaviour. Between 4 and 8 months of age, babies are easily distracted, for example when they hear a noise. They may suddenly stop suckling. It is a sigh that they are alert. After the age of 1 year, a baby may wean himself. This is usually gradual.

How to help a family with a baby who refuses to breastfeed or cries a lot?

Look for a cause

Listen and learn

- Help the mother to talk about how she feels. Empathize with her feelings.
- She may feel guilty and angry
- Other people may advise her to give the baby complements or pacifiers.

Take a history

- Baby's feeding and behaviour
- Mother's diet, coffee, smoking and drugs
- Pressures from the family and other people
- Job work and general health of the mother.

Assess a breastfeed

Check the baby's suckling position, skin of the breast, nipples and the length of a feed.

Examine the baby

8

- Make sure he is not ill or in pain. Check his growth
- If the baby is ill or in pain, treat or refer as appropriate.

Build confidence and Give Support

- Accept what the mother thinks about the cause of the problem
- Accept what she feels about the baby and his/her behaviour.

Praise what the mother and baby are doing right

- Explain that her baby is growing well, he is not sick
- Her breast milk is providing all that her baby needs. There is nothing wrong with it or with her.

Give relevant information

- Her baby has a real need for comfort. He is not sick but he may have real pain
- The crying will become less when the baby is 3–4 months old
- Medicines for colic are not now recommended. They can be harmful.
- Complementary feeds are not necessary, and often do not help. Artificially fed babies also have colic. They may develop cow's milk intolerance or allergy and becomes worse.

Make one or two suggestions

What you suggest depends on what you have learnt about the case of the crying. Common causes may be different in different countries.

If she has an oversupply of breast milk.

Help her to improve her baby's attachment to the breast. Suggest that she lets him suckle from one breast only at each feed. Let him continue at the breast until he finishes by himself. Give the other breast at the next feed. Explain that if her baby stays on the first breast longer, he will get more fat-rich hindmilk.

Give practical help

- Explain that the best way to comfort a crying baby is to hold him close, with gentle movement and gentle pressure on his abdomen. Offer to show her some ways to hold and carry her baby.
- Sometimes it is easier for someone not the mother to carry the baby so that he cannot smell the breast milk.
- Show her how to bring up her baby's wind (called as burping). She should hold him upright, for example, in a string position or upright against her shoulder.
- Offer to discuss the situation with her family, to talk about the baby's needs and about her need for support.
- It is important to help to reduce family tensions so that she does not start giving unnecessary complements.

Treat or remove the cause if possible

Illness
- Treat infections with appropriate antimicrobials and other therapy
- Refer if necessary
- If a baby is unable to suckle, she/he may need special care in hospital
- Help his/her mother to express her breast milk to feed to him/her by cup.

Pain
- *For a bruise:* Help the mother to find a way to hold the baby without pressing on a painful place.
- *For thrush:* Treat with gentian violet or nystatin.
- *For teething:* Encourage her to be patient and to keep offering him her breast.

8

- *For a blocked nose:* Explain how she can clear it. Suggest short feeds, more often than usual for a few days.

Sedation

If the mother is on regular medication, try to find an alternative.

Breastfeeding technique

Discuss the reason for the difficulty with the mother. When her baby is willing to breastfeed again; you can help her mother with her technique.

Changes which upset a baby

Discuss the need to reduce separation and changes if possible. Suggest that she stops using the new soap, perfume, or food.

If it is a distraction

Suggest that she try to feed him at a quiet place. The problem usually passes.

If it is self-weaning

Suggest that she makes sure that the child eats enough family food; give him plenty of extra-attention in other ways; continues to sleep with him because night feeds may continue. This is valuable at least up to the age of 2 years.

INADEQUATE MILK

Introduction

Almost all mothers can produce enough breast milk for one or even two babies. Usually even when a mother thinks that she does not have enough breast milk, her baby is in a fact getting all that she/he he needs.

Sometimes, a baby does not get enough breast milk. But it is usually because she/he is not suckling enough or not suckling effectively. It is rarely because his/her mother cannot produce enough milk.

So it is important to think not about how much milk a mother can produce, but about how much milk a baby is getting.

Signs that a baby may not be getting enough breast milk
Reliable

- Poor weight gain (<500 grams a month) (< birth weight after 2 weeks)
- Passing small amount of concentrated urine (< 6 times a day).

Possible

- Baby not satisfied after breastfeeds
- Baby cries often
- Very frequent breastfeeds
- Very long breastfeeds
- Baby refuses to breastfeed
- Baby has hard, dry or green stools
- No milk comes when mother tries to express
- Breasts did not enlarge (during pregnancy)
- Milk did not "come in" (after delivery).

How to find out if a baby is getting enough breast milk or not

Check the Baby's Weight Gain

This is the most reliable sign. For the first 6 months of life, a baby should gain at least 500 g in weight each month or 125 g each week (one kilogram per month is not necessary and not usual). If a baby gains less than 500 g in a month, she/he is not gaining enough weight. Look at the baby's growth chart if available, or at any other record of previous weights. If no weight record is available, weigh the baby. If the baby is gaining enough weight, she/he is getting enough milk. However, if no weight record is available, you cannot get an immediate answer.

Check the Baby's Urine Output

This is a useful quick check. An exclusively breastfed baby who is getting enough milk usually passes dilute urine at least 6-8 times in 24 hours. A baby who is not getting enough breast milk passes urine less than 6 times a day (often less than 4 times a day).

Reasons for baby not getting enough milk

Breastfeeding factors

- Delayed start, poor support
- Poor attachment
- Feeding at fixed times
- Infrequent feeds
- No night feeds
- Short feeds
- Bottles, pacifiers
- Other foods
- Other fluids (water, teas)

8 *These are common*

Mother: Psychological factor
- Lack of confidence
- Worry, stress
- Dislike of breastfeeding
- Rejection of baby
- Tiredness.

Mother: Physical condition
- Contraception pill, diuretics
- Pregnancy
- Severe malnutrition
- Alcohol
- Smoking
- Retained piece of placenta (rare)
- Poor beast development (very rare)

These are not common

Baby's condition
- Low birth weight
- Nose block illness
- Cleft lip or palate
- Other abnormalities
- Oral thrush

Factors that do not affect the breast milk supply
- Age of the mother
- Sexual intercourse

- Menstruation
- Age of baby
- Caesarean section

If a baby passes lot of urine, it usually means that she/he is getting plenty of breast milk.

Breastfeeding in Special Situations

Introduction

There are some breastfeeding challenges. These are special situations. They are not problems. Twins, cleft lip and palate, working mother, implants, pregnancy induced hypertension (PIH), adopting, mother sick, baby sick, and yes you can do it. It may be a "challenge" but you can do it if (i) you do not quit and (ii) find a good support system.

Breastfed twins

Best thing is to contact someone who has breastfed twins. Breastfeeding twins require more work, dedication, responsibility. Mother may worry that she would not produce enough milk for two. Or she may be afraid that nursing twins will take too much time, common problems such as sore or cracked nipples, engorement and low milk supply, and worry. Mother needs support from baby's doctor, lactation specialist, family and friend.

Breastfeeding and working mother

Work and breastfeeding can happen at the same time. She can exclusively breastfeed her baby if she knows how to do it and she has a desire. A good start is important. Proper breastfeeding should be established in first 6 weeks. Success at expressing and storing is all that maters. She has to express and store every 2–3 hours, if she wants to exclusively (100%) breastfed. It does not have to be all or nothing. Mother should ask for a 6-month breastfeeding leave, a place to express every 2–3 hours on job, a facility to store the expressed milk. Working and breastfeeding, it is worth it.

8

Breastfeeding and cognitive development (brain development)

Children who are breastfed have better neurodevelopment outcomes, and the duration of breastfeeding also effects a child's intelligences. There are three substances, which may explain the association between breastfeeding and higher scores on intelligence tests. There are two fatty acids associated with the development of nerve cells, retina and the brain, and are present in breast milk but are absent in infant formula and cow's milk. These, decosa hexaenoic acid (DHA) and arachidonic acid (ARA), have been shown in experiments to improve eyesight and some motor responses in infants and young children. The third lactose, a carbohydrate, is a readily available source of galactose, which is essential in the production of the galactol acids including cerebroside. The amount of lactose in the milk of a species and the relative size of brain varies and is highest in human milk.

The studies done over the last few years prove the point that breastfeeding enhances the neurodevelopment of infants and their intellectual and scholastic ability in later life.

Increasing duration of breastfeeding was associated with significant increases in both verbal IQ and performance IQ.

Babies who were preterm and were fed breast milk in early years of life had an 8.3 point advantage in intelligence quotient over those who had artificial milk.

Longer the duration of breastfeeding better the developmental milestones.

Breastfed infants showed greater motor activity than those fed with formula.

Breastfeeding is associated with enhanced stereoscopic vision.

Advantages of proper complimentary feeding

The young child should be made accustomed to eating family foods. Complementary feeding should be started when baby can no longer get enough energy and nutrient from breast milk alone. For most babies, this is after 6 months of age. If young children do not have energy and good food, they will not have energy to grow and be active. Adequate complementary feeding prevents undernutrition, anaemia, vitamin deficiencies, and illness and promotes proper growth and development.

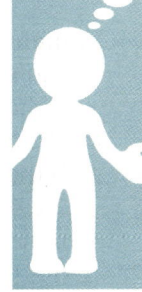

Points to remember

1. Exclusive breastfeeding is best feeding for 1st 6 months
2. Breastfeeding has several advantages
3. No pre lacteal feed should be recommended
4. Exclusive breastfeeding by mother for 1st 6 months will give a healthy and brainy child.

8

FURTHER READING

1. Clinical Management of Breastfeeding. By Dr Anil Mokashi, Dr Santosh Nimbalkar
2. Breastfeeding and complementary feeding—Guide for Parents, By B.P.N.I.
3. Baby Breastfeeding within minutes after birth.
4. Breastfeeding a cleft child.
5. Breastfeeding in public
6. Breastfeeding—cradle hold

Faulty Feeding Leads to Smaller Brains and Weaning Readiness

Hemant Joshi, Anil Mokashi

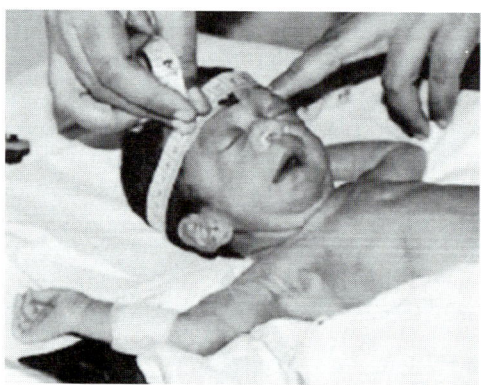

MALNUTRITION IN FIRST YEAR OF LIFE IN INDIA

Table showing head size (circumference)
At birth and at one year

	Indian children	American children
	Head size	*Head size*
Age	90th centile	95th centile
At birth	35 cm	37.5 cm
At 1 year	46.5 cm	49 cm

Above figures are taken from standard childcare textbooks.
This table shows that

1. The big Indian children from good families and big American children have same head circumference at birth that is 37.5 cm

2. At 1 year brain growth and head circumference of Indian children is 2.5 cm less than that of similar American children. It is 46.5 cm in Indian children and 49 cm in American children.

Reason? Faulty weaning with liquid foods in best of homes.

Weaning Readiness

WHO, UNICEF recommend waiting until six months of age before starting a child on food. However, individual babies differ greatly because of their unique developmental progress. A good way to know when to introduce baby food is to watch signs of readiness in the child.

9

Signs of readiness include

1. The ability to sit without help,
2. Loss of tongue thrust, and
3. Display of active interest in food that others are eating.

Baby may be started directly on normal family food if attention is given to choking hazards; this is referred to as baby-led weaning. Because breast milk takes on the flavor of foods eaten by the mother, these foods are especially good choices

Lesson

1. Teach proper weaning. With thick homemade foods.
2. In India, true malnutrition occurs in first year of life in best of the people.
3 Teaching proper weaning is the most important step in eliminating malnutrition.

Parenting
Newborn to Six Months

Monideepa Banerjee

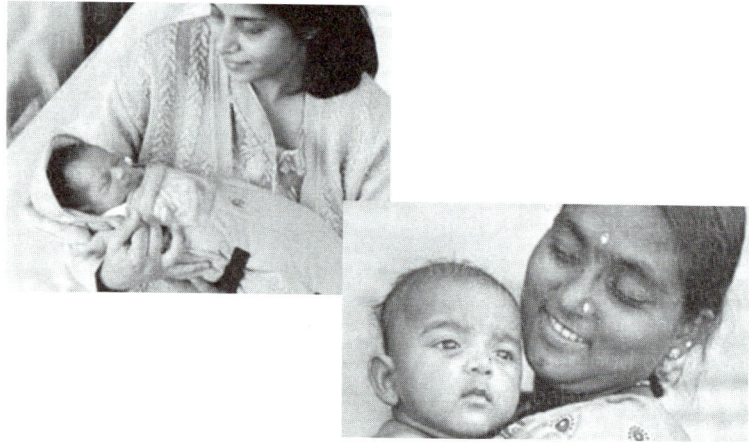

Holding your newborn in your arms can be the most wonderful and yet the most unnerving experience of your life.

Your Baby is Unique

Babies are all very different

All recommendations and routines act as a guide only. Have faith in nature, as most problems ease out with time.

Initially all your child does is feeding and sleeping with plenty of wet nappies in between. Your child is strongly influenced by the environment, daily activities and routines. A predictable routine helps your child establish good sleep patterns. The feed, play, sleep routine is the core structure of a baby's day at any age. As your baby matures, day playtime increases and night patterns continue but without playtime. Your baby is unique therefore their need for sleep and the time of waking varies. Some days things will go smoothly but illness, disruption to the family environment and extra busy days out can all affect your baby's routine.

0–3 months

Establishing breastfeeding is very important at this stage. Besides providing nourishment and immunity it creates wonderful bonding. It makes babies feel secure and settled. Exclusive breastfeeding is recommended till 6 months of age.

In the early weeks, you are getting to know your baby as your baby engages in activities, such as feeding, sleeping, listening and focusing, moving and vocalising. Feeding is an essential task which also provides you with an opportunity to interact. In the early days babies need a minimum of 6–8 feeds in a 24–hour period. This includes overnight feeding. Although a sleep between each feed is ideal, babies of this age often have long crying periods and may not settle between feeds.

10

3–6 Months

It takes time for your baby to develop a predictable routine. This can be a fun time as your child develops new skills such as exploring their world. As your baby becomes more mobile it is important to ensure your home and play areas are safe. Once the child starts rolling do not leave the child unattended in high places like beds without railings.

Babies become more predictable in their routine by 3 to 4 months. From 3-4 months most babies know the difference between day and night. They generally settle well overnight but may still need 1–2 milk feeds. Awake time is becoming longer. Time spent playing with and talking to your baby is very important for their development. Sleep times can vary, with some having three longer sleeps per day and others needing only short naps. If your baby is generally alert and happy your baby is probably getting enough sleep.

Some ideas for interacting during awake/playtime include:
- Tummy time (floor play)
- Using rattles and soft toys

- Taking baby for a walk in the pram
- Telling stories using soft books
- Having a relaxing bath time or baby massage
- Singing songs or playing music

By 6 months your baby can commence taking solid foods. It is also a good time to commence feeding your baby cooled boiled water from a cup.

10

Early morning	Milk feed
	May return to sleep
	or have some playtime
SLEEP	
Mid morning	Milk feed
Awake time 1½ to 2 hrs	Play
SLEEP	
Lunchtime	Milk feed
Awake time 1½ to 2 hrs	Play
SLEEP	
Mid afternoon	Milk feed
Awake time 1½ to 2 hrs	Play
SLEEP	
May only require a short nap	
Evening	Milk feed
	Bath
	Quiet time
	Cuddle
Settle for night	
SLEEP	
1–2 milk feeds may be needed overnight	

Settling your baby comfortably

Crying babies can be very frustrating for the parent and make him or her feel inadequate. Learning how to go to sleep is a skill babies usually develop during the first year of life with help from their parents. Like most skills, it takes time and varies for each baby.

Why do babies cry?

Crying is normal and is your baby's way of communicating. Babies have individual crying patterns which can vary from 20 minutes to 5 hours a day. Babies cry because they are hungry, thirsty, hot or cold, wet or soiled, overtired, excited, frightened or in need of a cuddle.

10

To soothe your baby try:
- a cuddle or holding your baby close (this may include skin-to-skin contact)
- rhythmical movement
- walking using a pram or sling
- soft music
- a "top up" breastfeed within 30 minutes of the last feed (up to 3 months)
- a dummy
- baby massage; or
- warm bath.

Babies sleep patterns vary however by the end of the first month. Most babies sleep 13 or 14 hours spread across both day and night. As your baby grows he/she will sleep for longer periods through the night with 2–3 shorter sleeps during the day. If your baby is happy during wake periods during the day, he/she has had enough sleep.

Babies show tired signs, when they are getting tired and need sleep such as grimacing, yawning, grizzling, frowning, sucking, staring, snuggling in, turning head away, jerky movements, becoming over active, clenching fists, rubbing eyes, squirming, fussiness or crying. Responding early to these tired signs prevents your baby becoming distressed and makes it easier to calm for sleep.

Wrapping often helps babies settle down. Use a light material (cotton) making sure that the arms are above waist level and there is room to move the legs. Ensure your baby is not over dressed and your baby's head is uncovered. However consider environmental temperature and make sure your baby is not uncomfortably warm. Stop wrapping your baby when he/she is able to turn onto their tummy during sleep or play (from 3–6 months).

Soothing in arms is usually done in the early weeks: Hold your baby in your arms until they fall asleep. You can use gentle rhythmic patting, rocking, stroking, talking, or softly singing before putting your baby into the cot asleep. The repetition of soothing sounds and actions are comforting and signals relaxation and sleep. If your baby wakes after a sleep cycle you may need to re-settle to ensure enough sleep.

10

When babies are 4 to 6 weeks old?

1. Wrap baby comfortably.
2. Talk quietly and cuddle your baby which makes baby calm
3. Put your baby on their back in the cot when awake but also calm or drowsy
4. Comfort your baby with gentle 'ssshhh' sounds, gentle rhythmic patting, rocking, or stroking until baby is calm or asleep
5. If your baby becomes distressed pick your baby up for a cuddle until calm or asleep before putting baby back in the cot
6. Stay with your baby until he/she is asleep

When to worry?

Parents worry about unrecognised illnesses in their babies. Common conditions that affect babies are cold, vomiting and loose stools.

A cold will affect a baby more than it will affect an older child—that's because babies' immune systems aren't used to fighting off infections. But be prepared: babies can get anywhere from 6 to 10 bouts of minor infections, mostly viral, in their first year, so make sure you pay extra attention to his/her symptoms.

Some red flags for seeing your doctor

- Your baby shows any signs of illness if she's less than 3 months old
- Your baby has a >100°F fever and is 3 months or younger; has a 101°F degree fever and is 3 to 6 months, or your baby has a 103°F degree fever and is over 6 months
- Your baby has a persistent cough or nasal mucus
- Your baby's lips or nails turn blue
- Your baby has breathing difficulties
- Your baby is excessively fatigued or cranky

Keep your baby's nasal passages clear by suctioning out mucus with a rubber bulb or applying saline nasal drops.

If your baby is vomiting, make sure to keep up fluid intake by offering short but frequent feedings of breast milk or formula, or half an ounce ORS every 10 to 15 minutes. If your baby has a mild fever but otherwise is eating, drinking and playing, monitor his temperature for 24 hours.

- The vomiting continues beyond 24 hours, or if it is high in volume and frequency (meaning she's persistently throwing up everything she's consumed)
- There is blood or bile in the vomit
- Your baby cannot keep any amount of food or liquid down
- Your baby appears lethargic or dehydrated, marked by decreased urination, dry mouth, absent tears, and sunken eyes or fontanels (the "soft spot" on an infant's skull)
- A high fever accompanies vomiting. High fevers include:
  - >100°F in 3 month-old or younger
  - 101°F in 3 to 6 month olds
  - 103°F or higher in babies 6 months and above

If your baby has diarrhoea, make sure to keep him hydrated with breast milk, formula or a rehydrating drink.

Call your paediatrician if

- Your baby is 3 months or younger
- The diarrhoea continues for more than a 24 hours
- Your baby shows signs of dehydration (this includes decreased urination, sunken eyes or soft spot, decreased energy and absent tears)

- There is blood in the diarrhoea
- A high fever accompanies diarrhoea. High fevers include:
  - >100°F in younger than 3-month-old
  - 101°F in 3 to 6 month old
  - 103°F or higher in babies 6 months and up

10

Points to remember

1. For 1st 6 months exclusive breastfeeding is important.
2. Parents should understand sleep cycle of babies below 6 months.
3. Parents must know alarming signs.

Crying Child

Anil Mokashi

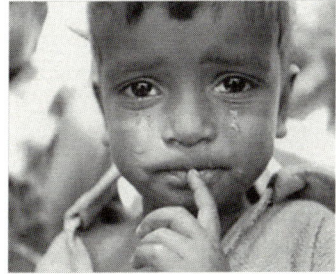 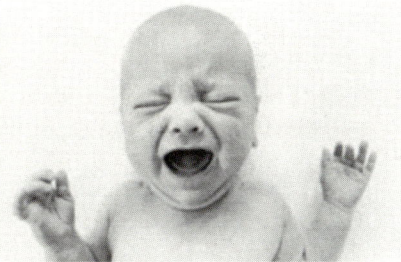

All babies cry. Some cry more, some cry less. He is trying to tell you something. It is his language. It is his means of communication. It is natural for a baby to cry. He may cry even when nothing is wrong, crying is healthy. It is an activity. It is an exercise for the baby. Cry only means that the baby needs help.

Learn the Meaning behind Cries

Knowing the meaning behind baby's cry is important. You have to get used to your baby's cry. And to learn what it means. Initially, all crying sounds the same. After a few weeks of listening closely and responding to your newborn's needs you will an idea of what your baby is trying to tell you.

Babies Cry Differently

Not all babies cry the same. Cry depends upon personality the baby is born with. Some babies just cry more than others. The crying is part of a baby's natural development. It won't last forever! Eventually, all babies outgrow their crying.

Why babies cry?

- Hunger
- Fatigue/tired
- Too hot or too cold
- Wet or soiled diaper
- Need to be burped
- Need to be held
- Abdominal gas discomfort
- Need to suck
- Need to feel secure
- Sensitivity to bright lights or loud noises
- Over-stimulation
- Boredom
- Frustration
- Clothing too tight or uncomfortable
- Stress
- Temperament (some babies simply cry more)
- Stressful home environment
- Drugs. Anti-histaminics in cough formulas, bronchodilators oral and inhaled.
- Cry-Startle-Cry vicious cycle (cry is a part of Moro's reflex)

What to do when your baby cries?

Respond quickly and try to meet baby's needs. Baby is not spoiled if you pick her up. Give her attention. She will cry less overall. Longer a baby cries, the more upset she becomes, and the more difficult it becomes to calm the baby.

Change the diaper, feed, burp, or change position of baby. Provide reassuring contact and a pleasant environment. Provide skin-to-skin contact and a relaxed environment. Try one or another of the following to calm your baby:

- Rocking a baby gently in your arms, while standing or sitting in a rocking chair

- Gently stroking baby's head
- Patting back or chest
- Wrapping baby snug in a blanket
- Singing or talking
- Playing soft music
- Walking (in arms, stroller, or carriage)
- Riding in car
- Burping to relieve gas
- Giving a warm bath
- Changing locations (from light to dark)
- Changing locations (from quiet to less quiet or *vice versa*)

11

Dealing with Frustration

Bouts of endless crying, high-pitched shrieks, test the nerves. Nothing seems to work. Do not get frustrated, feel helpless, get mad at the child and shake her. Do not lose control. You need a break. Change hands. If you have a "chronic crier," accept it. Check with your pediatrician to see if there is a medical reason for crying.

When to go to a doctor?

- Illness
- Nothing works and you are concerned
- Fever, not sucking, not accepting feeds
- Passing less urine, less than 6 times a day
- Watery loose motions
- Breathing fast
- Help

Final Thoughts

Crying baby is a great challenge for a new parent. Don't worry. Recognize that a baby's cries have special meaning to you. Babies are given the ability to cry for a reason. It is her first attempts to talk to you. Stay calm. Crying is just a part of her healthy development. Learn to care. Prevent stress in baby and you. Prevent child abuse by controlling your emotions.

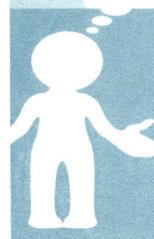

Points to remember

1. Crying child is real challenge to parents and pediatrician.
2. Physical and emotional causes must be identified.
3. Management of crying depends on the cause

11

Parenting Styles

Shrikant Chorghade

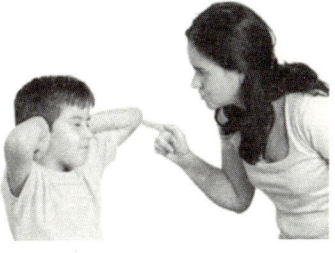
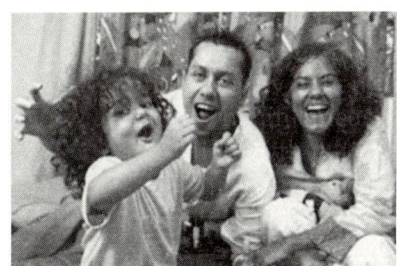

As a child grows physically from birth onwards, it's personality also start taking shape. Erik Erikson, a psychologist of yester century had postulated that "Growth and development of a child is epigenetic, viz. genetically determined but, its personality is shaped by its environment".

For every child the environment is constituted by the family it lives in. The family may be constituted by parents and the older siblings in a nuclear family but in a joint family there may be grant parents, uncles and aunts and cousins, etc.

Every child learns by imitation of the people around it. The quantum and quality of learning depends upon the genetic abilities for learning and the enriched favorable loving environment. Parents are the source of genetic abilities, they also a role models for the learning process. The parental behavior and parenting style decides the behavior and quality of learning of every child. In a nuclear family parental style has maximum impact on a child's learning process and the behavior which ultimately decides the personality development.

Some other factors in the environment related to the family also influence the shaping of child's personality. These include the social and economic status of the family in the community, size of the family and outsiders in a family. These include elderly relatives, guests, domestic servants and paid and unpaid caretakers. The social environment in the surroundings also has an influence on the personality development of the child.

The factors described above have secondary role to play shaping of the personality of the child. The primary role is played by the parents and their parenting styles.

Five major types of parenting styles are observed.

1. Authoritative
2. Authoritarian
3. Permissive
4. Uninvolved
5. Inconsistent

1. **Authoritative style:** This style of parenting is ideal and conducive to the physical, mental and personality development of the child. The authoritative parents are able to give tender loving care to the child. They accept their child in spite of its size, shape, color, disabilities and behavior. Such parents are warm in their approach. They are patient and sensitive to the needs of the child. They are responsive and attentive and have close interaction and warm communication with their child. They establish mutually enjoyable emotionally fulfilling parent child relationship. While disciplining a child these parents use adaptive control technique. Their demands on the child are reasonable and are decided according to the age maturity and ability of the child under their care. They consistently force these demands without duress or threat. The parents believe in positive communication, they give reason for their demands and expectations. Their disciplinary technique implies teaching moments when the child goes wrong or makes mistake. Authoritative technique promotes self-regulatory behavior in the child.

12

The children under care are given choices to make decisions appropriate to the age and maturity of the child. They encourage the child to express its thoughts, feelings and desires in mattes of conflicts. They resort to joint decision making whenever possible. These parents are willing to accept and accommodate child's opinions, perspectives and desires. This is usually a reciprocated by the child to value, respect and accommodate parent's perspectives and opinions.

This technique makes parenting enjoyable and rewarding. The child under care is likely to have a self-controlled motivating, happy and healthy personality. Such children are likely to accept the vagaries and difficulties in life and face challenges effectively. Such children can achieve maximum benefits out of their genetic endowment and learning opportunities and likely to reach maximum heights in the pursuit of their aspirations.

12

2. **Authoritarian:** This parenting style involves old and rejecting attitude of parents. These parents demean and degrade their child by mocking and putting down. Their focus is on the control of child's behavior by coercing, yelling, demanding, commanding and criticizing "you must do eat because I say so" is the diction. If the child makes mistake or disobey, these parents resort to force and punishment. The children under care are not given liberty to make decisions. Parents enforce their own wishes and desires and decisions. Childs self-expression and independence are suppressed.

This parenting style result into negative changes in the personality of the child under the care of these parents. These children are unhappy, anxious, indecisive and dependent and lack exploration. They are scared of unexpected situation and challenging task. When frustrated they react with hostility. This behavior is likely to make them mutually hostile to their teachers, classmates and playmates. The boys particularly show higher rate of anger, defiance and aggression. Such children have difficulty in adapting with their friends, partners and spouses. They are not able to achieve their desired goals in life and are always unhappy with the life they lead.

3. **Permissive style:** Parents who resort to this style are warm and accepting. They don't insist on proper behavior. They are not concerned and inattentive to the child's behavior. They don't guide, neither have they made demands on the child. They don't teach the limits to their children's. The liberty given to these children to make decisions is likely to be inappropriate for the age and maturity of the child and the moral and social values of the community they live in. they have full freedom to eat whatever and whenever they want. They can watch the television whenever they want for whatever time they like to watch. They have full liberty about the time to go to sleep or to get in the morning. These parents don't guide the children on socially acceptable behavior.

These children are likely to be disobedient, disorganized, impulsive and over demanding. They are under achievers in their academic and nonacademic pursuits.

During adolescence such children are likely to show defiant antisocial behavior and under performance in schools and colleges. When they grow up this behavior doesn't lead them anywhere and making themselves a burden on the parents, family and the society.

4. **Uninvolved parenting style:** These parents are hardly concerned about the child beyond minimal efforts for feeding and clothing. They are emotionally detached and uninvolved in the child. Parents are likely to be over involved in other aspects of their life. They might be paying more attention to their career, profession and prospects in life. The affluent parents may be more interested in partying, merrymaking and socializing. Such parents may over provide the child and fulfill child's reasonable and unreasonable demands. They are not aware about any parenting techniques or strategies which will provide guidelines for their children.

Uninvolved parenting amounts to maltreatment to the child called neglect. The children brought up with this style are turn out to be having poor cognition, scholastic problems, and poor emotional and social skills. They are likely to have lower self esteem. They are likely to indulge

12

in antisocial activities during late childhood and adolescence.

5. **Inconsistent style:** Ideal parenting involves uniform strategies to be used in parenting style by both parents in concurrence with each other if a child is exposed to dichotomy in parenting style. It disrupts the social , moral and personality development of the child. In a joint family this dichotomy may be due to conflict between the parenting styles of grant parents and the parents. In a nuclear family the father and mother may have totally different attitudes towards parenting. In such situations there may be occasions of criticisms on the sides of each other and indulgence into blame game. The child is likely to be confused whom to listen. Such a child will not be able to develop self-respect and self-confidence. The conflicting attitudes in a family will affect the ability of the child in decision making and problem solving. Child will not be able to develop social and moral values as the child grows up. The child may favor one parent and may emotionally blackmail the other and learn to play them against each other. These children are likely to be poor performers in academic pursuits and careers. They may get involved into aggressive, rowdy and antisocial behavior. They may have emotional breakdown and psychotic tendencies.

12

Well-designed research has revealed that relation between parenting and child's personality development is sometimes substantial. Parenting intervention in behavior problems show that when child rearing improves child's behavior changes accordingly.

What can precisely be advised in the best interest of their children is as follows

a. Parents should teach social and moral values to the children who will help them to make choices in the face of their genetic inclinations and peer pressures particularly during adolescence.

b. Parents should adopt their parenting strategy to overcome unfavorable depositions, coercive control and overprotection. This will prevent maladaptive behavior in children.

Rational firmness and encouragement favors healthy personality development.

c. Parents should foster positive capacities in children through exposure to rich experiences in academic, social, athletic, artistic, musical and spiritual fields.

d. Warm supportive parent child relationship permits children to explore ideas and social roles. It fosters autonomy, high self-reliance, work orientation, academic competence and high self-esteem.

e. Intrusive, coercive psychologically controlling attitude of parents interferes with the development of autonomy and self-motivation. It leads to low self-esteem, depression, anti-social behavior and psychotic problems in children.

CONCLUSION

Tender loving care which gives sense of security and feeling of being loved to the child leads to healthy personality development in a child.

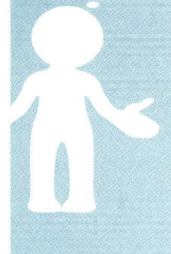

Points to remember

1. For every child the environment is constituted by the family it lives in. The family may be constituted by parents and the older siblings in a nuclear family but in a joint family there may be grant parents, uncles and aunts and cousins, etc. Every child learns by imitation of the people around it.

2. Five major types of parenting styles are observed. (a) Authoritative; (b) Authoritarian; (c) Permissive, (d) Uninvolved; (e) Inconsistent.

3. Tender loving care which gives sense of security and feeling of being loved to the child leads to healthy personality development in a child.

Parenting—Myths and Facts

Anjan Bhattacharya

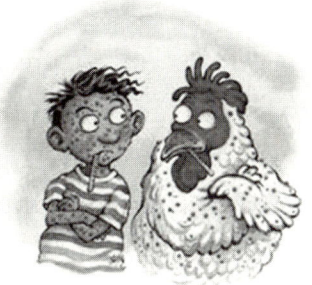

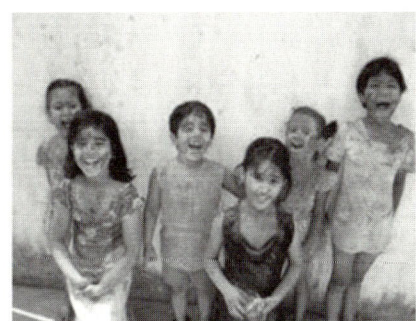

INTRODUCTION

Every parent wants their children to do their best. But not everyone succeeds in the pursuit. There is a strong sense of personal failure associated with an offspring's lack of expected level of achievements. Seldom parents realize that a lot of it is because, they went about rearing their children in an amateurish way, where expert help is just round the corner.

Knowledge is power. Separating folklores from facts on parenting issues give parents similar power over their children to guide them to achieve their best.

Let us take you through some of these so that as parents and as the first line of defense, you as a professional is not falling prey to the strongholds of the myths, thereby inadequately dishing out ineffectual or sometimes dangerous anticipatory guidance to parents.

13

Myths	Facts
Newborn Period	
They should not cry	Cry is their first communication mode and should only be attended to, if they need tending
If they wake up and cry, they must be picked up and soothed	Let them fall back to sleep on their own, if they feel sleepy (*i.e.* let them develop their own "self soothing" developmentally healthy skill)
If they cry, they should be picked up every time	Neonates see this as biofeedback for gratification by being held by an adult, i.e. a secure base. This may rob them on self reliant skills and produce dependency
If they cry, they must be rocked gently	This gives biofeedback, that "if I cry, I get what I want" i.e. crying is good for me. Moreover, what is gentle to you may not be gentle to the babies. They may develop abnormal sensory processing patterns, constantly needing stimuli habit of being rocked can be addictive with risk of addictive behavior in later life
Crying will psychologically weaken them	Repeated and immediate gratification will develop poor behavior management skills
It is cruel to let the baby cry	Be "cruel to be kind". Let him have the opportunity of learning that crying in real life will not fetch him everything in life
If a newborn breaks his voice by hard crying, it is calamity	It may be a sign of later difficulty in managing his emotional outbursts, rage attacks or difficulties to change, i.e. it may be a red-flag sign of EBD* problems later in life. If doctor does not find any obvious physical problem, e.g. obstructed hernia, testicular torsion, there is no need to worry immediately though. Follow-up for emotional dysregulation
"Colic" must be given decolics!	Antispasmodic medicines have a number of side-effects and possibility of hiding a real calamitous pathology. "Colic's" are harmless. Therefore, paediatricians should refrain from treating parents and family

Contd.

Contd.

	members/neighbors by prescribing potentially risky medications for the baby
Breast milk is inadequate	Colostrum is adequate, although it does not feel so to the parents and family members. Professional support may be incompetent instead of natural flow of milk being inadequate!
"Surma" will make eyesight better	Soot or any other crude substance application on newborn eyes have potential to infect and occasionally cause even blindness
Oil massage is beneficial	Physical activity is. Normal bathing, walking around doing regular chores without having to do much extra for the baby is beneficial. Massages may be overzealous and may cause micro-tears in baby's muscles and ligaments. Oil used may have potential to harm, especially the scented ones. For example, mustard oil is a potent allergen and baby may develop allergy proneness in later life!
Baby must be always wrapped around, especially if premature	Babies have poor thermoregulatory mechanisms, especially if premature. Over wrapping may lead to over heating. Abnormal rise in core temperature has shown to lead to 'Cot Death' or SIDS**
Babies should not be disturbed	Babies need to be exposed to the hustles and bustles of the real world to acclimatize. Common sense needs to be applied. But, stimulating them and engaging them of activities of their interest help them develop

Infancy

They need 14 to 18 hours of sleep daily	Like you and me, they vary in their daily sleep requirement. Find out what it is for your baby by the end of neonatal period and strive to achieve that. Regularity at this age helps but any unavoidable shift from the norm is not calamitous. Accept some discomfort. Allow time for more sleep next night, if necessary

Contd.

13

Contd.

Daytime sleep is good	Often unnecessary but children vary. Early to bed and early to rise is most often best physiological sleep pattern instead of day time sleeping pattern. Find out your child's own.
Putting hand to mouth is bad or it means he is hungry	Baby is self-booting to acquire hand-to-mouth skills, which would be essential to feed self, following successful weaning. Disrupting it may push them towards skewed developmental trajectory. Keep the hands clean though
Infants need to be sanitized in sterilized baby environment	They need to be clean but NOT squeaky clean! NB: Hygiene Hypothesis—every needs a healthy dose of germs at a developmental window of acquiring immunity.
They are growing fast, so they need to eat more and more	If they did, they will swell up and burst eventually, as some of them do. Endemic of obesity, metabolic syndrome, NAFLD[§] and NASH[§§] are not that uncommon anymore!
They will gag, if they chewed	While learning to chew, normal infants will have initial difficulties. Get your doctor to check your child. If okay, a bit of gagging in your presence is not a risk. Do a BLS[d] course.
They touch everything being naughty	If they did not, they will not learn basic facts about objects and their property. Adults MUST make the home environment child safe by removing harmful items out of reach.
They put everything in their mouth as they are naughty	They are going through their 'oral exploratory' phase of their natural development. Just keep clean large, non-sharp objects around, which they can happily goggle
They are so naughty that they throw things away just to irritate us	They are going through their 'casting object' phase of their natural development

13

Contd.

Contd.

They make so much noise with their toys by banging them as they are silly and irritating	Banging toys' phase is to acquaint them with fundamental sounds around their stages of speech and language development

Toddlers

Does not listen to any instruction	Toddlers are 'self-directed' developmentally
Disobedient	They are yet to be developmentally so mature as to be able to act on adult's agenda
Always playing, no discipline	Parents are having unrealistic expectation from a child. Play is their earliest learning tool. Play has different stages to train them step by step through play, e.g. container play, role play, pretend play, etc. Also, they need to burn their energies.
Shouts unruly as they are brutes	Either they are very happy and squealing or they are role modelling adults who shout at them or to each other

13

Pre-school years

Naughty child, stubborn	Opposition defiant. Either parents are asking too much of him exasperating him, finally turning him against parents' wishes or child has ADHD[dd] or its variations or comorbidities.
Hits others	Either they are very happy and expressing their exaltation in an odd way or they are role modelling adults who hit them or hits each other. It justifies violence as a means of solving a problem to a child by role modelling
Throws tantrums, if I do not give him what he wants	Permissive parenting is a subtle form of emotional child abuse. He throws tantrum *because* YOU give in, if he does. He feels more and more unhappy for not having proper behavioral boundary laid down by adults
Exploring genitalia must be a terrible child. He	Natural for the age. But child sexual abuse needs to be ruled out. Watch, if acts

Contd.

Contd.

must be stopped, punished exemplary	sexualized or not. Simple exploration can be managed by distraction techniques. Punishment will only make it worse or hidden.

School Age—Junior School

Crying when starting school, my boy will be a failure at education and a disappointment to me	Natural separation anxiety varies in children. If excessive, i.e. more than two weeks, you need professional help, even if that is just to rule out and reassure. Who knows, if it is a red-flag sign of Asperger syndrome or not?
Afraid to go to school. He is doomed to fail in education	School may be archaic. Most often the fault lies with the school and parents being too meek. But this may herald dyslexia, dyspraxia, depression or even autism
Gets in to fight, naughty child	Rule out bullying, child abuse, ADHD, autism
Does not mix with other children, moody	Rule out autism spectrum disorders, hypothyroidism, neurodegenerative disorders, sensory impairment or social problems like witnessing domestic violence

School Age—Senior School (Teenage)

Using slangs! Urchin!! People are going to raise fingers at us as bad parents	Going through natural experimentation. He will soon find out, if using slangs help him or hinder him, if ignored for a while. If persists, seek professional help. Rule out Tourette's
Reported to have tried to smoke with friends. He must be a junky type!	Opportunity for emotional coaching. Parents can discuss and share their experiences. They must set personal examples. No lecturing please! Lecturing is often counter-productive.
Lying, stealing, thieving brat! How could our	Avoid 'small lies' from infancy. Avoid 'tricking' him into eating or getting him to do your things. These are signs of low self-esteem and the child would love the guidance to get out of

13

Contd.

Contd.

such state although may put up resistance/ fight in the beginning. Set personal examples by paying all your taxes, even when you could have not declared all your earnings and got away with it!

Caught watching porno-graphic images. Must have inherited from my spouse's family!	This is the age for curiosity towards the opposite sex. Opportunity for emotional coaching. Find out why he has to peep? Use your own life saga but without frivolous affect. He needs one or two opportunities. But specify what consequences he can expect. Do not use false threats or false promises.
Day dreams too much! Romeo-type?	Most likely EBD problem. Needs professional help, if you cannot find quick and permanent remedy. Do not wait for too long.

13

All ages!

Doctors are useless, of no real help	Doctors need training and education in EBD problems in children to advocate efficiently

NB: The comments are generally gender neutral, i.e. equally applicable to a boy child or a girl.

Happy parenting!

---

* EBD = Educational/Emotional, Developmental and Behavioral
** SIDS = Sudden Infant Death Syndrome
§ NAFLD = Non Alcoholic Fatty Disease of the Liver
§§ NASH = Non Alcoholic SteatoHepatosis
dBLS = Basic Life Support
ddADHD = Attention Deficit Hyperactivity Disorder

Points to remember

1. Every parent wants their children to do their best.
2. Knowing myths and facts they will help to bring best out of their children.

FURTHER READING

1. Nelson's Text Book of Pediatrics, 19th Edition
2. Meichenbaum D. Cognitive Behavior Modification. New York: Plenum Press. 1977.
3. Piaget J. Play, Dreams and Imitation in Childhood. New York: Norton Company, 1962.
4. Rutter M. Helping Troubled Children. Penguin Books. Harmondsworth. 1975.
5. Patterson GR and Forgatch MS. Parents and Adolescents Living Together. Part 1 & 2. Eugene OR: Castalia Publishing Company, 1987 and 1989.

13

Section

3

Growth and Nutrition of Child

14

Nuclear Family *vs* Joint Family

Shrikant Chorghade

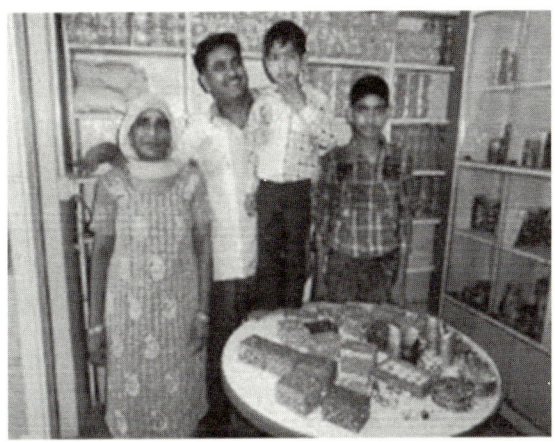

Child in a Nuclear Family

over last few years with industrialization and education, large joint families are gradually becoming rare. Nuclear family is the order of the day, which consists of the child, the parents and one or two older or younger siblings. A smaller family enhances parent child interaction. Parents of fewer children are likely to be more patient and less punitive. They are likely to have more time to spend with the child. In such families the children are likely to be widely spaced, with at least two years difference between two children. This gives more time to parents to look after individual child and pay more attention and better resources to be invested in each child. Children in such families are likely to be healthier having higher intelligence test scores and likely to do better in schools and attain better level of education. These children are likely to get engaged in anti-social behavior.

However these findings will depend on the parental style and availability of parents with the child. A very busy father or both, who are working parents are not likely to give quality time to the child. Their energy level will shrink and hence their participation in parenting will suffer. Child in such a family may feel insecure and emotionally deprived and will have lesser opportunities for learning directly or indirectly from the parents. If their care is left to the caretaker, their development depends on the social and intelligent status of the caretaker.

Joint Family

Family size per se is not alone responsible for relationships that develop amongst family members. Addition of each new member in the family increases the proportion of relationship. Larger the family, greater is the interactional system and greater the friction in home, as multiple egos and multiple expectations are involved. Increased friction results into unhealthy home climate which is detrimental to the emotional development and learning process of the child. Many times in larger families the head of the family has to use authoritarian style of parenting to minimize the friction. Composition of family also decides the friction. Statistic shows that presence of more female members is likely to increase the friction as their interaction is longer and frequent in a home setting. Family relationship is also decided by the attitude of family members and the parents of the child toward the family size. If larger family size is favored the emotional climate is likely to be healthy and possibility of friction will be less. To minimize friction in a family, every adult member has to make personal and financial sacrifices to keep the friction under control. When grandparents are part of the family the effect of family relationship on emotional climate will depend upon the type of role they play.

a. **Noninterference:** Some grandparents stay in the family without interfering in parenting style. They play role of a givers, by offering gifts and treat. Such grandparents are not likely to increase friction.

b. **Loving grandparents:** Some grandparents enjoy interacting and playing with the children, giving quality time and love to them. Such grandparents are likely to increase and enrich emotional atmosphere in the family.

c. **Substitute grandparents:** When both parents are busy the grandparents take over the role of parents in care and discipline of child. Their parental style and parents' cooperation in executing the style, will decide the emotional climate and friction in the family.

d. **Wise and mature grandparents:** These grandparents concentrate on teaching special skills and general knowledge to the children in the family. They do not interfere in the parenting strategies and the academics of the children. Such grandparents are an asset for the family and enrich the emotional climate in the house and enhance the personality development of the child.

14

e. **Nagging and demanding grandparents:** Some grandparents are self-centered are narcissists. They always seek attention and own comforts. They are unhappy and demanding. They criticize and interfere in the working of the family, including parenting strategies. Instead of being a help for the family they insist on fulfilling their demands and desires from the family members and the children. They nag and criticize and they are always unhappy and grumbling. Such grandparents increase the friction in the family spoiling the emotional climate. Children in such a family are likely to lose the feeling of security which is essential for the healthy personality development.

CONCLUSION

Size of any family does not necessarily ensure favorable emotional climate in home. It is the attitude of the members of being helpful and cooperative to each other which enriches the emotional climate in the home, which is conducive to the personality development of the child.

Points to remember

1. Size or type of family is not responsible for child's development but attitude matters.
2. Role of grandparents and parents need to be identified and they must understand the child as a person.

14

– growing too rapidly and climbing centile lines on growth chart

The cut offs for normal on height chart are 3rd and 97th percentiles, for BMI chart are 23 adult equivalent for overweight and 27/28 for obesity and below 5th percentile for underweight. There is no specific weight percentile cut off. Overweight, underweight and obesity can only be detected with BMI.

If the answer is "no", it is abnormal and should be investigated. Children grow in short bursts and therefore readings taken too frequently might give a false impression of a pathological slowing. Short children born to short parents, a phenomenon of familial short stature may continue to cruise along the same line below the 3rd percentile but as per the mid parental centile.

15

An exception is catch-up growth seen in children born with a low birth weight (small for gestational age) wherein they cross up the height centiles in the first 2–4 years to regain their genetic potential. Phenomenon of catch down growth with babies born larger than their genetic potential that cross centiles downwards have also been described.

- There is a wide range of normality in children both below and above the average for their age. Your child is normal as long as he/she is in the normal range for age.
- Do not compare your child to other children around him/her. They are all from different genetic backgrounds. Your differing height and genetic background may be the cause of the difference. Check your child's height and weight on the growth chart provided to you by your pediatrician.
- Get over the common belief that a chubby child is a healthy child. Your child may rather be slim with an appropriate weight centile rather than be an unhealthy overweight or obese child.
- If your child was born preterm, remember that he/she has come early into the world and therefore should not be compared to counterparts of same age until two years. Always take into account the corrected age of the child.
- If your child was born small for gestational age (underweight) at birth and is still growing along the lower centile in terms

of weight and height, do not get desperate and overfeed your child to try and catch up to the "normal average 50th centile". Studies have shown that when children born small for gestational age catch up rapidly, they tend to have a higher risk of obesity, diabetes and hypertension in later life.

- Get your child's height and weight measured regularly and plot them on growth charts (WHO charts for up to 5 years and IAP charts by Khadilkar committee/CDC/Agarwal beyond 5 years).

- Do not measure readings too frequently, readings taken at short intervals have higher chances of error and are difficult to interpret. Readings taken at 3 monthly in infancy, 6 monthly in childhood and even annual readings later on suffice.

- It is important for your child to cruise along the same centile line on the growth charts. Jumping of lines either upwards or downwards both for weight and height needs to be brought to notice of your doctor and any underlying pathology should be looked for.

WHO growth charts can be obtained from: http://www.who.int/childgrowth/standards/en/

Recently published Indian growth charts by Khadilkar et al can be obtained from: http://www.indiachildgrowth.com/growth-charts.html

Growth is one of the best signs of general health and development.

Growth patterns are different for each individual child.
-8- Growth may reflect family growth patterns.

What affects growth?

Nutrition (protein, minerals, iron)

Height of the parents

Level of physical activity

Hormones (growth hormone, thyroid)

15

> **How can I improve my growth?**
>
> Sports for at least one hour daily
>
> Don't watch TV for more than 1 hour
>
> Color your plate
>
> Have junk food only once a month

How IAP growth charts will be publish in Jan 2015. They are prepared by committee headed by Dr Vaman Khadilkar

Growth patterns over time are more important than one single measurement.

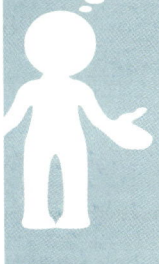

Points to remember

1. Every parents wish to ensure that they should give best care to their children
2. A wide variation exists in the heights and weights of children of the same age and also in their growth pattern.
3. Numerous factors such as genetic background, nutrition, intrauterine and extra uterine environment determine child's growth.
4. Measurement of height and weight properly is essential.
5. Plotting of growth charts, knowing growth potential and BMI helps child to achieve best.

FURTHER READING

1. Patel L, Clayton P. Normal and disordered growth. In: Brook C, Clayton P, Rosalind Brown, editors. Brook's Clinical Pediatric Endocrinology. 5th ed. India: Blackwell Publishing 2005; p. 90–112.
2. Keane V. Assessment of Growth. In: Kliegnan et al. Nelson Textbook of Pediatrics. 19th ed. Philadelphia: Elsevier 2012; p. 39.

3. Bhatia V. Normal and Abnormal Growth. Pediatric Endocrine Disorders. Editors: Meena P. Desai, P S N Menon, Vijayalakshmi Bhatia. 3rd ed. Chennai: Orient Blackswan 2014æ P.41–84.

4. Khadilkar V, Khadilkar A, Choudhury P, Agarwal A, Ugra d, Shah N. IAP Growth Monitoring Guidelines for Children from Birth to 18 Years. Indian Pediatr 2007; 44:187–97.

5. Khadilkar V, Khadilkar A. Growth charts: a diagnostic tool. Indian J Endoc Metab 2011; 15(Suppl3):S166–71.

6. Khadilkar VV, Khadilkar AV, Borade AB, Chiplonkar SA. Body Mass Index cut-offs for Screening for Childhood Overweight and Obesity in Indian Children. Indian Pediatr 2013; 49:29–34.

15

Approach to A Short Child

Anurag Bajpai

Management of growth failure involves comprehensive assessment and timely initiation of growth promoting interventions. Given the limited duration of growth the process should be expedited in children presenting at an older age.

INDICATIONS FOR EVALUATION

Extensive evaluation is reserved for children with height below –3 SDS. In children with milder growth failure (height SDS between –2 and 3 SDS) evaluation should be done if growth velocity is compromised. Children with slow growth rate resulting in crossing two percentile lines between the age of two years and puberty need to be evaluated even if height is in normal range.

ETIOLOGY

Familial Short Stature

A short normal child born in a short family will continue to grow near the 3rd centile or just under it, parallel to the line. This child is growing as per genetic potential and therefore has familial short stature. It is important to realize that this is not a disease and does not need treatment.

An exception would be a family wherein parents are affected with a medical disorder leading to short stature such as growth hormone deficiency or skeletal dysplasia that has been transmitted to a child.

Constitutional Delay in Growth and Puberty

This common scenario is usually seen in boys wherein they slow down in the pre pubertal years, have delayed puberty and delayed growth spurt. Thus they look much smaller and physically immature as compared to their peers. They eventually have a growth spurt and changes of puberty at a later age and attain their final height. History of delayed puberty in the father is often present. This is a physiological variation and may be treated with a short course of testosterone to start puberty. With the onset of puberty, pubertal growth spurt sets in thus improving their stature and physical appearance.

16

Pathological Short Stature

Primary bone disorders such as skeletal dysplasia and osteogenesis imperfecta are uncommon and appear striking with their clinical features.

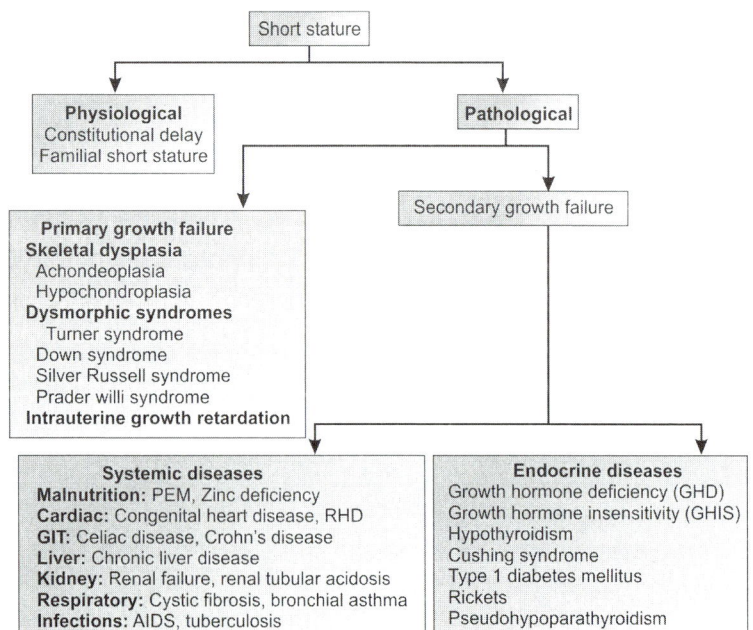

EVALUATION

History

- Age of onset
  - *Prenatal:* Genetic syndromes, intrauterine infections
  - *Infancy:* Congenital growth hormone deficiency, hypothyroidism
  - *Early childhood:* Malabsorption (celiac disease), RTA
  - *Late childhood:* Acquired GHD, hypothyroidism, systemic diseases
- Perinatal history
  - Birth weight, length, head circumference (IUGR)
  - Mode of delivery (breech delivery associated with GHD)
  - Jaundice (intrauterine infection, hypothyroidism, hypopituitarism)
  - Hypoglycemia, micropenis (hypopituitarism)
  - Lymphedema (Turner syndrome)
  - Feeding difficulty, hypotonia (Prader-Willi syndrome)
- Puberty
  - *Delayed:* Hypothyroidism, hypopituitarism, CDPG, celiac disease
  - *Advanced:* Hypothyroidism (girls), untreated precocious puberty
- Family history (familial short stature, GHD, GHIS, skeletal dysplasia)
- Onset and progression of puberty in parents (constitutional delay)
- History suggestive of urinary tract infection, tuberculosis, HIV infection
- Features of steatorrhea (cystic fibrosis, malabsorption)
- Features of liver disease, renal failure, cardiac disease, hypothyroidism
- History of exposure to steroids, radiotherapy, chemotherapy
- Developmental delay—PHP, hypothyroidism, genetic syndrome

Examination

- Upper segment to lower segment ratio

16

- *Increased:* Achondroplasia, Turner syndrome
- *Decreased:* Spondylo-epiphyseal dysplasia
- *Arm span:* Decreased in achondroplasia and hypochondroplasia
- *Metacarpal shortening:* Turner syndrome, pseudohypoparathyroidism
- Pubertal status (delayed in CDGP, hypopituitarism, Turner syndrome)
- Diagnostic clues, features of common disorders

16

Table 16.1: Clues to etiology of short stature

Clue	Etiology
Mid line defect (cleft lip, palate)	Hypopituitarism
Micropenis	Hypopituitarism, Prader-Willi syndrome
Blindness (optic dysplasia)	Hypopituitarism
Single central incisor	Hypopituitarism
Rickets	Renal failure, malabsorption, RTA
Pallor	Renal failure, malabsorption
Malnutrition	Protein energy malnutrition, malabsorption
Metacarpal shortening	Turner syndrome, pseudohypoparathyroidism
Cardiac murmur	Turner syndrome, CHD, intrauterine infection
Deafness	Turner syndrome, intrauterine infection
Tetany	Pseudohypoparathyroidism (PHP)
Mental retardation	Hypothyroidism, genetic syndromes, PHP

Table 16.2: Comparison of familial short stature and CDPG

Feature	Constitutional delay	Familial short stature
Weight	Decreased	Normal
Growth velocity	Normal	Normal
Skeletal maturation	Retarded	Normal
Family history		
Short stature	No	Yes
Delayed puberty	Yes	Variable
Puberty	Delayed	Normal or early
Final height	Low normal	Compromised

16

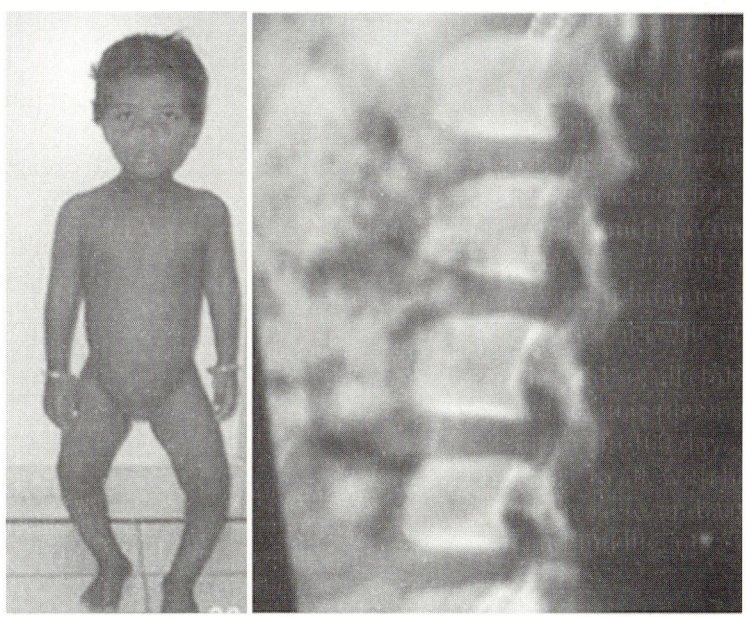

Fig. 16.2: An eight-year-old girl with disproportionate short stature. She had large head, bowing of legs and short limbs. X-ray of the lumbar spine showed cuboid lumbar vertebrae confirming achondroplasia.

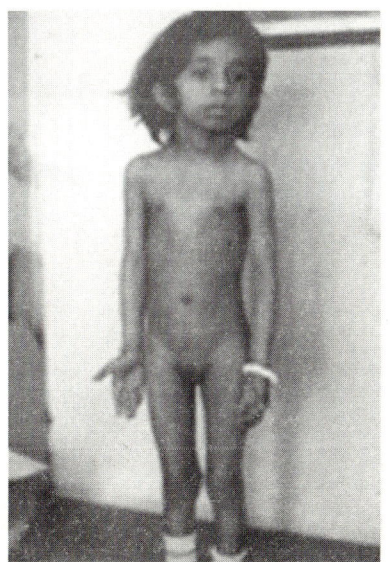

Fig. 16.3: A nine-year-old girl with Silver Russell syndrome. Please note severe growth retardation (height SDS < –3), asymmetrical body habitus and triangular facies

16

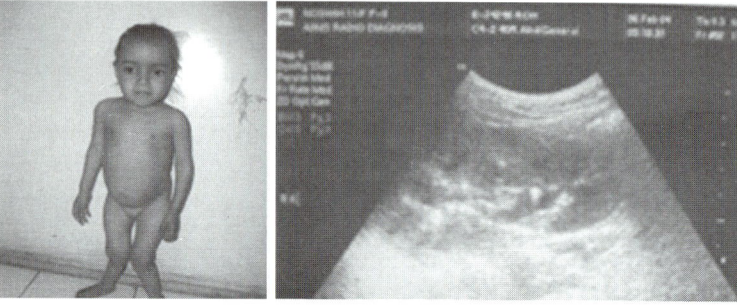

Fig. 16.4: A six-year-old girl with severe growth retardation (height SDS –7) and rickets. Investigations showed severe hyperchloremic acidosis and nephrocalcinosis suggesting distal renal tubular acidosis.

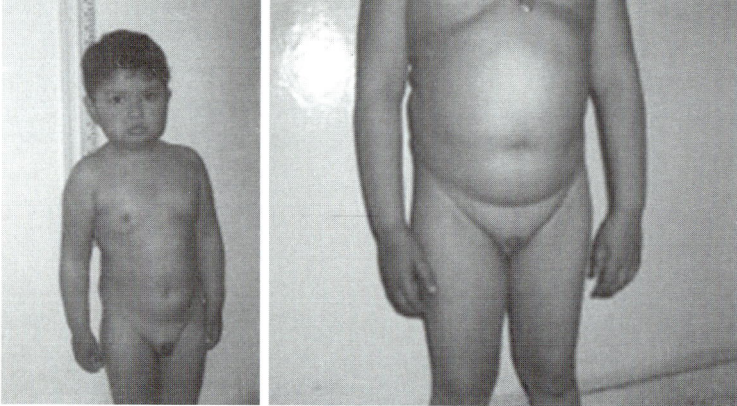

Fig. 16.5: A six-year-old boy with severe growth retardation (height SDS –3.4), central obesity, micropenis and cryptorchidism. Peak GH after clonidine stimulation test were 0.4 ng/ml confirming growth hormone deficiency.

APPROACH

No evaluation is required if height SDS is greater than –2. Children with height SDS between –2 and –3 SDS should be followed-up for six to twelve months for assessment of growth velocity. Assessment is indicated if height SDS is below –3 SDS or in those who have reduced height SDS between –2 and –3

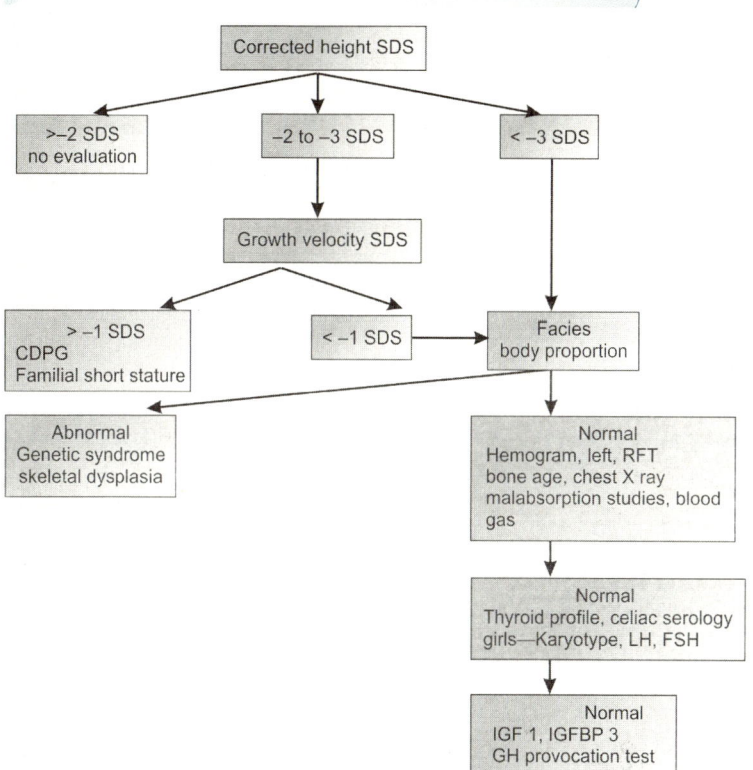

16

and growth velocity less than 25th percentile. Initial evaluation of short stature should include complete blood count, liver function test, renal function test, blood gas and bone age. Thyroid profile, celiac serology and karyotype in girls should be done if these investigations are normal. Evaluation of the GH-IGF-I axis should be done only if all these investigations are normal.

MANAGEMENT

Nutritional Therapy

- Correct iron deficiency (3 mg/kg/day iron for three months)
- Zinc supplementation (10 mg/day for 3–6 months)

Specific Treatment

- *Hypothyroidism:* Thyroxin supplementation
- *Celiac disease:* Gluten free diet
- Constitutional delay of puberty and growth
  - Androgens after bone age is greater than 12 year
  - Testosterone 50 mg once a month intramuscularly for 6 months
- Experimental therapy
  - Delay of epiphyseal fusion: GnRH agonist, aromatase inhibitors
  - Limb lengthening (Ilizarov technique): Skeletal dysplasia

16

Growth hormone therapy				
Condition	*Indication*	*Dose*	*Gain*	*Status*
GHD	All	25–50 µg/kg/d	2–3	Recommended
Turner	Ht < 5th percentile	50–100 µg/kg/d	1–2	Recommended
Renal failure	Growth retardation	50–100 µg/kg/d	1–2	Recommended
SGA	No catch up**	50–200 µg/kg/d	2–3	Recommended
PW syndrome	Growth failure	25–50 µg/kg/d	2–3	Recommended
ISS	Growth failure***	50–100 µg/kg/d	0.5–1	Experimental

* In height SDS, ** by four years of age, ***Height SDS < –2.5, GVSDS < –1

- Growth hormone deficiency
  - Exclude or treat ACTH and TSH deficiency
  - Minimum period of two years after treatment for malignancy
  - Treatment—growth hormone—25–50 µg/kg/day
  - Increase in growth velocity to 8–12 cm/year during first year
  - Growth velocity of 6–8 cm/year during subsequent years
  - Overall improvement in height by 2–3 SDS
- *Turner syndrome*
  - Indications

- Height less than fifth percentile
- No need of GH provocation test
- Dose 50–100 µg/kg/day
- Concomitant treatment
- Oxandrolone (non aromatizable androgen)
- Pubertal induction after 13 years or five years after GH
- *Chronic renal insufficiency (CRF)*
  - *Indication:* Growth retardation on renal replacement program
  - *Prerequisite:* Correct metabolic acidosis, anemia, hyperparathyroidism
  - *Dose:* 50 µg/kg/day
  - *Expected benefit:* Increase in height by 1.0–1.5 SDS

16

Small for Gestational Age (SGA)

- Indications
- Birth weight less than –2 SDS
- Height less than –2.5 SDS by four years of age
- Growth velocity less than 0 SDS
- *Dose:* 50–200 µg/kg/day
- *Prader-Willi syndrome*
  - *Indications:* Growth failure
  - *Pre-requisite:* Exclude obstructive sleep apnea (risk of death)
  - *Dose:* 25–50 mg/kg/day
  - *Follow-up:* Height SDS, BMI SDS, glucose tolerance
  - *Response:* Improvement in growth, body composition, obesity
- *Idiopathic short stature*
  - *Indication:* Height SDS < –2.5 and growth velocity SDS < –1
  - *Dose:* 50–100 µg/kg/day (for at least six months)
  - *Expected benefit:* 5–6 cm

Prognosis

However medical conditions causing short stature need treatment. Achievement of final height depends on condition and timing of onset of treatment. Generally, younger is the child at diagnosis and well monitored therapy will produce better final height results.

Short stature

Why worry?
Marker of serious disease Lower self-esteem

When to worry?
Shortest in the class Growth less than 6 cm/year Short girl at 10 and boy at 12 yr

16

Fact

Hormone disease likely in short and plump child

Fact

Growth hormone is secreted during sleep so sleep early to grow more

Important causes (serious disease in one in three)

Familial short stature

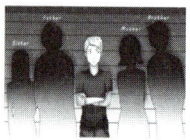

Celiac disease

Allergy to gluten (wheat)
Damage to intestine
Diarrhea and anemia
Respond to stopping wheat

Growth Hormone Deficiency

No growth hormone
Height 30 cm below
Treat with GH

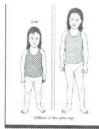

Hypothyroidism

Low thyroid
Weight gain
Poor attention

Points to remember

1. Management of growth failure involves comprehensive assessment and timely initiation of growth promoting interventions.
2. Proper investigations and diagnosis is necessary.
3. Younger is the child at diagnosis and well monitored therapy will produce better final height results.

FURTHER READING

16

1. Growth hormone research society. Consensus guidelines for the diagnosis and treatment of growth hormone (GH) deficiency in childhood and adolescence: summary statement of the GH Research Society. GH Research Society. J Clin Endorinol Metab 2000; 85; 3990–3993.
2. Bajpai A, Menon PS. Growth hormone therapy. Indian J Pediatr 2005; 72; 139–144.
3. Rosenfeld GR, Cohen P. Disorders of growth hormone/insulin like growth factor and action. In: Pediatric Endocrinology Eds: Sperling MA. WB Saunders, Philadelphia, 2 nd Edn. 2002, 211–288.

Micronutrients Deficit

Hemant Joshi, Archana Joshi

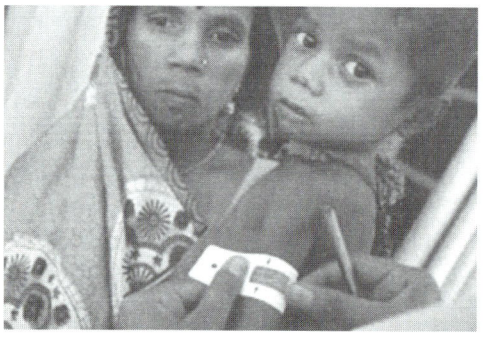

Micronutrients are those food items that we need in small quantities daily in our food. Like vitamins and minerals. Their deficiency in daily diet leads to malnutrition. It makes us miserable.

World Health Organization says that most people in developing countries do not get enough micro nutrients in diet daily. It advises that governments should add 5 micronutrients to salt or wheat floor, etc. so that all get them. These are iodine, folic acid, vitamin D, iron, and vitamin B_{12}. Of these our government has already added iodine to common salt. Let us ask government to add others. Till then, let us see how we can give remaining 4 to ourselves and kids and family. Do this today.

1. *Iron:* Use iron utensils to cook food. Buy iron *Kadhai* (pan) today. While cooking iron gets added to food. That makes vegetables cooked in iron utensils black. That increases their nutritional value. Thus, we get iron free. Studies show that 85% children (and people) are iron deficient. We all are ion

deficient (unless proved otherwise), that makes us anemic, that reduces out efficiency, ask your doctor and take ferrous sulphate one tablet daily for 100 days. Half tablet for small children. Ask doctor to give iron syrup to kids who cannot swallow iron tablet. Government clinics give it free. All students should take this. It improves their studies. Doctor or chemist can give a tablet or liquid having iron, B_{12} and folic acid.

B_{12} and folic acid are needed for cell division and growth.

2. *Folic acid:* We get folic acid from green leafy vegetables. Eat them liberally daily. We can get a tablet of 5 milligrams of folic acid in chemist shop. One needs about 1 milligram of folic acid. A family can divide a tablet and take.

3. *B 12:* Our brain needs B_{12}. Lack of B_{12} spoils brain function and gives rise to many complaints, like leg cramps, and many brain dysfunctions. Only nonvegetarian food gives it. There is no B_{12} in plants. Most vegetarian Indians are deficient in B_{12}. Our studies confirm this. Those who take nonvegetarian food as good as vegetarians. Milk has B_{12}. It increases when we make curds. It is wiser to eat curds in place of milk.

Many Indians in Western countries are given this by their doctors as most Indians are B_{12} deficient. One can take B_{12} as methylcobalamin from doctor as tablet. Or one can take a one thousand microgram injection of Methylcobalamin every 6 months or every year. Ask for most economical brand as prices have big difference.

4. *Vitamin D:* Studies show that vitamin D is needed for general illness fighting power. All get cough and cold but those who have less vitamin D can get pneumonia. We need it to make our bones. Less vitamin D makes us short/dwarf. Studies show that most of us are vitamin D deficient. When afternoon sunlight falls on our skin, for 1 to 2 hours daily we make enough vitamin D for ourselves. For this we must wear such respectable clothes that allow maximum exposure of skin to sunlight. We should do all outside jobs in afternoon sunlight. We should allow kids to play in sunlight. A T-shirt and a half pant make a good dress for

17

gents and kids. Women and girls should wear similar respectable dress.

Vitamin D is available as 60 000 units' sachets in medical shops. Take them with doctor's advice.

5. *Calcium:* Those who eat Pan (betel leaf) get calcium with it. Egg shells are made of calcium. They can be washed, roasted, crushed and stored and added like common salt to food items like vegetables, etc. This is most economical way of getting calcium. Nonvegetarian food and milk also gives calcium.

At the time of marriage a woman should visit a doctor. With doctor's advice she should take iron + B_{12} + folic acid. Deficiency of B_{12} and folic acid leads to babies with birth defect. Deficiency of all the three leads to having smaller babies.

17

> Points to remember
>
> 1. Micronutrient deficiencies are well known hurdles for growth.
> 2. We must know sources, daily requirement and treatment of deficiency.

Eating Disorder and Picky Eaters

Upendra Kinjawadekar, Vikas Alure

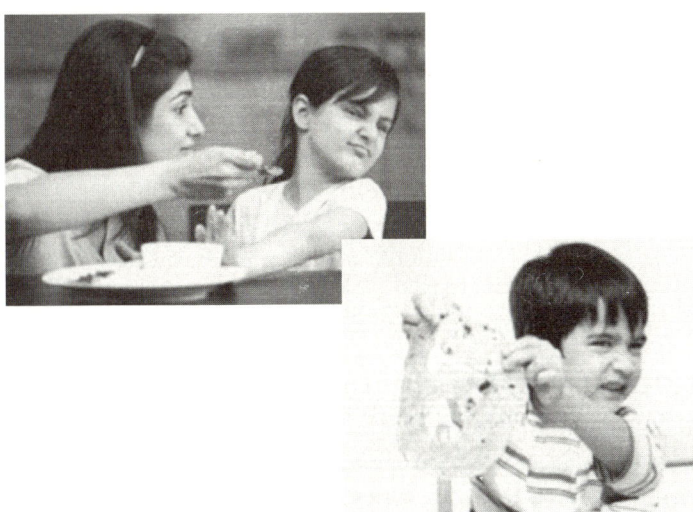

INTRODUCTION

The incidence and prevalence of eating disorders in children and adolescents has increased signicantly in recent decades, making it essential for paediatricians to consider these disorders in appropriate clinical settings, to evaluate patients suspected of having these disorders, and to manage (or refer) patients in whom eating disorders are diagnosed.

Diagnostic and Statistical Manual of Mental Disorders, fourth edition, Text Revision (DSM-IV-TR) classifies them as anorexia nervosa or bulimia nervosa (AN or BN) and some other disorders are labelled as having "partial syndromes" or "eating disorder not otherwise specied" (ED NOS). There are many more patients with ED NOS than there are patients with AN or BN; Anorexia Nervosa and Bulimia Nervosa are not so common in day-to-day practice hence not discussed in details over here. Instead an overview of feeding disorders in infants and very young children which are not commonly discussed elsewhere would be given. The prevalence in India is estimated to be around 1.25%, depending on the denition used.

ETIOPATHOGENESIS

18

Genetic predisposition to various trait disturbances such as behavioural rigidity, perfectionism or harm avoidance may be more salient than genetic influences on eating, hunger or satiety. Dieting has also been implicated as a potent proximal risk factor in the development of disordered eating and eating disorder. Neuroendocrine abnormalities like leptin concentrations are sensitive to the acute metabolic effects of decreased intake and energy deficits, and decreased circulating leptin concentrations reflect depleted stores of body fat.

Current Diagnostic Criteria for Feeding Disorders

Feeding disturbances are much more common in very young children as manifested by persistent failure to eat adequately with significant failure to gain weight or significant loss of weight over at least 1 month. The criteria before diagnosis are:

A. The disturbance is not due to an associated gastrointestinal or other general medical condition (e.g. esophageal reflux).

B. The disturbance is not better accounted for by another mental disorder (e.g. rumination disorder) or by lack of available food.

D. The onset is before age 6 years.

Chatoor's (2002) Subtypes

Feeding disorder of reciprocity (neglect)

A. Infant shows lack of developmentally appropriate signs of social responsively (e.g. visual engagement, smiling, babbling) during feeding with primary caregiver.

B. Infant shows significant growth deficiency.

C. The growth deficiency and lack of relatedness are not solely caused by a physical disorder or a pervasive developmental disorder.

Infantile anorexia

A. Child refuses to eat adequate amounts of food for at least 1 month.

B. Onset of food refusal often occurs during the transition to spoon and self-feeding, typically between 6 months and 3 years of age.

C. Child does not communicate hunger and lacks interest in food but shows strong interest in exploration and interaction across caregiver contacts.

D. Child shows significant growth deficiency.

E. The food refusal did not follow a traumatic event.

F. The food refusal is not caused by an underlying medical illness.

Sensory food aversions

A. Child refuses to eat specific foods with specific tastes, textures, smells, or appearances.

B. Onset of the food refusal occurs during the introduction of a different type of food.

C. Child eats better when offered preferred foods.

D. Child must have specific nutritional deficiencies or oral motor delay or both.

Feeding disorder associated with concurrent medical condition

A. Child readily initiates feeding but over the course of feeding shows distress and refuses to continue feeding.

B. Child has a concurrent medical condition that is believed to cause the distress.

C. Medical management improves but does not fully alleviate the feeding problems.

D. Child fails to gain adequate weight or may even lose weight.

Post-traumatic feeding disorder

A. Food refusal follows a traumatic event or repeated   traumatic insults to the oropharynx or gastrointestinal tract that trigger intense distress in the infant.

B. Consistent refusal to eat manifests in refusal of the bottle and/or refusal of solid foods.

C. Reminders of the traumatic events cause distress.

D. Food refusal poses an acute or long-term threat to nutrition.

INITIAL EVALUATION OF THE PATIENT WITH DISORDERED EATING

18

When screening raises suspicion of an eating disorder, initial evaluation includes establishing the diagnosis, evaluating medical and nutritional status, determining severity, and performing an initial psychosocial evaluation.

Most laboratory results will be normal in patients with eating disorders; however, normal laboratory results do not exclude serious illness or medical instability in these patients. The patient's social functioning at home, in school, and with friends should be assessed. Psychiatric comorbidity is common with eating disorders and is often previously undiagnosed.

Patients who are more ill often require more intensive services, ideally delivered by a specialized multidisciplinary team, and sometimes in day-treatment, hospital, or residential settings.

TREATMENT CONTINUUM FOR CHILDREN AND ADOLESCENTS WITH EATING DISORDERS

Most adolescent patients with eating disorders will be treated in outpatient settings.

Collaborative Outpatient Care

Most children and adolescents with eating disorders will be managed in an outpatient setting by a multidisciplinary team comprising of pediatricians, nutritionists, child counsellors, child psychologists, teachers and of course with active participation of parents.

GUIDANCE FOR PEDIATRICIAN

1. Pediatricians need to be knowledgeable about the risk factors and early signs and symptoms of disordered eating and eating disorders.

2. When counselling families on preventing obesity, paediatricians should focus on healthy eating and building self-esteem while still addressing weight concerns. Care needs to be taken not to inadvertently enable excessive dieting, compulsive exercise, or other potentially unhealthy weight-management strategies.

3. Paediatricians should be encouraged to calculate and plot weight, height, and BMI by using age- and gender-appropriate charts and assess menstrual status in girls at annual health supervision visits.

4. Paediatricians should screen patients for disordered eating and related behaviours and be prepared to intervene when necessary.

5. Paediatricians should monitor or refer patients with eating disorders for medical and nutritional complications.

6. Paediatricians need to be familiar with treatment resources in their communities so that they can coordinate or facilitate multidisciplinary care.

7. Paediatricians can play a role in primary prevention during office visits and through school-based and community interventions.

18

PICKY EATING

The patients come to pediatricians for various reasons. Some come for fever, some for cough and cold, and some for loose motion, vomiting and some for routine check up. Whatever may be the primary complaint, some questions which usually pop up at the consultation time are

A. My child doesn't eat; can you please write a tonic?

B. My child eats only sweets

C. Neighbour's child is of the same age and eats so wonderfully

D. My child takes 2 hours just to finish a bowl of rice!

"Picky" eating is when a child (or adult) refuses foods often or eats the same foods over and over. Picky eating usually peaks in the toddler and preschool years. Many parents worry that their picky eater is not getting enough nutrition to grow. But in most cases, he is. Keep a food diary for a day—writing down everything your child eats—and you will probably find that he is eating more than you thought. Food preferences have a lot to do with genes (though not entirely). Children's taste buds are much more sensitive than adults and their food dislikes may seem strange to us but may be very strong for them.

What to Do About Picky Eating

18

- Don't stress…
  If your child is growing normally and is not lacking in energy, he or she is most likely getting the nutrients he or she needs for healthy development, even if he or she is picky. You can always check with your paediatrician if you have concerns. Too much stress at meal time doesn't help anyone out, least of all you!

- But still encourage them…
  You can still have an impact on how your children think about food. It important to help them form good habits and learn to make good choices, even if it doesn't always result in them eating what you want right now. Children can learn that it is expected of them to behave a certain way at the table and that they are expected to eat certain foods, even if it's a future goal. One day your child is likely to grow out of it, and you want him or her to have the opportunity to make a good choice, rather than thinking of himself or herself as a picky eater forever.

- Picky eating: Strategies
  1. Involve your children in preparing meals. Even a simple step like helping to wash produce or set the table can help
  2. Be a good role model! They will be more likely to try something if they see you eating it and enjoying it.
  3. Try setting a rule that they have to have a little bit of vegetable (or whichever food is a problem) on their plate

at each meal. Tell them that they don't necessarily have to try it, but it has to go on the plate

4. If your child says she's hungry, but then only wants dessert or other treats, have a conversation with her about whether they're really hungry or not.

5. Try using fun names for food, or having your children make edible fruit and vegetable art.

6. Try serving vegetables or problem foods first, before other foods appear on the table. If it's not competing with a more familiar food, a child will be more likely to try it.

- Reducing your stress

  18

  It's late, you are tired, you have to cook dinner and your child is refusing to eat. It's hard not to get upset or stressed when your child is digging in his or her heels about food. But remember, getting stressed about mealtimes and picky eating isn't going to help anyone out, least of all you! Here are a couple things to keep in mind to help you

  1. Plan your meals ahead of time as much as you can. Then you will not be strapped for time with shopping and planning.

  2. Your child is in a stage where he or she is figuring out limits, and knows how to push your buttons! If you find yourself getting in a tug of war over food, remember to take a deep breath and stay calm. Remember that you are the parent and you set the limits, not your child.

  3. Keep in mind that children may be resistant to eating when they're not hungry. If your child is being really picky at lunch or dinner, take a look at how often he or she is eating. Spacing out meals more or serving less for snack can help make a child ready to eat main meals

- Some things to avoid

  1. Using sweets as a reward for eating a vegetable. While this may work in the short term, it ultimately makes your child less likely to develop a liking for vegetables. It also makes the sweets even more desirable—so brownies become more appealing than before!

2. "Hiding" vegetables in comfort foods. It's great to incorporate chopped or pureed veggies into pasta, soup, or meatloaf, but it's important your children know what they're eating. Otherwise, they are not going to learn to choose to eat vegetables. And anyway, most recipes that "hide" vegetable purees in comfort foods are not adding very much to the nutrient content of the food.

3. Remember that you're not a shortorder cook! make the same meal for adults and children that way, children will not get the message that they can always eat whatever they want.

18

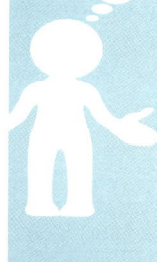

Points to remember

1. Eating disorder like anorexia nervosa and bulimia needs proper diagnosis and management.
2. Picky eaters is very common worry of parents but if your child is growing well you should not be worried.
3. Proper eating habits and firm parenting to inculcate good habits is necessary part of management.

FURTHER READING

1. Identification and Management of Eating Disorders in Children and Adolescents-David S. Rosen and the Committee on Adolescence: Pediatrics 2010; 126: 1240
2. Prevalence of Eating Disorders and Psychiatric co-morbidity among Children and Adolescents: P. Mammen, S. Russell and P.S. Russell : Indian Pediatrics: Vol. 44 may 17, 2007.
3. Picky Eaters Hand-out–Rudd canter for food policy and Obesity-Yale Uni.
4. Gibbs, J. (2006, Jan–Mar) Working with picky eaters: The Toddler years. Family and Consumer Sciences Quarterly Media Packet, Michigan State University Extension, East Lansing, MI.
5. Lerner, C, & Parlakian, R (2007). Healthy from the start: How feeding nurtures your young child's body, heart, and mind. Zero to three: Washington, DC.

Parenting Lessons from Our Gods for Nutrition

Hemant Joshi, Archana Joshi

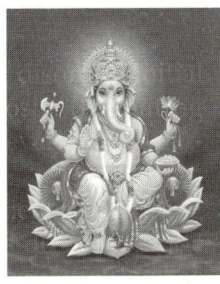 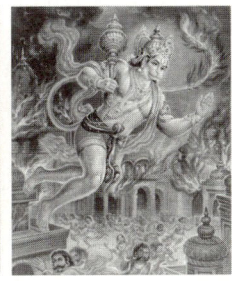

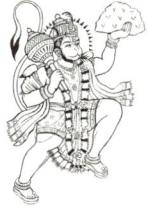

Coconut day keeps malnutrition away both Lord Ganapati and Hanumanji are offered coconuts. Give 1 coconut to each child daily and malnutrition will disappear. No exercise no games and only eating will make them" Lambodar" obese Ganpati. Make food liberally available and let children exercise and play outdoor games one hour daily. They will become strong Hanumanji.

We love Hanumanji. Immortal most intelligent, powerful and works at the speed of thought.

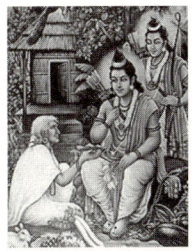

Shabari and Lord Ram

Shabari tasted fruit and then gave them to Lord Ram "We must taste food and medicines before giving to babies. Western studies show that on adding *breast milk* to medicine and food children take them better. "

19

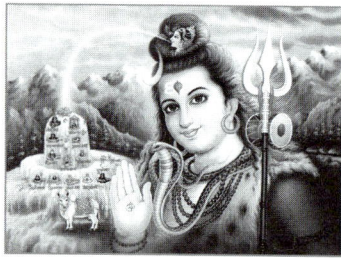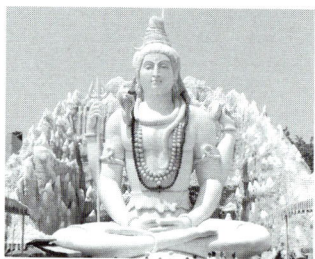

"Gangajal" is better name for ORS

Improves acceptance—success of treatment

Sit in Padmasan which is one of the yogasans. Learn Ashtangyoga Patanjali yoga.

Patanjali sutra by PATANJALI. Indian text of psychology and mind control makes you superman/superwoman. Yoga will teach you control over the mind and body.

Karna

We can learn many lessons from Karna. He grew in an ordinary house. By his hard work he became King. Karna forgot Bramhastra in war and died. To avoid such tragedy in our life we must keep learning all the time. Wheel of his chariot got jammed in ground at the time of war and he was killed.We must every minute maintain our instruments well so that they do not fail us in emergency.

Karna and Shalya: Shalya his driver cursed him all the time and spoiled his mental peace. We must not do this to our people. Forgive them if they are wrong, and correct their error. Teach your people all the time. Treat them like your children. Love and care for them will reap huge dividends. Karna's Father God Surya gave him KawachKundal. Vaccines are modern KawachKundal. Be god Sun and give all vaccines to all kids all the time. Karna was born of unwed mother. To avoid such pregnancies, give sex education to children.

Krishna and Karna were "adopted "immediately after birth. Promote adoption as soon after birth as possible. Let us make "Give baby take baby clubs" for such adoptions.

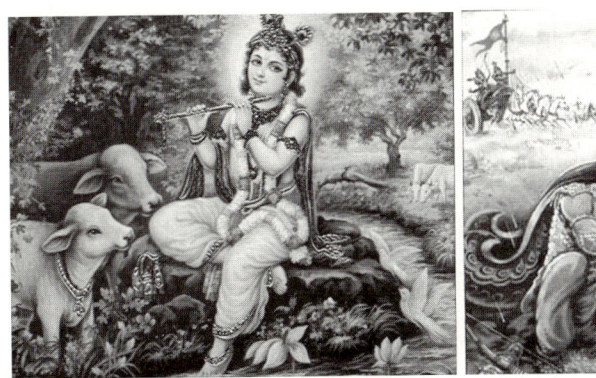 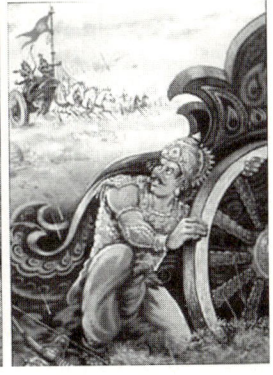

19

Karna was a great donor. Let us donate all our knowledge to all.

20

Nutrition: Story Therapy
Best to Educate and Improve Child Survival and Children Started Eating

Hemant Joshi, Archana Joshi

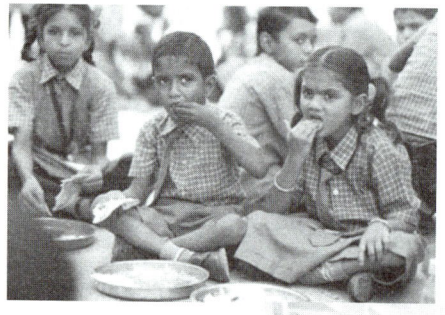

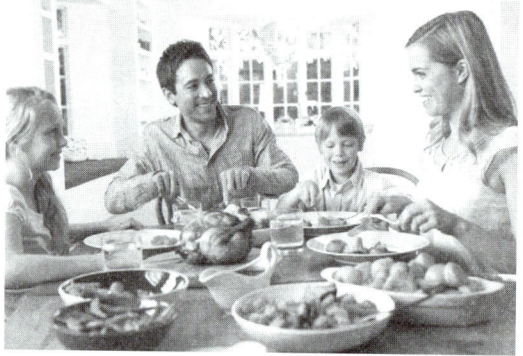

Once there lived a lovely family in India. They had a son and daughter named A and B. The family was happy except that A and B never ate properly. Hence, both become pale white, weak, irritable and never slept well. They passed plenty of urine. They had hard stools. They were constipated. The parents sought doctors' help. A and B were given milk, tonics, tinned food, and medicines. But it was of no use.

A and B got fed up with the treatment. They ran away from home in forest outside the city. They ran until they got exhausted. They fell fast asleep.

A childless couple in the forest saw A and B and took them to their hut. They gave them food. But both A and B ate nothing.

The couple said, "Sitting is sickness. Playing working is wellness."You run, play, work, and dance. Then you will be hungry. Then you will feel good, eat well and sleep well.

A and B followed their advice. They helped all to collect fruits and firewood, did household jobs, ran, played and danced with all. And for the first time in life A and B felt very "very good" and "very hungry". That night they had very good dinner and very sound sleep. With this routine in 100 days both gained weight and became very healthy and handsome. There was a town fair. A and B and friends visited the fair. Both won prizes in the healthy children contest. Their city parents had come to the fair. A and B had changed so much that city parents could not recognize them. Finally A and B went back to the city with the parents.

20

The parents gave a party on their return. In the party A and B told the secret of how they started eating sleeping and growing well. They said, "Earlier you gave us tea, milk, fruit juice, rice water and dal water. All these liquid foods have more water and less food. They filled our stomach but starved us. We had to eat when you wished. We got everything in our hands. We had no exercise either. So we became weak. In jungle, we had the freedom of eating as per our wish. There were no liquid foods. We did lot of physical work. We danced, played, worked and had lot of fun. So we were happy and we grew well.

DO AS FOLLOWS AND YOUR CHILDREN WILL GROW WELL

1. Give one corner of the house to kids. Call it child fruit snack water corner. There on the floor keep a plate or a transparent plastic jar. Call it Akshaypatra. It should be always full of fruits and snacks that children like. Children may eat some and spill some. None should shout. All neighboring kids should also be allowed to eat from this as well.

2. All children's all clothes must have pockets. The pockets must be full of snacks all the time.

3. Liquid foods have more water and less food. They starve children. Nobody will give tea, or milk to children. The money saved will be used to for snacks.

4. Best donation for children is donation of playground. Every child must play on ground in evening for at least once hour. "Do this and tell all."

5. Wear minimum clothes. Clothes increase warmth and reduce appetite and growth.

20   They did so; all children started eating round the clock. They started singing, playing, studying, and growing better and made all happy. In 100 days, all became better. Let us right now tell this story to all, with help of TV, Radio, Newspapers, speeches, email, sms, etc. and save lives and make our children stronger, tall, and intelligent.

Points to remember

1. "You run, play, work, and dance. Then you will be hungry. Then you will feel good, eat well and sleep well.

2. Give one corner of the house to kids.

3. All children's all clothes must have pockets. The pockets must be full of snacks.

Section

4

Toddler

Recommendations for Pre-School Education

MKC Nair, Suchit Tamboli, IAP Pre-school Committee 1994

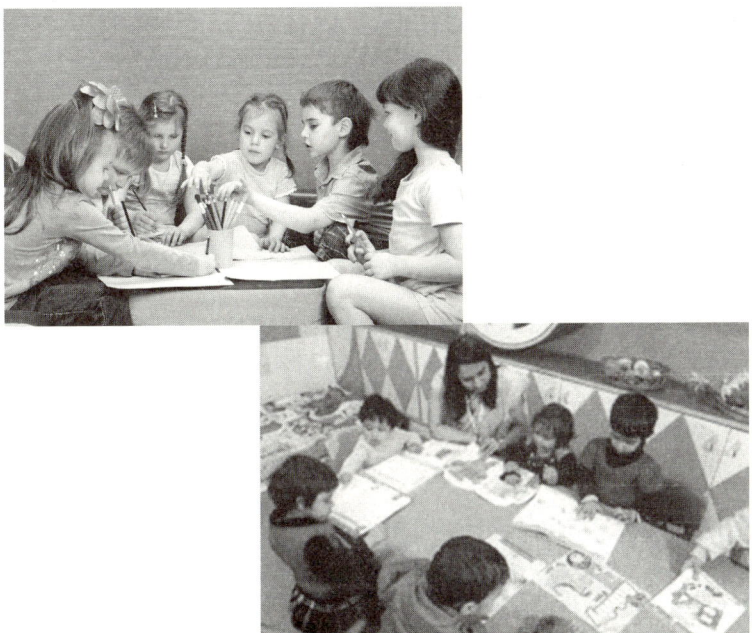

GENERAL RECOMMENDATIONS

1. The pre-primary age is crucial one in the development of the child and hence a developmental approach rather than an educational approach must be adopted.
2. Pre-primary education is not a downward extension of primary education and hence only non-formal educational method must be adopted.

3. Pre-primary child can express herself best in her mother tongue and hence the medium of communication in the nurseries

4. Some of the apparently normal looking children who may have developmental disabilities need to be integrated into normal nursery system with special attention.

5. Pre-primary period is the most vulnerable period of childhood and hence all efforts should be made in assuring quality in the training of teachers.

6. There is no uniformity in the pattern and academic content of pre-primary teacher's training of various Government departments and private sector in India and hence the State units of NCERT (SCERT) may be entrusted with the academic content of teachers training program.

7. Although universalization of pre-primary education is an accepted policy of the Government, finances often come in the way and hence Panchayats and other local bodies may be encouraged to come in a big way into the field of pre-primary education.

8. The public and a large number of parents are not aware of the advantages of promoting non-formal pre-primary education and its vital role in overall development of the child and hence all efforts may be to enlighten the public on this concept.

SPECIFIC RECOMMENDATIONS

1. Minimum age for entry into LKG should be "FOUR YEARS COMPLETE" on the day of admission.

2. The selection criteria for admission should not be based on interview and testing the child.

3. Medical fitness and immunization certificate should be a must for admission.

4. Mother tongue should preferably be the medium of communication in pre-school education.

5. The undue emphasis on reading and writing is detrimental to the development of a pre-school child and it should not be practiced.

6. The pre-school activities should be based on the recommendations of the NCERT, New Delhi.

7. Pre-school activities should be subjected to formal examination and homework. Grading should be preferred to ranking or marking.

8. R.T.O. Safety regulations should be strictly followed while transporting children to and from a school.

9. Pre-school education should not be a must for admission in 1st standard.

10. The Indian Academy of Pediatrics should be involved in formulating guidelines for pre-primary education at all levels as had done in Kerala.

21

IAP SUB-COMMITTEE ON "PRE-SCHOOL EDUCATION"

(Recommendations Approved by Executive Board of IAP,1994)

Parenting— From Cradle to Crayons

Pramod Jog

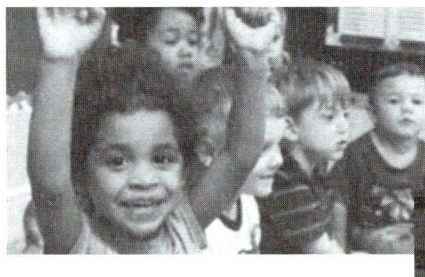

If I had my child to raise all over again,
I'd build self-esteem first, and the house later.
I'd finger-paint more, and point the finger less.
I would do less correcting and more connecting.
I'd take my eyes off my watch, and watch with my eyes.
I'd take more hikes and fly more kites.
I'd stop playing serious, and seriously play.
I would run through more fields and gaze at more stars.
I'd do more bugging and less tugging.

— Diane Loomans

For most of us, becoming a parent has been easy. All of a sudden we had a baby in our hands not knowing what to do with him or her.

"Parenthood is a lot easier to get into than out of"
—Bruce Lansky.

The rearing of a child or children, especially the care, love, and guidance given by a parent is parenting; parenting can also mean the care and upbringing of a child. Parenting is the art and science by which the parents are able to equip the child under their care with skills to lead a life in this world without being dependent on adults for ever.

"The most important thing that parents can teach their children is how to get along without them"
—Frank A. Clark

22

Parenting is an art that has been passed on for generations without much of thought about the same. We have learnt the competence to parent from how we were treated by our parents and from how we have seen others treat their children. The skills have been imbibed predominantly by observing, experiencing as well as by noticing certain obvious flaws in the techniques that have resulted in behavioral disturbances in the children.

Parents are those who provide significant care for a sizeable period of time to children without being paid for the same. Parents include biological parents, foster parent, adoptive parents, grandparents and other relatives.

Parenting in a joint family is different from the parenting that is being done in a nuclear family where there are only two parent figures.

We all as parents have a common agenda in our minds when we start our journey on parenting. All of us want our children to be happy, well looked after and cared for and we also want our children to inculcate the right values and progress ahead in an acceptable manner so that they are appreciated by all significant members of the community including the members of the small microcosm in which they are brought up.

We all are keen on knowing the best parenting techniques to provide the best for our children. Parenting is an art as well as a science but it is not a standard tool that one recommendation applies to all children. There is nothing like good parenting and bad parenting practices. Certain practices have been encouraged as they help in the nurturance and maintenance of self-esteem in our children. This enables our children to become independent adults in this world.

A child who is offered encouragement, appreciation and unconditional love evolves into a confident, self reliant, lovable, respectable adult.

As pediatrician, we all have an excellent opportunity to interact with parents during almost all consultations. We have the prospect of meeting parents while they harbor different emotional states. We have the chance to relate with parents when they are excited at the sight and feel of their newborn baby, or when they are anxious to see their little one receive his or her immunization, or when they are disturbed that their baby has developed the first febrile illness. We also have the likelihood of encountering parents when they want to complain about their children's mis behavior at home or school or outside the home environment. We also have the possibility of sharing the moments of success enjoyed by the child and the family at various stages of the child's journey in this world.

Common Discipline Mistakes and the Solutions

1. Not being respectful

We parents ask our children to respect us, but we sometimes forget that respect should be a two-way street.

One of the most common mistakes parents make disciplining children is yelling, speaking in harsh and angry tone, or even insulting their children.

Giving and asking for respect in return is one of the cardinal tips to remember about disciplining children.

The solution

Think about how you would like to be spoken to if you were working out a conflict with, say, a family member or a friend or co-worker. Get down to your child's eye level, and discuss the problem at hand in a gentle (but still firm) and respectful manner. And no matter how angry you are, try to remain calm; do not yell, and never belittle your child.

2. Disciplining while angry

There are some things that just should not go together, like drinking and driving or writing a heated email to someone who's made you angry before you've had a chance to cool down. Disciplining a child while angry is definitely in that category of dont's. When you reprimand your child while you are mad about something they did, you are more likely to shout or say something you don't mean.

The solution

Take a few minutes to calm down and collect your thoughts before talking to your child about his bad behavior. Remove yourself or your child from the immediate situation by, say, taking a walk.

22

In fact, giving you and yourself some time to reflect on the conflict may help you both deal with the situation in a calmer manner.

3. Being inconsistent

If you reprimand your child for not cleaning his room one day then not bother to talk to him about it when his room is messy for days on end, only to scold him again for not keeping his room clean, your child is getting a very inconsistent message. One of the best ways to help children correct their behavior is by giving them clear instructions about what is expected of them.

The solution

Give your child clear and simple directions. For instance, if you want her to clean her rooms every week mark it on a calendar and make that "room clean-up day". Set her up for good behavior, and if she does not follow through, give her a consistent set of consequences (by, say, taking away a favorite toy for a set amount of time). Be constant and consistent in enforcing the rules.

4. Talking/explaining too much

While it's a good idea to talk to your child about why something she did was not appropriate so that she can have a clear sense of what she did wrong and how she can behave differently the next time, going into lengthy and detailed explanations about her behavior is not a good idea.

The solution
With younger children, simply state what the behavior was and why wrong ("you went into your brother's room and played with his toy without his permission, and that made him feel like you didn't care about his feelings"). Be as direct as possible and break it down into basics for your child. With older children, talk about what went wrong and discuss possible scenarios that could have been better choices.

22

5. Going negative

Hearing a string of "don'ts" and "no's" isn't any fun for anyone, especially a child.

Focusing on what a child did wrong or what he should not do instead of emphasizing what a child should do can put a negative spin on things and set the tone for your interaction.

The solution
Approach things from a more positive perspective by talking about what can be done better. If your child is whining or talking back to you, show her some examples of how to speak in a nice and more friendly manner. After tempers have cooled on both sides, try a lighthearted game of speaking nicely to each other to express yourselves better. If your child is fighting with a sibling, suggest some ways they can build a good sibling relationship, such as by having them work together on a project.

6. Thinking disciplining means punishing

Often, parents forget that the point of disciplining children is to give them firm guidelines and limits so that they do not need to be punished. Disciplining means setting up boundaries and expectations so that kids know what is expected of them. The primary goal is to have kids learn to eventually regulate themselves so that they do not need to be punished.

The solution

Re-think the way you view discipline. When you discipline a child, you are showing him how to make good choices and choose behaviors that are positive and ultimately good for him. And by showing him how you handle his misbehavior—in a loving and constructive manner that emphasizes learning rather than punishment —you are teaching him how they demonstrated bad behavior.

7. Not practicing what you speak

You tell your child not to tell lies but routinely to get out of things you don't want to do like join that school volunteer committee or attend an unimportant meeting at work. Or you yell at your children & angrily tell them to speak nicely to each other.

22

The problem is that we often do not see our own behavior, and forget that our children are watching our every move and learning how to behave by using our example.

The solution

As much as possible, try to live up the example that you are setting up for your child. And if you do occasionally break one of your own rules, explain to your child the particular circumstances and why you behaved the way you did. Admit to how you could have handled it better, and talk about how you may do things differently the next time.

8. Not fitting the discipline technique to your child

When it comes to child discipline, one size does not fit all. What technique worked for one child may be the wrong approach for another child. Instead of repeatedly trying to fit a certain approach to correct or guide a child's behavior, try different techniques to see what might work best on an individual child.

The solution

Remember that children, like adults, have their own personalities, temperaments, and quirks. One kid may be more stubborn than others or be more likely to have a meltdown when things don't go to his way. Try different approaches to tailor discipline techniques to each individual child. For instance, while one child may be able to focus after just about 1 or 2 reminders, another child may need charts and schedules and more. Moreover, while one child may stop misbehaving after a warning that he will lose privileges (a toy or an activity), another child may actually need to have those things taken away and experience the consequences of bad behavior before learns.

9. Not disciplining children at all

Among the many important reasons why we need to discipline children is the fact that children who are raised with clear limits and guidance are more likely to be happy, pleasant people who have good self-control. When children are not disciplined, the effects are clear, and in most cases, quite catastrophic. Children who are not given any limits or consequences and are spoiled are often selfish, unable to self-regulate, and unpleasant to be around.

The solution

Give your child rules and limits and clear and consistent consequences when they don't do what they are supposed to do. If you are worried that disciplining your child may make them angry with you, keep the bigger picture in mind: Not disciplining a child is not good for him. As long as you handle his misbehavior with love and firm guidance, your child will learn and grow from his mistakes.

Parent these days are very keen on providing their best to the children with respect to the basic needs of food, clothing and shelter. In the process of fulfilling this desire of many parents are in tightly placed employment that makes it difficult for them to give time to their children.

Love for the child to establish connection, setting limits to control behavior, respecting individuality, effective role modeling to imbibe values and habits and providing safety and protection are the key dimensions of parenting...

Effective parenting during early childhood definitely helps in the development of a capable, independent young adult.

Here are 3 unbelievably simple parenting ideas that work

1. Children need a minimum of eight touches during a day to feel connected to a parent. If they're going through a particularly challenging time, it's a minimum of 12 a day. This doesn't have to be a big deal; it could be the straightening of a collar, a pat on the shoulder or a simple hug.

2. Each day, children need one meaningful eye-to-eye conversation with a parent.

   It is especially important for babies to have that eye contact, but children of all ages need us to slow down and look them in the eyes.

3. There are nine minutes during the day that have the greatest impact on a child:

   The first three minutes right after they wake up

   The three minutes after they come home from school

   The last three minutes of the day before they go to bed

We need to make those moments special and help our children feel loved.

These are simple, right? Nothing really earth-shattering here.

But try it. For a month.

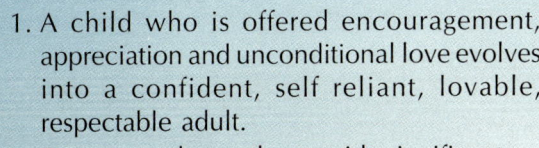

Points to remember

1. A child who is offered encouragement, appreciation and unconditional love evolves into a confident, self reliant, lovable, respectable adult.

2. Parents are those who provide significant care for a sizeable period of time to children without being paid for the same. Parents include biological parents, foster parents, adoptive parents, grandparents and other relatives.

23

Behavioral Problems in Toddlers

Sunil Godbole

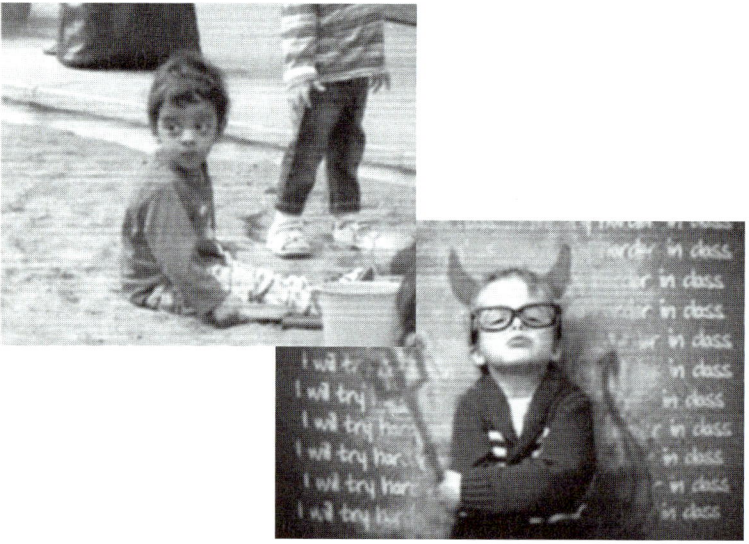

I. INTRODUCTION

The term behavior refers to the way a person responds to a certain situation or experience. Behavior problems usually peak at around age three and start to decline as language develops. Toddler behavior can be very confusing. When toddlers misbehave; it's not planned, it's not deliberate and they are not doing it to hurt somebody. It's more like experimenting with emotions and finding out the responses from the people around. As the emotional brain is immature in toddlers; behavioral issues are just similar, to those falls an infant experiences when it learns to walk!

Though behavioral disturbances are normal in a toddler; when these behavioral problems occur regularly it can impact on a child's progress at school and their social–emotional development. It is the right age to educate the child about 'good, socially acceptable norms of behavior'. Especially the fast life-style, working parents, grandparent laden family, electronic media (the 3 idiots: Television, Computer and Mobile) and early schooling—all make the toddler vulnerable for behavioral problems. As a pediatrician; we nowadays face lot of anxious parents coming with behavioral problems of their tiny toddlers; and asking advice (sometimes medicines!) for the same. The growing awareness of developmental problems like autism, ADHD and learning disorders also sensitize parents to over-react to the behavioral problems of the toddlers.

23

II. DEFINITION OF CHALLENGING BEHAVIOR IN TODDLERS

The Center on the Social and Emotional Foundations for Early Learning's definition of challenging behavior for children from birth to 5 years old is:

- Any repeated pattern of behavior that interferes with learning or engagement in pro-social interactions with peers and adults, and
- Behaviors those are not responsive to the use of developmentally appropriate guidance procedures.

This definition of challenging behavior applies to infants and toddlers as well as pre-schoolers. Challenging behavior is often caregiver-specific. In other words, what is challenging to one caregiver may not seem challenging to another caregiver.

III. THREE TYPES OF BEHAVIOR

1. Behaviors that are wanted and approved. For example being polite, doing homework and chores. These actions receive compliments freely and easily.
2. Behavior is not sanctioned but is tolerated under certain conditions, such as during times of illness (of a parent or a child) or stress (a move, for instance, or the birth of a new sibling). For example not doing chores, regressive behavior (such as baby talk), or being excessively self-centered.

3. Behaviors that should not be tolerated or reinforced. They include actions that are harmful to the physical, emotional, or social well-being of the child, the family members, and others. They might include very aggressive or destructive behavior, overt racism or prejudice, stealing, truancy, smoking or substance abuse, school failure, or an intense sibling rivalry.

IV. RISK FACTORS FOR BEHAVIOR DISORDERS IN TODDLERS

1. *Parental factors*
   - Marital conflict
   - Parental mental illness, aggressive behavior
   - Poor communication between parents or parent and child
   - Poor parenting skills
2. Family factors
   - Parental rejection of child
   - Inconsistent management including harsh discipline
   - Large family size
   - Single parent family
   - Parent with anti-social personality disorder and alcohol dependence
   - Death of close family member.
3. Social or economic environment
   - Poor quality and quantity of maternal social contacts with relatives or friends outside the home (influences mother–child interaction within home)
   - Socioeconomic disadvantage

V. CAUSES OF BEHAVIOR DISORDERS IN TODDLERS

1. **Developmental:** Infants and toddlers have immature cortical brain, which means that they cannot control their primitive impulses like pushing, biting, beating or running around!
2. **Emotional:** Toddler's emotional development is also incomplete. This makes them vulnerable for emotional out-bursts and hence problematic behavior.

23

3. **Under-stimulation:** The toddler; in fact all the children; need some or other stimulus to keep them busy. If they cannot get one; they make their own—such as hitting a sibling, head banging or throwing a temper tantrum!

4. **Attention seeking:** We all have an innate desire to be recognized; to have an impact on people around! Most of the times a good behavior of a child is not well appreciated. In such case the child resorts to bad behavior. The angry parental reaction is also appreciated by the attention seeking child.

5. **Lack of structured environment:** Lack of clear rules and routines makes a toddler vulnerable for bad behavior. But too rigid discipline is also responded by a tantrum!

23

6. **Inadequate language development:** Toddlers are yet to develop adequate vocabulary and fluency of verbal communication. This leads to limitation of verbally expressing their needs and emotions. As a result they become physical!

7. **Stressful family environment:** Parental conflicts, chronically ill person in the family, death of a near one— are all the reasons of stress and hence the miss-behavior in a child.

8. **Parental emotional disturbances:** An angry father, a weeping mother, an irritable grandparent—all make a child unhappy. Even parental emotional reactions to the child's behavior can trigger primitive rage and fear responses in toddlers.

9. **Physical causes:** Lack of sleep, tiredness, hunger, diseases (fever, earache, stomach-pain, skin rashes, nose block...) can trigger bad behavior.

10. **Sugary food plays havoc in child's brain:** Sudden rise in blood sugar due to chocolate or candy eaten on empty stomach is responded by insulin release. This in turn drops the blood sugar rapidly; even lower than normal. This hypoglycemia releases stress hormones (cortisol and epinephrine) which leads to anxiety, aggression, panic and confusion. The child becomes restless, throws a tantrum!

11. **Food additives:** Some food additives—sweeteners, benzoates, artificial colors and many more—can reduce levels of dopamine, norepinephrine and tryptophan in brain. This results in hyperactive behavior in some children.

VI. COMMON TYPES OF BEHAVIORAL DIFFICULTIES IN TODDLERS

Researchers and psychologists have tried to enumerate and analyze different types of behavioral problems in toddlers. Even DSM–V and DSM–PC criteria also enlist a long list of behavioral problems. For practicing pediatricians the classification by Gardner and Shaw appears simple and clear! They group toddler behavioral problems under two major groups—the term "**disruptive problems**" to refer to a group of oppositional or attention related symptoms, and the term "**emotional problems**" to refer to depressive and anxious-type symptoms.

A. Disruptive Behaviors

Sometimes referred to as externalizing or "acting-out" problems, include attention related, oppositional and conduct problems and their corresponding disorders, ADHD and ODD. Disruptive behaviors have a driven quality that is expressed either in the intensity, the frequency, or the duration of the behavior.

1. **Attention related disorders:** Toddlers present with multiple issues related to inattention, impulsivity and motor over-activity which later in children above 7 years age are referred to as attention deficit hyperactivity disorder (ADHD). Core features of ADHD include inattention, impulsivity and hyperactivity. ADHD requires detailed discussion separately.

2. **Oppositional defiant disorders (ODD):** These include defiant, angry, annoying, non-compliant and sometimes aggressive behaviors.

3. **Conduct disorders (CD)** include more serious forms of aggression, property destruction and theft, which are rarely applied to toddlers.

   Some examples of disruptive or acting out behaviors are:
   • Frequent or intense tantrums,
   • Fussing,

23

- Inconsolable crying,
- Fighting, pushing,
- Biting,
- Hitting,
- Frequently throwing things, knocking things down, or destroying property,
- Persistent refusal to participate in activities, and
- Harm to self or others.

Temper tantrums are common in toddlers!

A temper tantrum is a loss of control which emerges as an expression of frustration. Toddlers want to make decisions; but they don't know how to compromise, how to express their feelings in words. So instead they act out their anger or frustration by crying, throwing on the floor and even throwing a breath holding spell! Interestingly temper tantrums happen only when parents are around. Temper tantrums have a purpose—this emotional explosion serves as a kind of energy release; which often ends in exhaustion and a long, delightful sleep.

The pediatrician's role is effective counseling of anxious parents by few simple and reassuring sentences:

1. In toddlers temper tantrums are normal and unavoidable
2. Stay calm, don't shout, and let the child know that the parent is in full control of situation.
3. Don't neglect the tantrum; but do not bow to the demands of the child.
4. Don't discuss rules and discipline when the child is disturbed. It's useless!
5. Be gentle, firm and consistent.
6. Whole family should act in unison.

Biting, hitting, hair-pulling, fighting, throwing objects, destroying property and similar violent acts are also extremes of 'Normal Emotional Outbursts' in toddlers. These violent acts are impulsive and are usually without any purpose. Still violent behavior is NOT socially acceptable and should be addressed immediately and directly. Frustrated parents reach pediatrician's clinic when these violent behaviors are frequent, and are disturbing either school performance or social interactions. The counseling of such parents should aim at:

1. Reassurance that such behaviors are common in toddlers and do not last long!
2. Honor the emotions of the toddler, look for the intent and respond to the impulse!
3. Declare simple and brief verbal limit. Let the child know that parents disprove this behavior.
4. If dangerous; physical restrain is a must for 'Child safety'. If necessary, remove the child from the hostile environment.
5. Don't ever label the child with the problematic behavior! It will increase the problem.
6. Provide better alternatives. Educate the child when in cool, listening mode.

23

B. Emotional Behaviors

Sometimes referred to as internalizing or "withdrawn" problems are more intense and challenging due to the inability of toddlers to communicate about their emotions, or for adults to notice them as problematic. Furthermore, there are difficulties in distinguishing developmentally normal emotions (e.g. fears, crying) from more severe and prolonged anxiety or depression that might constitute a disorder. The classification of these behaviors also includes other developmental disorders with behavioral issues.

1. Anxiety disorders; which include:
   a. Separation anxiety disorder (common in toddlers!)
   b. Obsessive compulsive disorder
   c. Post-traumatic stress disorder, social phobia, selective mutism—Rare in toddlers.
2. Depressive disorders: rare in toddlers
3. Feeding disorders which include feed refusal, excessive fussiness over food and pica.
4. Elimination disorders; which include enuresis and encopresis—ill-defined in toddlers.
5. Autism spectrum disorders sometimes present with behavioral issues first; and later these children are identified as autism spectrum disorder.

Some examples of emotional or withdrawing behaviors include:

- Pulling away while being held,
- Rarely talking, poor, low volume speech,
- Looking sad,
- Not showing preference for a caregiver,
- Not making eye contact,
- Whining (to complain in an annoying way), and
- Being overly compliant or avoidant with the caregiver, and anxiety, loneliness, fears and phobias, depression

Though in toddlers 'withdrawing behaviors' are uncommon as compared to the 'disruptive behaviors', these behaviors warrant immediate parental attention. As an empathetic pediatrician; we should listen to these parents as they are also anxious along with the anxious child! We can help these parents and their child by some assertive suggestions like:

1. Acknowledge child's fear—don't dismiss or ignore it.
2. Gently encourage the child to do things he/she is anxious about, but don't push to face situations the child doesn't want to face.
3. Wait until your child actually gets anxious before you step in to help
4. Praise the child for doing things she/he is anxious about, rather than criticizing for being afraid.
5. Avoid labeling your child as 'shy' or 'anxious'.
6. Don't compare with peers and siblings.

VII. MANAGEMENT OF BEHAVIORAL PROBLEMS IN TODDLERS

Every child and its behavior is 'Unique'. Still a basic management plan can be followed.

A. Assessment
1. Detailed interview of parents and caregivers
2. Talking to the child
3. Play way observation of the child
4. Structured questionnaire to know 'Parenting style'

5. Structured questionnaire to be filled by schoolteacher/crèche manager

B. Child directed intervention
1. Praise appropriate behavior
2. Active listening
3. Describe, demonstrate, imitate appropriate behavior.
4. Playing with the child—let the child lead, learn to take turns, understand how to interact with others, appreciate appropriate behavior
5. Spend 'Quality Time' with the child

23

C. Parent directed intervention
1. Simple, clear and direct commands/instructions. One instruction at a time.
2. Tell the child what to do rather than what not to do.
3. Instructions should be given politely and respectfully. Do not yell. It teaches toddlers to listen better and obey politely.
4. Avoid rewarding bad behavior. Parent's attention is a powerful reward for the child. Avoid giving it when the child is doing something wrong.
5. Parents should be trained to 'control' their own emotions and behaviors!

D. Environment modification
1. Analyze the family environment, closely associated families and the society with which the child usually reacts!
2. Try to make the environment soothing, non-threatening and comfortable.
3. Discuss the intervention plan with all the family members and act in unison.
4. Develop clear, predictable and simple daily routines
5. Set aside defined time for 'family interactions'

Ten Tips for Positive Parenting to Manage Terrible Toddler!
1. Children do as you do. Watch your own behavior.
2. Stay calm. Choose your battles. Plan ahead.
3. Show your child how you feel.

4. Toddlers are naturally curious about the world. Allow exploring.

5. Keep your expectations realistic.

6. Offer limited, reasonable choices. Teach ways to make choices.

7. Avoid rewarding bad behavior. Your attention is a powerful reward for your child.

8. Keep instructions simple, short, clear and positive. Avoid negative personal remarks.

9. Be positive! Try to say six positive comments (praise and encouragement) for every negative comment (criticisms and reprimands).

10. Most habits go away by themselves. Disprove the habit, NOT the child!

23

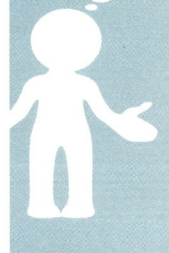

Points to remember

1. Behavior refers to the way a person responds to a certain situation or experience.

2. When toddlers misbehave; it's not planned, it's not deliberate and they are not doing it to hurt somebody. It's more like experimenting with emotions and finding out the responses from the people around.

3. Behavioral problems in toddler needs understanding by parents regarding the problem.

4. Toddlers need good role models.

5. Psychiatric disorders are rare in this age.

6. Management depends on environmental modification, acceptance of child by parents and firm and loving parenting.

FURTHER READING

1. Watson C, Hawley V, Addressing Challenging Behaviors in Infants and Toddlers, Center on the Social and Emotional Foundations for Early Learning, University of Minnesota, 2010

2. Lutz Ericka. A Well-Behaved Child, Alpha books, Division of Macmillan Company; 1999

3. Jain Sugandha, Jain Neeraj. Handling Behavior Problems in young children, Scholars Hub, New Delhi, 2006

4. Shelow S. Behavior. In: Caring for your baby and young child, American Academy of Pediatrics, 1998; 507–518

5. Neary E, Eyeberg S. Management of Disruptive Behavior in Young Children, Infant and Young Children 2002; 14(4): 53–67.

6. Gardner F, Shaw D. Behavioral Problems of Infancy and Preschool Children (0–5), Rutter's Child and Adolescent Psychiatry, 5th edition. Edited by Rutter M., Bishop D, Pine D, Scott S, and A. Thapar. Blackwell Publishing, 2008; 53: 882–893.

7. Behavior Problems: Practice Resource, Centre for Community Child Health 2006, Downloaded from www.rch.org.au/ccch, Accessed August 6, 2014.

23

Approach to Behavioral Disorders

Suchit Tamboli

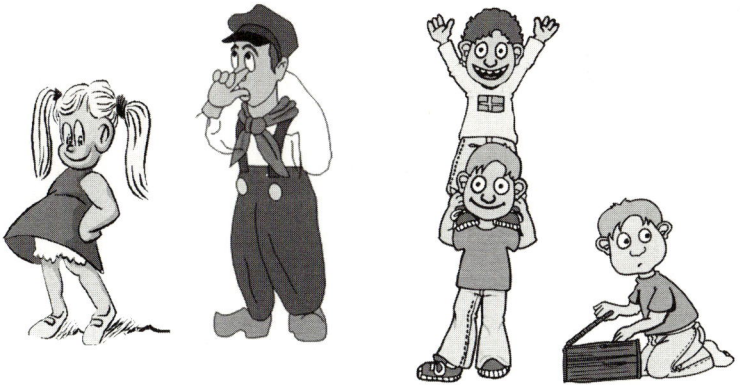

- To **"Behave"** is to conduct oneself and **Behavior"** is manners or conduct act.
- The child's behavior is the end of result of a wide variety of factors operating before pregnancy, during pregnancy, during delivery and in his subsequent environment.
- His behavioral problems are the result of the conflict between his developing personality and attitude of his parents, teachers and peer's.
- 'Normal' or 'abnormal' based on developmental age of the child depending on Personality of individual child, parental responses, and environmental factors.

Normal developing behavior in which no treatment is required except reassurance and counseling are as follows:

1. At **three month** old baby hand-mouth coordination and **thumb sucking**

2. High level of **negativism** is characteristic of late **infancy and toddlers**
3. Development of 'ego' a part of normal growing, e.g. **Refusing to eat**
4. **Stammering** at 2–4 years of age
5. Expression of **fear** 3–6 years
6. **Over-aggression** 2–4 years of age
7. **Jealousy** 3–5 year
8. **Bedwetting** before 6 years

All these problems need only assurance as most of the children outgrow from them

24

School Going Children

1. Sudden changes in body proportions, appearance of secondary sexual characters development of 'self-esteem'.
2. Increasing separation from parents and acceptance in the peer group.
3. Fears of being 'subnormal'.
4. Masturbation, sexual experimentation, interests in pornography.
5. Lying and stealing may be seen in some children as features of heroism and fantasy.
6. Some phobias.

All needs just understanding parents. **Academic performance and classroom behavior have great impact on personality development**

PROBLEM BEHAVIOR

"Problem" depends on

a. Type
b. Frequency
c. Duration
d. Severity of the behavior in question
e. Threshold of tolerance of the caretakers.

- **Parents do not pay attention to the needs of the child unless child shows behavioral changes. Negative behavior gets reinforcement; and such a behavior**

becomes a habit. Pediatrician has to learn to identify early try to break this vicious cycle.

The Joint Commission in USA on Mental Health of Children had defined an emotionally disturbed child as one who is impaired in:

1. Accurately perceiving the world around him or her
2. Controlling impulses
3. Achieving satisfactory relationships with others
4. Learning
5. Combinations of above four

The commission had observed about 8 to 10%, needed specialized services. 2–3% severely affected, 0.6% were psychotic. Data in Indian children is not available.

24

Common Behavioral Problems in OPD

Thumb sucking/nail biting: Manifestation of feelings of insecurity

1. **Thumb sucking—Facts:** Onset can be from 6 to 8 months following are the most important **Causes**:
   1. Feeling of insecurity
   2. Boredom, loneliness, frustration, and fatigue
   3. Hunger, warmth and physical contact satisfies
   4. Parents with less eye contact

   Results: malocclusion, mucosal trauma, callous

   Acts:
   1. Assurance, reinforcement, motivation
   2. Counseling, behavior modification
   3. Give alternatives continuously
   4. Make more eye contact

2. **Nail biting** or onychophagia, biting on or chewing one's own nails of the hand
   - Preschool age to adolescence ; prevalence is as high as 45–60%, Common in females

   Facts: Etiology
   1. Imitation from other family member
   2. Heredity

3. A transference of thumb sucking habit

4. Poorly manicured nail

Nail biting: Associated factors

1. Extremely short fingernails
2. Paronychia
3. Oral herpes
4. Herpetic whitlow
5. Damaged dentition
6. Apical root resorption
7. Fractures to the incisors and gingivitis

24 *Acts*

1. More parental affection, sympathy
2. Care of nails
3. Behavioral modifications techniques
4. Positive and negative reinforcement are important for management

3. Breath holding spell: Facts

It is benign, involuntary phenomenon. It occurs in children between 6 months and 6 years of age. Commonest cause is due to pain, fear or in anger frustration. Usually the child cries and then holds the breath.

- 5% children between 12 and 18 months out of 5% usually (80%) disappear by 4–5 years of age. Boys and girls are equal. There is a positive family history seen.

  2 ways: (i) Cyanotic spells, (ii) Pallid.

  Cyanotic spells in breath holding spells:

- Provoked by an upsetting situation, in anger or in frustration. Cries, screams loudly and then the cry gradually becomes noiseless as child open the mouth and holds the breath in expiration for about 20–30 seconds.

- The child turns blue (cyanotic) and then the child may again start breathing or may proceed to lose consciousness. He will have seizure like activity or loss of consciousness, in a cyanotic spell loss of consciousness is due to centrally mediated inhibition of respiratory center. It lasts less than one minute and regains full activity within a few minutes.

I. Pallid spells in breath holding spells

• Painful and fearful experience, pale and often loses consciousness within, vagally mediated bradyacardia. Diagnosed clinically. Differential diagnosis: seizures and syncope. Crying is prior to spell. Inter-ictal EEG normal. Usually investigations are not necessary in a classical case.

Acts: Breath holding spasms:

1. Parental support and reassurance
2. Relieve parental fear and anxiety
3. Explain involuntary nature of the attacks
4. Reassure that breath holding spells are not dangerous
5. They do not lead to epilepsy or brain damage.

24

• While trying to attempt to control environment, the parent should not hold the child upright, instead they should make him lie down flat or floor to prevent head injury. Nothing should be put in the child's mouth as it could cause choking or vomiting.

To prevent a spell: Child is distracted from their breath holding if intervened before they become blue by distracting them or making them look at something interesting.

• Parents are cautioned against running and picking up the child every time he cries to decrease the number of attack.
• **Behavior modification program** are applied. Parents are reassured that long term prognosis is very good.
• Most of the episodes resolve by the time the child is 4–5 years old.
• **Pharmacological treatment**: Atropine sulphate, iron therapy.
• **Anticonvulsants have no role**

4. Stubborn: Give or act immediately if you can , once refused do not accept, firm uniform parenting (when mummy says no all says no like that) will stop stubborn behavior in 3 months.

5. Pica—Facts

1. Compulsive eating of non-food substances over a sustained period is termed as pica
2. It is eating disorders

3. Commonly seen in 2nd half of infancy and may persist up to 18 months of age
4. Pica after 2nd year of life needs investigations.
- **Pica can lead to stomach complaints, poisoning, damage to the teeth**.
  Following screenings are indicated for pica:
  1. Iron deficiency anemia
  2. Worm infestations
  3. Lead poisoning
  4. Family dysfunction
  5. The exact cause of pica is not known
  6. Autism
  7. Sickle cell disease and malnutrition

Predisposing factors for pica:
a. Lack of parental nurturing
b. Mental retardation
c. Family disorganization
d. Lower socioeconomic class

Pica can lead to parasitic infestation and lead poisoning
Acts for pica:
1. Treatment of predisposing factors
2. Treatments of iron deficiency anemia, lead poisoning
3. Rule out underlying psychiatric disorder like depression and separation anxiety.

6. Bruxism (teeth grinding): Facts
Forcible gnashing, grinding, clicking, clenching of teeth. Nocturnal bruxism occurs during sleep, unaware of the problem. Brief lasting 8–9 seconds with audible grinding noises. Pain and dysfunction of mastication.

Diurnal (daytime) bruxism, clenching of the teeth and generally does not produce audible noises. Related to other oral habits, such as nail biting or lip chewing.

It is seen in 5–30% of children. It begins in first 5 years of life. Peaking at 7-10 years of age and decreasing after. It is found more in females than males.

24

Effects of bruxism
1. Chronic dental pain, dental fractures, wearing down of dental enamel
2. Thermal hypersensitivity of the teeth
3. Hyper mobility of teeth
4. Injury to the periodontium, dental occlusion and pulpitis.

Acts for Bruxism: Help child find ways to reduce anxiety
- Parent reads relaxing stories at bedtime
- Parent daily reviews fears and angers experienced on that day.
- Praise child
- Emotional support.

24

Persistent bruxism leads to muscular or temporomandibular joint pain.

7. Anxiety disorders in children
Types are as follows
A. Over anxious disorder
B. School phobia
C. Separation anxiety
D. Social anxiety
E. Selective mutism

Phobias
Can be attached to a
1. Specific non-threatening stimulus
2. Out of proportion to the demands of the situation
3. Cannot be reasoned or explained away
4. Beyond voluntary control
5. Leads to avoidance of the feared situation
6. Persists over an extended period of time
7. Un adaptive
8. Not age- or stage-specific
Acts: Counseling and if required medicines

8. Enocoparesis—Facts
Involuntary "fecal soiling", who have usually already been toilet trained. Leak stool into their underwear. More common in boys.

Causes
- *Constipation:* Complication of chronic constipation, stool behind the impaction begins to leak around it, and eventually leaks out of the rectum.
  1. By deliberate withholding of stool (meningomyelocele, muscle disease).
  2. Oppositional defiant disorders.
  3. Conduct disorders.
  4. "Parental control" attempt by the child.
  5. Fear of the commode, simple reluctance
  6. Symptom of child sexual abuse.

24

Diagnosis of encopresis
1. Repeated passage of feces into inappropriate places (e.g. clothing or floor) whether voluntary or unintentional.
2. At least one such event a month for least 3 months.
3. Chronological age of at least 4 years (or equipment developmental level)
4. The behavior is not exclusively due to a physiological effect of a substance (e.g. laxatives) or a general medical condition, except through a mechanism.

Two subtypes
  i. With constipation and overflow incontinence
  ii. Without constipation and overflow incontinence.

Acts of encopresis
  i. Cleaning out
  ii. Using stool softening agents
  iii. Scheduled sitting times, typically after meals
  iv. *Diapers:* Sit on the toilet at a regular time each day and 'try' to go for 10–15 minutes, usually soon after eating. Proper elimination pattern.

9. Speech problems
1. Unclear speech
2. Disarticulation
3. Stammering

Remedies
1. Early detection of hearing problems if any by testing BAEP
2. No interference or anxiety during speech problem.
3. Mother's anxiety should be allayed.
4. Ignore completely the behavior which you do not want
5. Shadowing, mirror talk, imitation, word practice, pranayam

10. Habit disorders
A. Trichotillomania
Involves hair-pulling episodes that result in noticeable hair loss of scalp, eyelashes, and eyebrows. Hair-pulling can occur without the individual's awareness, but is frequently processed by a sense of increasing tension, sense of relief or gratification.

Untreated trichotillomania can result in impaired social functioning and medical complications. More females than males present. The mean age of onset is 13 years.

Following conditions must be present for a diagnosis of trichotillomania
1. Noticeable hair loss (alopecia) due to recurrent hair-pulling.
2. Tension immediately before hair-pulling, or when attempting to resist hair-pulling.
3. Reduction of tension, or a feeling of pleasure or gratification, immediately following hair-pulling
4. Significant distress or impairment in social, occupational, or other important areas of functioning.

Causes of trichotillomania: The etiology of trichotillomania continues to be unknown
1. Serotonin deficiency
2. Structural brain abnormalities
3. Abnormal brain metabolism by positron emission tomography
4. Psychological theories. These four theories are hypothesized.

Diagnosis of trichotillomania:
Other possible causes of symptoms must first be ruled out. Dermatological condition. Delusion or hallucination in schizophrenia.

24

Treatments of trichotillomania: Determining the current frequency and severity of symptoms by

a. Self-report
b. Reports from significant others
c. Objective measures, such as saving pulled hairs, video tapes, or measuring areas of hair loss
d. A combination of these methods.

Acts for trichotillomania: *Psychoanalysis:* Medications—antidepressants. Behavior therapy has reported long-term success rates of 90% or better. Follow-up sessions are encouraged to prevent relapses.

B. Tics:

- A part of the body moves repeatedly, quickly, suddenly and uncontrollably.
- Lip smacking, grimacing, tongue trusting, eye blinking, throat clearing, etc.
- Suppressible by child for short periods if made conscious or reprimanded.
- Never associated with transient inability to interact.
- Tics disappear when child is asleep.
- Rarely tics precipitated in child on stimulant medication.
- They are tension relieving habit disorders.
- Vocal tics are involuntary sounds produced by moving air through the nose, mouth, or throat. Usually they are mild and hardly noticeable. They can be frequent and severe.
- No direct cause known to reason tic disorders, but anxiety, tiredness, and some medications may provoke tics.
- Punishment by parents, teasing by classmates and scolding by teachers will not help the child to control the tics but will hurt the child's self-esteem and increase their distress.
- Opinion of pediatric neurologist and psychiatrist is necessary in some cases.
- Medications, diazepam and clonidine help to control the symptoms, emotional support, and appropriate educational environment.
- To provide emotional support and the appropriate educational environment for the youngest.

C. Rhythmic habits

Head banging and rocking are tension release phenomena, a kind consolation for the child.

Causes of rhythmic habits: Neglected or have developmental delays

Treatment of rhythmic habits: Inhibited automatically particularly in social situations. Keep patience and understand the need of the child and to provide optimum environment to the child. Children with mental retardation may be more refractory to treatment.

Adolescent Problems

24

Conduct disorder

Clinical features—ADDS

Aggression
Destruction
Deceitfulness/theft
Serious violation of rules

If they are present ≥ 3 in last 1 yr, then impairment is present. There are 2 types—*childhood onset* and *adolescent onset type.*

Treatment

Non-pharmacological treatment: Rapport, target symptoms, avoid situation, reinforcement of problem solving skills, family therapy, parent training, to look into educational needs of the child. Encourage self-esteem.

A. **Behavioral intervention:** Family therapy, Promotion of learning at home and at school.

B. **Pharmacological:** In severe cases drug are used.

   Drugs: Stimulants—methylphenidate, nonstimulant— Atomoxetine

   Antidepressant like fluoxetine, clonidine.

Counselling: Guidelines for the parents on ways to alleviate stress

- *Acceptance*: Accept the child as it is
- *Love:* Convey to the child in words and actions that they love good behavior, appreciate in words and actions like hugging,

caressing, kissing; use the words **'I LOVE YOU'**, **'I LIKE YOU'**

- *Touch*: Physical touch on lap, hugging, caressing
- *Communication*: An exclusive time for the child is desirable on one to one basis. For a walk or a vehicle ride. A good listener is a good communicator. Exchange of thoughts or ideas and not advice. Child is intelligent enough to understand why parents are angry or resort to punishment earning praise or reward depend on the desirable behavior.
- *Structuring of time*: Set a routine for their child. Time of getting up, toilet, bath, school, studies, play and extra-curricular activities, etc. Time of free play, time for viewing TV also included. Time to go to bed
- **Structuring of activities:** Encourage to do house chores complemented and praised. Assigning small tasks, encouraging the child to complete. Positive way of educating re-enforcing desire to indulge into activities which parents like. Resulting in a sense of security
- **Rewarding the positive:** Child's positive, constructive and creative activities parents approve. Reward need not costly, pat on back. "Star" likes a story book, coloring pastels. A scooter or a car ride, visit to an eating joint, "Please", "Will you please" avoiding shouting and using harsh words helps in two ways. It does not add to child's stress and child learns not to shout and to speak softly.
- It is the counseling of the parents and their compliance to the counselor's suggestions, and changes they make in the response to child's behavior, which are likely to show the desired changes in child's behavior.

24

Points to remember

1. Behavioral problems need early identification to prevent personality changes.
2. Assurance, counseling, proper environmental changes solve mild problems.
3. Some problems need medicines and counseling.

Pre-School Education: ABCD or Skill-Based

Sunil Godbole

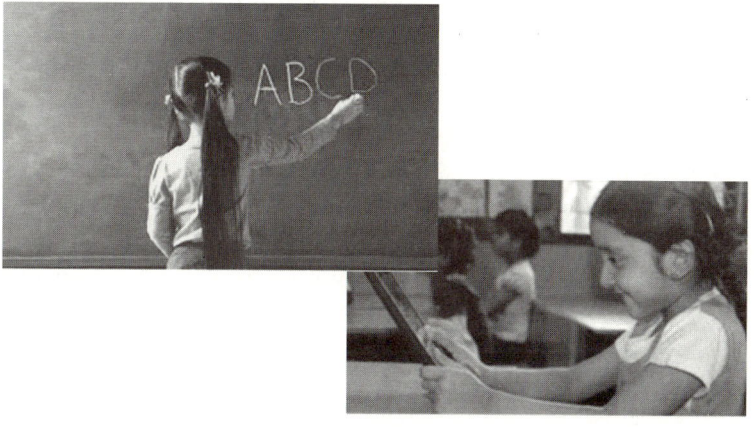

There is a growing debate about the goals of early childhood education. Traditionally, academic success depends upon a child's basic ability to read, write, spell, and do math equations (arithmetic's)—abilities commonly known as the three Rs. With growing pressure of early education, soaring expectations, bombardment from media, explosion of knowledge due to internet and glamorous advertisements of new generation pre-schools—the parents tend to push their tiny tots at an early age in 'the rat race' as early as 18 months! (If this continues; don't be surprised if you read an advertisement of 'In utero Schooling'!)

Various researchers, teachers, psychologists and even pediatricians have expressed the necessity of pre-school education (though the earliest age to start remains a matter of debate) to have strong 'Learning Foundation'. The real issue is

– to choose between 'Academic Learning' or 'Skill-oriented Play-based learning'?

In a well-designed study Rebecca A. Marcon from University of North Florida, it was observed that by the end of their sixth year in school, children whose pre-school experiences had been academically directed earned significantly lower grades compared to children who had attended child-centered pre-school classes. Children's later school success appears to have been enhanced by more active, child-initiate dearly learning experiences. In many other studies, children who attended more "academic" pre-schools instead of play-focused pre-schools were found to be more anxious, less creative, and less enthusiastic about learning than the children who had learned primarily through play.

25

Limitations of "Academic Pre-schools"

Early childhood programs that implement a directed academic curriculum often replace essential, hands-on learning activities with structured, formal instructions, work sheets, skill drills and rote-learning tasks. This leads to multiple learning issues:

1. Forces children to use immature neural pathways to complete tasks. The normal growth and development of the brain can be distorted by such practice;

2. Forces the child to tackle a problem that is unrelated to his or her environment or concrete experiences, and leaves gaps in the development of reasoning and logic;

3. Does not allow the child to use intrinsic motivations to engage in learning;

4. Risks placing inappropriate expectations and pressure on young children;

5. Decreases the development of the intuitive foundation of knowledge needed for complex abstract thinking in the future;

6. Limits opportunities for a child to practice and develop essential nonacademic abilities;

7. Lower in conduct and work-study habits; and

8. More distractible, less willing to follow directions.

Developmentally Appropriate Skill-based Play-school!

Many child-development experts say toddlers learn better through play than through direct instruction. Here are some reasons for the same

1. Play is how children begin to understand and process their world;
2. Children's play unlocks their creativity and imagination;
3. When playing with other children or adults, child will listen and learn the language he/she hears without even realizing;
4. Children can solve complex problems that arise as they play and learn a few mathematical concepts as well;
5. Play can provide many opportunities to work on strengthening muscles without your child even being aware of it!
6. Play-school focuses on 'Learning within context' rather than learning meaningless, disembodied facts. A toddler can remember 'Tables' in an 'academic—pre-school' but the application of 'Tables' is missed! But in a 'Play-school' the child will device a 'Table' while sorting or grouping blocks and balls!
7. In a 'Play-school' a child may not learn alphabets or numbers; but he/she will learn to engage in give-and-take with children and adults, to negotiate, and to start and maintain social relationships.Ultimately, the child is ready to socially and emotionally handle primary school and through that, more prepared for academic success.
8. When toddlers master abilities through play, they exhibit a higher language level, more innovation, greater empathy and cooperation, better problem-solving strategies, and longer and greater attention spans—all essential characteristics of learning readiness.

The Three 'Is of Pre-school Education

Mari Blaustein; an early childhood content and curriculum designer; in 'The Basics of Learning Readiness' strongly recommends use of three 'Is of intrinsic motivation as the backbone of pre-school education over the three 'Rs of primary/secondary school education.

1. **Interaction:** All children; right from infancy up to adolescence; want to socialize; interact with other children and adults. Successful interactions not only expand a child's personal knowledge base, social skills, and language abilities but also build self-esteem and create the confidence. But this needs freedom and free time to interact with other children—this is possible only in play based pre-schools; that too when the teachers are aware of these concepts.

2. **Imagination:** According to Mari Blaustein, creative and imaginative play opportunities motivate toddlers to imagine, wonder, and explore ways to organize and use new knowledge, test the learning environment, seek possible explanations, and practice new skills safely. Rather than focusing on an activity with only one correct outcome, the imaginative play motivates children to consider alternative possibilities by applying organization, logic, and symbolic thinking.

3. **Integration:** In play-based pre-schools; toddlers integrate acts of sight, sound, and touch with language as they experience, explore, question, and use new knowledge. This integration builds understanding and insights into the concrete world; generates new ideas; and allows children to wonder about, discuss, and explore different outcomes. For 'Integration' children require an open—frame environment, opportunities to interact and try their new skills and most importantly motivated facilitators—the enthusiastic teachers!

The Craze of 'Fast Schooling'!

Parents are nowadays crazy about 'putting their tiny tots in an aggressive academic oriented pre-school, in spite of awareness of child-centered education, knowing the importance of 'learn through play' and advice by pediatricians and child-friendly educationists. Probably this attitude comes from our "immediate gratification"culture. We; in our modern, fast, computer based world; expect to change the world by 'a touch of finger'. Similarly the parents want their children to achieve great academic fits at an early age. This pushes the child on a wrong track; which ruins their beautiful childhood! Here we should remember a simple analogy—the artificially ripened mangoes may look more attractive than the mangoes which take time to ripe on the tree—but when you taste them; you know the difference!

Pediatrician's Job!

1. Educate parents right from infancy during well-baby visits
2. Help parents choose the right school appropriate for their family culture.
3. Discuss pros and cons of early schooling, 'play versus academic pre-schools'
4. Growth and development assessment of children at an early age may help the parents to know the potentials of their child and select the pre-school accordingly. A developmental pediatrician can help the parents with this assessment.
5. If pediatrician's can keep a registry of child-centered, play-based, skill oriented pre-schools we can direct the confused parents to the best possible option.
6. Most importantly; we should spare some time from our busy practice to counsel parents as these initiatives will make the better tomorrow!

25

Parenting Tips

The pre-school forms the foundation of education and career of the child. Parents should be careful about choosing the 'right' pre-school for their child. Parents should:

a. Visit the school before admission
b. Confirm whether the school has required permissions and license.
c. Talk with school authorities, teachers and even support staff
d. Talk with senior parents about their experiences of school.
e. Compare the school expenses with the financial status of the family.
f. Use following checklist to select the 'right' pre-school for your child.

The Checklist for Ideal Pre-school

1. *Child-friendly school:* Small group of children with more resource persons.
2. *Premises:* Open, airy, spacious, well-lit.
3. *Teachers:* Well educated, competent, affectionate, calm, lively, interested in children, positive attitude.
4. Philosophy of education should match with that of child's family. Promote problem solving, independence, creativity and encourage the child to try new things that help value learning and social skills.
5. *Learning material:* Building blocks; props for pretend play; picture books; paints and other art materials; and table toys such as matching games, pegboards, and puzzles.
6. Child safety, stringent health and hygiene norms
7. Cultural activities, field trips, projects, exhibitions, hands on learning activities.
8. *Outdoor play and activities:* Adequate space, dedicated ground and play-gym adhering to safety guidelines.
9. *Distance from residence:* School should be within 3 kilometers.
10. *Communication:* Free, transparent, supportive communication between school authorities, teachers, support staff and parents.

25

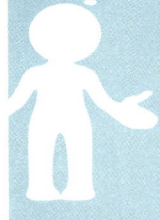

Points to remember

1. Growing pressure of early education, soaring expectations, bombardment from media, glamorous advertisements of new generation preschools—the parents tend to push kids in rat race.
2. Developmentally appropriate skill-based play-school accelerates learning through play.
3. Play helps child understand the world.
4. Play unlocks creativity and imagination.
5. Play can solve complex problems, few mathematical concepts, focus on contextual

learning, strengthen muscles without child even being aware of it.

6. The three 'Is' of pre-school education are—Interaction, imagination and integration.

7. Parents should visit school before admission, confirm whether the school has required permissions and licence, talk with school authorities, teachers, support staff and even senior parents.

8. Ideal pre-school should have teachers who are well educated, competent, affectionate, calm, lively, interested in children and positive attitude.

9. School should have good premises, learning material, etc.

10. Child safety, stringent health and hygiene norms.

11. School should be closer to the residence.

12. Effective communication between school authorities, parents, teachers and support staff.

25

FURTHER READING

1. Marcon Rebecca A.Moving up the Grades: Relationship between Pre-school Model and Later School Success, ECRP. Vol 4 No 1. 2002. Available at http://ecrp.uiuc.edu/v4n1/marcon.html

2. Blaustein, Mari, "See, Hear, Touch! The Basics of Learning Readiness" 2005 by the National Association for the Education of Young Children. Available at http://www.journal.naeyc.org/btj/200507/01Blaustein.asp

3. Geiser Traci,Play in Pre-school: Why it Matters, 2006, Available athttp://www.education.com/magazine/article/play-pre-school-matters/

4. Godbole Suneel, Godbole Ashwini; Smart Mool, Sakal Papers Pvt. ltd. 2013

5. Godbole Suneel, Godbole Ashwini, BalpanFulwitana, Anmol Publications, 3rd Edition; 2012; 207–221.

26 Positive Discipline

Atul Kanikar

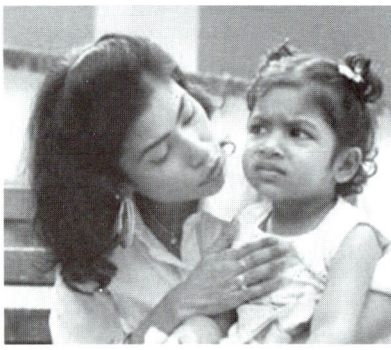
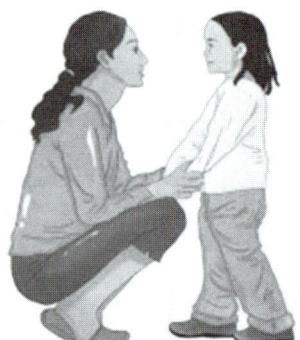

All of us, who care for children have a responsibility to guide, correct, and socialize our children toward appropriate behaviors. The process of discipline involves a series of well-intended efforts by parents and caregivers to inculcate "the art of controlling oneself." If properly learnt and consistently practiced, discipline becomes a very important foundation for the growth of children. It brings self-confidence, feeling of mastery over life and positive social experience for children even after growing as adults. The positive feelings themselves add up to bring out a well-behaved and confident parent of the future, who would in turn express positive discipline techniques successfully. The discipline process should act as "vaccination" against untoward effects of peers, media and other difficult to handle situations in life.

Discipline, by definition means, "to teach". How ever, by tradition, we equate this with punishment. Discipline also is, encouraging children, guiding them and helping them feel good about themselves. The root word of discipline is disciple—a person who leads others in the way they should go. Discipline is not what you do to the child, but what you do with and for the child.

The reality is however different. Discipline is easier said and suggested than practiced. It is very easy to read (and download) readymade recipes available on the net and in bookstores. To put this information everyday into practice is very painful and exhausting, needing lots of patience and consistency. Reading Nelson's textbook is one thing, practicing pediatrics is another.

Common Myths in Disciplining Children

26

1. Discipline means punishment.
2. Disciplining children is school's responsibility.
3. Mother has to be blamed, if child misbehaves. Father is anyway very busy.
4. Grandparents never understand what is "good" for children.
5. Children should never cry or feel unhappy. Costly gifts should be provided to win them back.
6. Quiet children are always well behaved.
7. Tomorrow onwards my children will behave well, because I have disciplined them today.
8. Readymade magic recipes are available for bringing up children.
9. I am the only one, who is in trouble.
10. Spare the rod and spoil the child.

The list is unending, and so are the efforts for improving misbehaviors in children. The possible reasons should be considered before taking any actions for child's misbehavior. The reasons could be a physical illness, feeling of rejection or insecurity (a typical "nobody understands me!" expression.), extreme hunger or sleep, post TV boredom and lethargy ("what should I do next?" irritation.). Many a times, children simply test the permissible limits of their misbehaviors, and see what happens if they break the rules. On another occasion, the misbehavior could be an attempt to attract the attention of parents, especially when they are busy talking to the guests, in whose presence, they can misbehave safely, because parents can't do any harm. Most commonly, children simply copy the misbehaviors of their parents, e.g. shouting, hitting, talking back, etc.

Most of us express all forms of parenting styles, sometimes or the other. Depending on our moods and priorities, we would be either a "cane wielding ring-master"—Authoritative type, "leave them alone"—Liberal type, "leave me alone"—Avoidant type, or "sit across the table"—Negotiator type. What is desired is a good and "time-appropriate" cocktail of these types.

26   The short-term goal of discipline is to guide everyday behavior and to protect children from hurting themselves and others, however the long term goal should be to bring out a confident, self-disciplined individual, responsible for his/her own behavior, who is relying upon self and is comfortable and happy about it.

Do's and Don'ts in Discipline

1. Learn to say "NO" to children, whenever you want to.
2. Communicate your expectations very clearly, use only few words. Avoid lectures.
3. Ignore minor/harmless behaviors.
4. The expectations should be appropriate for the age and developmental stage of the child, culturally acceptable, unanimous and negotiated well.
5. Use positive statements. Avoid saying, "don't". Save "No" or "Don't" for important situations, so the child takes "No" seriously. For example instead of saying, "don't shout", say, "use your quiet voice."
6. Hold a positive expectation and make children feel responsible and co-operative. The more trust and confidence you place in children, the more they feel worthy of trust and the more trustworthy they become. Never "label" them as bad.
7. Acknowledge positive behavior. Praise them ACTIVELY even for minor good behaviors. Children (even adults) tend

to repeat and improve the behavior that is positively noticed by others.

8. Lecturing, fighting, impatience, and being punitive, only leads to frustration and fatigue for both.

9. Be fair, firm, and flexible whenever you make a rule. Make the consequences absolutely clear if the rule is broken, and most importantly follow them.

10. Be consistent in whatever strategy is chosen, and involve all the family members.

11. Accept your child's feelings, but reinforce your expectations. Active listening is the key.

12. Try to separate the behavior from the child. We must give UNCONDITIONAL LOVE to our children. It is the misbehavior that needs correction.

13. Make a list of possible misbehaviors that you want to correct, but correct only one behavior at a time.

14. Anticipate failures and frustrations, at least initially. Don't give up early. Keep on trying different methods till the desired behavior is expressed.

15. Make rational use of positive and negative reinforcements. Never try to bribe children for desired behavior; the children would do the same to you.

16. Take actions before the situation is out of control. Be a role model for your children. Parents need to improve their behavior first.

17. Giving time out is very effective technique for punishment. In this, following misbehavior, the child is made to remain alone in a non-distracting environment, e.g. a chair facing the wall, for a specified time (usually, one min per year of age is sufficient). During this period, the child is left alone and asked to think about why he is given a time-out.

18. Spanking/hitting is best avoided for the reason that we never liked it when we were children. Spanking is blamed for teaching violence to children. Resistance to spanking is fairly common.

Spanking is like a nuclear bomb. Always keep, never use. The untoward effects of spanking however are over-emphasized nowadays.

19. Try to spend quality time with children. Let them know that you also talk to them apart from imparting discipline.

20. Be comfortable and consistent with whatever you decide, because whatever you do is right for your child.

There are so many suggestions made by other family members, guests, neighbors, friends, etc. that parents at time get confused whether they are doing well to themselves and their children. Is the idea of disciplining, interfering with the natural child–parent relationship? Our parents never attempted to learn about bringing up children but nothing went wrong, then why should we bother about it now?

The answers to these questions are difficult. The probable explanations could be multidimensional. The family norms are changing. There are only one/two children per family now, and all parents wish to give the best to their children, there is no another chance. Nobody wants to accept that quite naturally, according to normal distribution probability curve, every child cannot be at the top. What we are giving to our children is a "filtered" parenting. (I keep the troubles with me; my children should never face problems.) In addition, we have working parents who un-necessarily feel guilty for not giving time to their children, but at the same time want their children to win the everincreasing competitions, may it be studies, sports or debating.

There are other players in this game, such as grandparents (nowadays, rare), teachers, etc. They have both positive and negative effects and if parents are not unanimous and careful, disciplining soon becomes a topic of conflicts and clashes in the family. Everybody puts the blame on others and eventually avoids the basic aim. In addition, one has to consider the fact that grandparents as well as parents have problems related to their own ages—both physical and psychosocial. The physical capacities are going down; they are at the peak of their careers and have tremendous economic burdens as well. All these factors sometimes can lead to a mix-up of strictness and cruelty and liberal handling and false ideas of "modern" parenting may turn into irresponsibility and risk taking behaviors. All this happens far more rapidly than expected, and things may spin out of control.

26

When the going gets tough, discipline—in combination with bilateral understanding, is one of the most precious and lasting gifts, parents can give to their children. As they grow, children will learn the skills, necessary to discipline themselves. As parents, we have been practicing what we have experienced as children. There are many unpleasant memories of childhood. How we felt when we were ignored? We never felt happy, when somebody shouted at us or spanked us, then why do the same to our children? Adults as well as children are likely to show enthusiasm in what **they** and not others feel right. Hence it is better to stop using words and actions that hurt. Start using words that help.

The concept and meaning of positive discipline can be easily summarized as follows:

D Daily routine.

I Ignoring minor misbehaviors.

S Setting limits of unacceptable behaviors.

C Consistency.

26

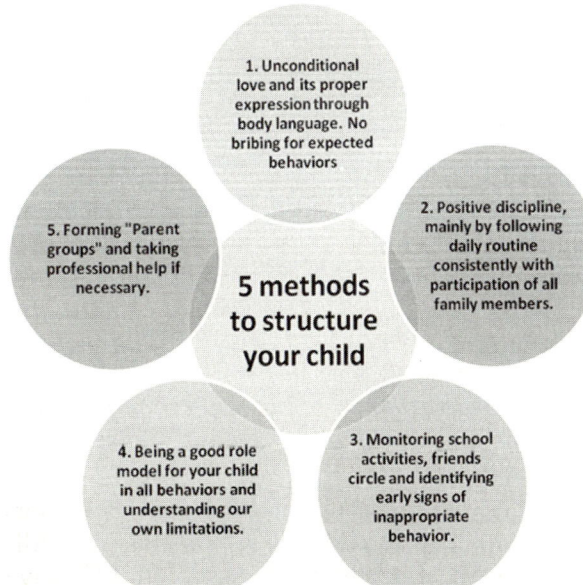

1. Unconditional love and its proper expression through body language. No bribing for expected behaviors

2. Positive discipline, mainly by following daily routine consistently with participation of all family members.

5 methods to structure your child

5. Forming "Parent groups" and taking professional help if necessary.

4. Being a good role model for your child in all behaviors and understanding our own limitations.

3. Monitoring school activities, friends circle and identifying early signs of inappropriate behavior.

I Informal talk and methods of disciplining children.
P Patience and persistence.
L Love (unconditional)
I Involving every family member.
N No nagging or lecturing.
E Education by being a good role model.

26

Nobody can be "the best parent" or "the most ideal child". Everybody does mistakes—parents and children alike, but with a lot of space and scope for improvement. Even psychologists face problems while handling their children. A pediatrician's child needs medicines occasionally. Unfortunately, there is no school or magic formula that will answer all the queries, nor is a perfect way to discipline. Every child and every parent is unique and so is every situation and discipline strategy. All that is needed is an unconditional love, little bit of patience, lots of consistency and comfort and peace with yourself. Disciplining children will soon become a pleasant task. Ultimately, we want our children to come to **us**, when in doubts and difficulties. In fact, that is what parenting means.

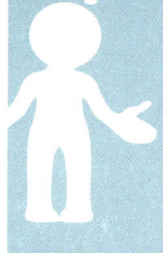

Points to remember

1. Being a good role model for your child in all behaviors and understanding our own limitations.
2. Unconditional love and its proper expression through body language should be done. No bribing for expected behavior.
3. No nagging or lecturing and patience, persistence and consistency is utmost important.
4. Monitoring school activities, friends circle and identifying early signs of inappropriate behavior.
5. Positive discipline, mainly by following daily routine consistently with participation of all family members.
6. Parent support group formation.

FURTHER READING

1. Atul Kanikar, Swati Bhave, Positive Discipline, Bhave's textbook of adolescent medicine, 854–859, Jaypee brothers.

2. Adolescent parenting. How and why it is different. Swati Bhave, Helen Pratt, Atul Kanikar. Bhave's Book of Adolescent Medicine 25.1 875–885

3. Communicating with your Teen. Shannon L, Sachs HYG 5158–96, http://ohioline.osu.edu/hyg-fact/5000/5158html

4. Fathering your adolescent; way to strengthen your relationship, http://www.ohioline.osu.edu/hyg-fact/5000/5158html

5. Monitoring: staying   involved in your teen's life. Shannon L Sachs HYG 5157–96, Ohioline.osu.edu/hyg-fact/5000/5157.html-9k

6. Parenting adolescents, parenting: preparing for adolescence, http://www.aacap.org/publication/fact/adolescence. Revised feb 2005

7. Parenting,   http://www.focusas.com/parenting.html

8. Parenting programs, Swati Bhave and Atul Kanikar, Course manual for adolescent health, 266–269

9. Parenting, Type of parenting, 137–138, Adolescent care 2000 and Beyond, Dr MKC Nairand Dr Ranjan Kumar Pejaver

10. Parenting adolescents, Indian Pediatrics 2004; 41:887–890, MKC Nair

26

Gifted Child! A Challenge

Sunil Godbole

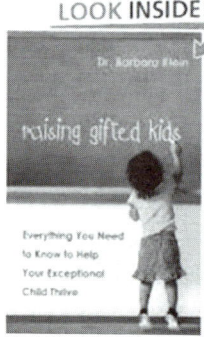
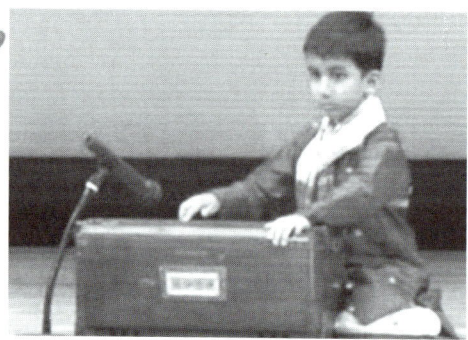

Some children are extraordinary. Chandrashekhar—a 12 year boy from our own India, is the smallest Microsoft Certified Computer Expert! Master blaster Sachin Tendulkar did his first century in International Cricket at the age of just fourteen! Abigail Sin (10 years old) is Singapore's most celebrated young pianist! And the list goes on.....! These children; popularly known as 'Gifted Children' pose multiple issues; right from identifying their giftedness up to managing them the best!

I. Definitions of Giftedness

Current literature contains a multitude of synonyms for giftedness, including bright, talented, high IQ, advanced, prodigy, precocious, exceptional, superior, creative, rapid learner, brilliant, genius, and so on. Similar to multiple names; researchers use different definitions to define 'Giftedness'. The Merriam Webster's College Dictionary defines the term "gifted" as: Having great natural ability and revealing a special gift."Gifted" children have also been defined as those children who by the nature of their outstanding abilities are capable of high performance.

Joseph Renzulli (1978) noted that people who have been successful in life possess three particular traits—high levels of ability, creativity,and task commitment.The interaction of these three basic clusters of human traits may result in gifted behaviors in general and specific performance areas. Howard Gardner (1983) identified 8 multiple intelligences suggesting that every child is 'smart' in one or either intelligence.

Robert Sternberg's Pentagonal Implicit Theory of Giftedness (1995): Sternberg's says that giftedness could not be possibly captured by a single number and has introduced a theory that describes a gifted person as one who meets the following five criteria:

1. *Excellence:* The individual is superior in some dimension(s) relative to peers.
2. *Rarity:* The individual possesses a skill or attribute that is rare among peers.
3. *Productivity:* The individual must produce something in the area of giftedness.
4. *Demonstrability:* The skill of giftedness must be demonstrable through valid assessments.
5. *Value:* The child shows superior performance in a dimension that is valued by the society.

Francoys Gagne (2004) believes that gifted people are born with a biological potential that will allow them to develop high ability in one or more of the areas of development. He provided a model of giftedness that expands on this idea. The natural abilities (intellectual, creative, socio-active and sensory-motor domains) in an individual with exceptional inter- and intra-personal intelligence; when nurtured by positive environmental influences will develop outstanding abilities or talent in various fields (academics, sports, arts, technology, etc.).

II. Identification of a Gifted Child

Various checklists are developed by researchers to identify a 'Gifted Child'. The 3 Ring model of Joseph Renzulli; now called

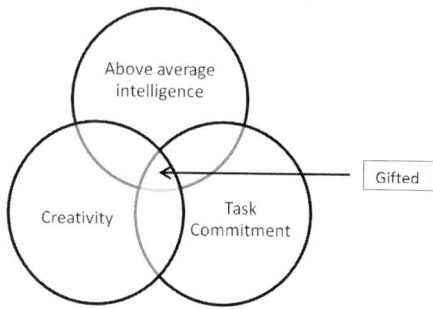

27 the School wide Enrichment Model, gives the simplest criteria to identify 'Giftedness'

Gifted

A. *Above average intelligence*
1. Advanced vocabulary: Start talking, walking early!
2. Has a good memory and remembers details of conversations or stories
3. Retains information easier and longer
4. Concentrates on certain activities much longer than other children of age
5. Large fund of information. Starts reading early and reads a lot.
6. Learns and comprehends quickly and easily
7. Generalizes, connects, synergizes and makes abstractions— diverging and converging.
8. Makes judgments and decisions quickly

B. *Creativity*
1. Curiosity
2. Has wide imagination
3. Transforms combines and elaborates ideas fluidly
4. Open, flexible and original
5. Problem solving ability
6. Sees consequences and implications easily
7. Provides multiple solutions or responses to problems

8. Finds subtle humor, paradox or discrepancies—intellectually playful!

C. *Task commitment:*
1. Sets own goals or standards
2. Intensive involvements in preferred problems and tasks
3. Enthusiastic about interests and activities
4. Needs little external motivation when pursuing tasks
5. High energy
6. Completes and shares products, however may not be able to follow through
7. Assumes responsibility
8. Leadership ability

27

III.Problems of 'Being Gifted'

Everything is not always 'Positive' with gifted children. They may have multiple problems; which make their life difficult:

1. **Asynchronous development** is relatively common among gifted children. This means that a child's intellectual, social, emotional and physical developments are at different stages. This uneven development results in academic and social maladjustment. Comorbidities like learning disability, ADHD are common in gifted children!

2. **Characteristics of giftedness** can vary greatly between children, even between children in the same family. So all gifted children are not alike. They possess exceptional qualities in different fields of life. But this makes extremely difficult for teachers to teach them.

3. **Social maladjustment:** Gifted children sometimes lack social skills. They are not accepted by friends and even teachers; because of high degree of perfectionism, adamant behavior and inability to accept discrepancies. Gifted children knowingly or unknowingly tend to challenge the authority, resist conventional approaches or responses, and criticize others. They make jokes or puns at inappropriate times. They often disagree with others in a loud, bossy manner. Obviously this is not accepted by the society.

4. **As these children learn faster:** They find school boring! They frequently daydream. They may be disruptive and inter-ruptive. Once they understand a topic, they lose the interest in it. This leads to—incomplete assignments and projects, resist completing rote or repetitive tasks.

5. **Emotional oversensitivity:** Gifted children are most of the times overly sensitive. Characterized by an intensity of feeling, a marked ability to empathize with others, and physical expression of feelings, these children can find it painfully difficult to make new friends, who cry at the smallest frustration.

6. **Sensory over-excitability:** Some gifted children may have sensory issues. They manifest themselves as extreme sensitivity to touch; delight with the aesthetic things in life, such as art, music, fabric, surroundings; extreme dislike or love for certain foods due to specific textures or tastes; sensitivity to odors or chemicals in the environment; or any other sensory-related experiences.

7. **Twice exceptional students:** Twice-exceptional students are identified as gifted in one or more areas of exceptionality (specific academics, general intellectual ability, creativity, leadership or performing arts). These students are also identified with a disability such as a learning disability, significant emotional disability, physical disability, sensory disability or ADHD. Twice exceptional students are difficult to identify because their strengths and weaknesses may mask each other, creating confusion between being gifted and having a disability.

8. **Vision problems:** Many gifted children become early readers because they are cognitively ready to decode the written word. However, eye sight and cognitive development may not progress at the same rate. Toddlers are far-sighted. Reading demands focusing on near objects causing visual disturbances!

9. **Associated physical issues:** Gifted children often show comorbities like clumsiness, lack of coordination, poor balance, delayed choice of handedness, poor pencil grip, slow handwriting speed, inability to cross the midline of the body

without switching hands, difficulty cutting or drawing simple figures, and avoidance of motor tasks.

IV. Assessment of Giftedness

1. Use of appropriate checklists to identify 'Giftedness'.
2. Academic performance and teacher's observations. Grade level assessment.
3. Analysis of intelligence quotient on standardized tests like ICIT, WISC, etc. But one has to analyze these children separately on subsets as 'gifted children' tend to do exceptionally well on one subset and falter miserably on another.
4. Behavior observations in different settings: school, family and social events.
5. Assessment of emotional quotient; especially in adolescent children
6. Assessment of 'Multiple Intelligences', especially creativity, art, music skills!
7. Analysis of comorbidities like Learning differences, ADHD
8. Physical, medical assessment—especially vision checkup.

27

High achiever	Gifted	Creative thinker
Strives for 'Marks' in exams	Not interested in 'Marks'	Not interested in 'Marks'
Enjoys school	Enjoys own way of learning	Enjoys new learning and creation
Hard worker	Requires less efforts to learn	Quickly grasps basic concepts
Good concentration	Concentrates only when decides	Remains in own world/ thoughts
Knows answers of known questions	Knows answers to unknown questions also. Asks questions!	Knows answers more than the expected one
Enjoys same age friends	Prefers adults or elder children	Prefers less friends
Likes to finish project	Enjoys process, not the result	May divert to some other project

V. Every Smart Child is not 'Gifted'!

Sometimes parents presume that a smart child or a high achiever child is 'Gifted'. There is a difference between being high achiever, being creative thinker and being gifted, and it has to do with the degree of a child's ability and talent.

VI. Management of a 'Gifted Child'

Managing a 'Gifted Child' is actually more difficult than a child with only learning differences or a child with ADHD or even a slow learner. Management plan for 'Gifted Child' is an IEP that is Individualized Education Plan developed by joint efforts of School teacher, Remedial Teacher, Psychologist, Parents and Developmental Pediatrician.

Developing an IEP involves six interrelated stages
1. *Identifying needs:* Assessment and interviews
2. *Setting the direction:* Short-term and long-term goal setting
3. *Creating a plan:* Team approach.
4. *Implementing the IEP:* Close monitoring, age appropriate cluster teaching in motivated schools aware of and ready to manage 'Gifted children'.
5. *Reviewing and revising:* Continuous process
6. *Transition planning:* Especially with respect to career guidance.

VII. Pediatrician's Job!

1. Identifying, understanding and reassuring 'gifted children' and their parents.
2. Watch for comorbidities. 'Being gifted' does not mean 'All is well!' Counsel the parents for the same. But 'Avoid labeling!'
3. Rule out associated physical problems; especially visual and sensory-motor issues!
4. Helping to build the team of necessary resource persons.
5. Suggesting 'Inputs' appropriate for 'Cognitive Level' rather than those for 'Age'.
6. 'Being gifted' is also troublesome and sometimes frustrating to the child and parents. We can reassure,

27

reward, remediate these children and build their confidence.

7. Suggest 'Higher level reading, Puzzles, software programming, word games' as these mental challenges keep 'Gifted Child' busy.

8. Planned introduction to 'Music, Arts, Sports and Nature Trails' will keep these kids busy.

9. Suggest 'Projects' in which the 'Process' is more challenging than the 'Result'. Accept if child leaves the project!

10. Help parents of 'Gifted Children' to form their own support group.

27

VIII. Parenting a 'Gifted Child'

Parents play an especially important role in developing the special capabilities of a young gifted child. To be effective, parents should:

1. Promote their child's growing need for independence;

2. Gifted child needs more praise when they succeed and 'more reassurance' when they fail!

3. Set clear limits and guidelines. Communicate clearly and with enthusiasm;

4. Expand vocabulary by using new words;

5. Provide a variety of learning materials, especially books;

6. Give puzzles and challenges to their brain!

7. Help develop special skills;

8. Find playmates who have similar interests (young gifted children sometimes enjoy the company of older children);

9. Promote creativity and encourage the child to try new things that help value learning and creativity;

10. Read to, and engage in, creative hobbies with the child.

"If we did what we are capable of doing, we would astound ourselves."

– Thomas Edison

Points to remember

27

- Gifted children possess three particular traits—high level of ability, creativity and task commitment.
- A gifted child should have the following five criteria:
  1. Excellence: In some dimensions relative to peers.
  2. Rarity: The child possesses a skill or attribute that is rare among peers.
  3. Productivity: The individual must produce something in area of giftedness.
  4. Demonstrability: Skill should be demonstrable through valid assessments.
  5. Value: Child shows superior performance that is of value to the society.

  Problem areas of 'Gifted child' could be asynchronous development, social maladjustment, emotional oversensitivity and sensory over excitability.
- Gifted children after show clumsiness, poor balance, delayed choice of handedness, poor pencil grip, slow handwriting speed, etc.
- Individualised Education Plan should be developed by school teacher, remedial teacher, psychologist, parents and developmental paediatrician.
- Parents of gifted child should promote independence, more praise when they succeed and more reassurance when they fail.
- Parents should help the child to develop his special skills, by providing him learning material, books, and thus promote creativity.

FURTHER READING

1. Gardener H. Frames of Mind: the theory of Multiple Intelligences, New York Basic Books, 1983

2. Silverman, L.K. What is Giftedness? The Boulder Parent, July, 1993, pp. 1, 13-14. Revised: March, 2007;50

3. The journey: a handbook for parents of children who are gifted and talented. Alberta Learning. Learning and Teaching Resources Branch. Available from www.learning.gov.ab.ca/k_12/ specialneeds/resource.asp.2004.

4. Alvino James, Arbor Ann, Considerations and Strategies for Parenting the Gifted Child, The National Research Center on the Gifted and Talented, Michigan, The University of Connecticut, September 1995.

27

Section

5

School Age

Parenting—6 to 12 Years

Anjan Bhattacharya

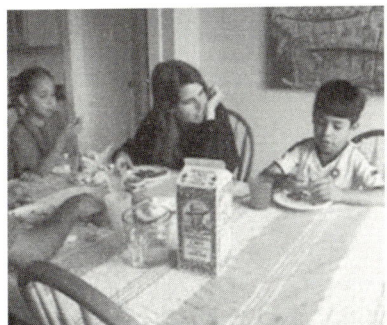

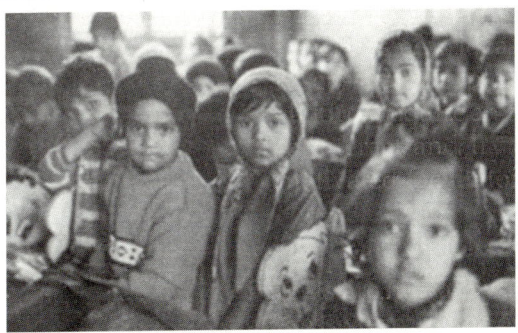

INTRODUCTION

Pre-adolescents bring fresh challenges for parents. In this chapter, we will try to see, what makes them tick, using available scientific evidence.

Every stage of human development has special needs. Therefore, we shall concentrate on the special developmental needs for this age group.

Special Needs

Wadsworth and Thompson in 2005, following Jean Piaget's theorem on human development, divided stages of cognitive development in to following four stages:

Stage 1: Sensory Motor Period (0–2 years)
> Coordination of sensory input and motor responses. Development of object permanence.

Stage 2: Preoperational Period (2–7 years)
> Development of symbolic thought marked by invincibility, centration and egocentrism

Stage 3: Concrete Operational Period (7–11 years)
> Mental operations applied to concrete events. Mastery on conservatism, Hierarchical classification.

Stage 4: Formal Operational Period (11 through to adulthood)
> Mental operations applied to abstract ideas. Logical, systematic thinking.

Since each child vary in their achievements of cognitive maturity, we can safely assume the Junior School Years (6–12) are that of Concrete Operations with Preoperational and Formal Operational thought processes operating in some candidates.

When this interface with varying parenting styles, special problems and opportunities of human existence explodes in front of our eyes in the form of troubleshooting in child rearing practices!

Parenting Styles

There are four categories of parenting with respective characteristics, as follows:

A. Dismissive parenting
   Understand child's demands but treat them as unimportant
   Ignore child's feelings
   Try to use distraction to get rid of the needs

B. Disapproving parenting
   Judge and criticize
   Reprimands, disciplines, punishes
   Believe child's opinion and needs are waste of time and need to be controlled

28

In short, they have a more negative approach towards raising children

C. Permissive parenting or laissez-faire parents

Freely accept all emotional expressions

Offer comfort to the child

Do not believe in limit setting and guiding the child

Do not help solve problems

These are ineffectual and inadequate parenting styles with following consequences:

Children do not learn to regulate their behavior

They have trouble concentrating, making friends and getting along with peers

They are self-centered/lack empathy/lack in ability to calm themselves

The desirable parenting methodology is:

D. Coaching parenting style

Accept and respect opinions/needs and use negative opinions as an opportunity for intimacy

Very patient and spend time with their sad, angry, fearful child

Use emotional moments as time to listen to the child, empathize, offer guidance, give choices, set limits and teach problem solving.

The effects of coaching style of parenting are:

Children learn to trust their feelings

Regulate emotions and solve problems

Learn well and get along well with others

High self-esteem

Normal Development and Deviant Development at Middle School Years

Now, if we combine these two important aspects, i.e. normal development in middle school going years (6–12) and parenting styles, the following issues emerge:

1. Children at this age normally have their developmental stage-specific needs, e.g.

a. Growth

i. At this age, pre-adolescents and just adolescents will naturally, first stretch and then fill up. The gangly and lanky lad and lassie are the norm. Trying to fill them up too early can lead to weight problem and subclinical and clinically manifest eating disorders.

ii. Hormonal spurts with accompanying behavior may be misinterpreted as rudeness, naughtiness or inappropriate.

iii. Physiological changes in sleep patterns may be mistaken for laziness.

iv. Tonsillar hypertrophy or bulging of neck glands are expected changes for this age. This is an age of exceptional healthiness. Therefore, caution must be taken not to take these custodians surgically taken out too promptly. However, protocols and guidelines should be followed stringently, so that the other way round, it does not harm by overdoing its job, creating obstructive sleep apnea.

b. Cognitive development

i. Children, at this stage, start assuming skills of independent thinking.

ii. They start realizing that the world around them are more complex.

iii. They start having their own views about such complexities.

iv. Therefore, they have lots of difficult questions for parents and figures of authority, e.g. teachers, elders.

v. It is important to address these questions with due care.

vi. Parents need to first critically appraise their own mental habits before discounting new approaches that their offspring bring. Please do not discount because these are new.

vii. Errors in judgment are opportunities to coach children.

viii. Asking odd questions, children try to find out their operational base in life.

28

ix. Therefore, honest answers, given in their individual developmentally age appropriate way, can coach a child to make smart choices in their lives.

x. Children will vary, so parents or parenting styles need to be varied.

c. Moral development

i. At this stage, for the first time, children start to see their own action and action of the others in moral and legal context.

ii. Questioning of existing moral conventions fosters the development of personal codes of ethics, which may be similar to or different from those of their parents.

iii. This is a great opportunity to coach moral values but it may need personal sacrifices. Influence of role modelling is high in this phase.

iv. Principles of cognitive development, described above, apply here too.

v. This is the stage for idealism.

d. Self-concept

i. Children start separating themselves from their parents as one entity

ii. They are more aware of self as a separate entity.

iii. For the first time, they start examining other individual's way of operating.

iv. Peer group starts assuming greater roles.

v. Philosophical frequently asked questions (FAQs) like "who am I?" and "Why am I here?" starts to crop up.

vi. Through this they start defining their own self-image, e.g. "I am a girl with close friends" (girls tend to focus more on relationships) or "I am good at sports" (boys tend to focus more on action). Designation of negative self-images imparts risk for future development, e.g. "nobody loves me because I am fat" or "I am naughty, so I cannot expect to make good friends" harbingers depression compounded with obesity or conduct disorders, delinquency or substance abuse in later life.

vii. Intense feelings and inner turmoil are common.

28

    viii. Coaching and not pushing children to problem-solve, where they feel the need can go a long way in preventing future difficulties. Dismissive, disapproving or permissive parenting styles may harm this process with life-long implications

e. Social development

    i. Socio-emotional development creates "stormy period" in 20 to 30% of children at this stage.

    ii. Some of these children will have an underlying neuro-developmental diagnosis.

    iii. Large majority of these diagnoses are easily managed either by parents themselves through appropriate coaching methods or through minimal professional support, where parents are not enjoying success.

    iv. Children will start exploring options for the future with some of them having the capacity of realistic self-assessments against available options. The presence or absence of realistic role models, as opposed to the idealized ones can be crucial.

    v. Sociopathic tendencies can be addressed best at this stage.

f. Sexual development

    i. This is a phase, where hormonal awakening interfaces with moral development.

    ii. Sexual orientation finds its way starting its journey, usually from this stage, working its way through its next stage of teen age years to adulthood.

    iii. It also tries to sort out other important aspects of sexual identity *viz.* beliefs about love, honesty and propriety.

    iv. Relationship at this age are often superficial, although could be intense, emphasizing on attractiveness and sexual experiments rather than genuine intimacy of the mature years.

    v. Homosexual experiments are common but these do not necessarily reflect the child's final sexual orientation.

    vi. Opportunity to discuss sexual identity related turmoil and confusions may help a child develop healthy sexual

28

behavior, especially if the coach is a responsible parent with healthy sexual behavior in themselves.

vii. Later in the course through adolescence, children chooses one of the three sexual identity: celibate, monogamous or polygamous which may include bisexuality.

viii. Knowledge regarding health risks of sexual experimentations including HIV and sexually transmitted diseases and its social fall outs are important for them to consider options in the light of reality rather than peer driven myths.

ix. But, knowledge, does not necessarily change behavior

x. Link with cognitive development and moral development are profound here.

xi. Unidentified special needs in such cases could spell profound implications for an individual at this juncture.

g. Special needs children

i. Children with EBD [Emotional/Educational, Behavioral and Developmental] problems may have core deficits in one or the other areas, which need appropriate attention to ensure healthy development.

ii. Most of these problems manifest in school. Therefore, having trained work force to alert through a standardized but robust School Health System is of paramount importance as a preventative tool, which should be based on the existing mountain of evidence (no reinventing the proverbial wheel in the pretext of Indian context must be avoided at all costs to save wastage of the borrowed time that we are already on).

iii. School curriculum will get more complex at this stage. Many EBD problems are about to raise their ugly heads. Since these are hydra-headed, i.e. symptoms are protean, adequate trained vigil must be maintained to nip these problems in the bud at the subthreshhold/subsyndromic/subclinical conditions.

iv. In out of school children, targeted assistance should be provided to include them in the ambit of school education as well as school health system.

28

2. Parenting does not have to come naturally to everybody but can be imparted
   a. Children vary, so the parent approaches need to vary, but all adults in the vicinity should try to adopt consistent method once the approach is agreed up on.
   b. Adults vary, so adults finding it hard to manage a child must seek anticipatory guidance from appropriate professionals.
   c. Single parents, foster or adoptive parents and *de facto* or *proxy* parents (nowadays, often grandparents) have special needs and may need extra support and/or top up training to avoid preventable (most often, unintentional) harm through their misguided parenting efforts (not always) unfit for present times.
   d. Teachers constitute a very important *proxy* parenting cohort during a child's waking hours and serves as a prime role model. Their input must therefore, be monitored with accountability through standardized procedures of appraisals and performance based management approaches.

3. Environment
   a. Social, moral and sexual development of a child interface with environment.
   b. There are studies to show that climatic conditions affect mood and can shape behavior.
   c. Microenvironment of home and school can shape a child's future development.
   d. Biological and cognitive development can depend on nutritional environment as well as opportunity for age and developmentally appropriate stimuli.
   e. Access to health and health consumptive patterns may influence through macroenvironment.

Do's and Don'ts

1. As parents and teachers
   a. Remain informed about their age appropriateness
   b. Avoid dismissive, disapproving or permissive parenting
   c. Try to become a role model for the youngster.

d. Never preach what you do not practice.

e. Never justify your weaknesses, they will learn to justify theirs.

f. Be truthful, avoid small lies and white lies, they cannot tell the difference.

g. Be fair in your approach, learn fairness.

h. Be consistent in your approach.

i. Be logical every time.

j. Do not give in to temptations.

k. Children need natural exposure to good things and bad things in life, try not to engineer everything for them, rather work hard towards a conducive environment, not protective from the day to day realities. Children are very resilient.

l. Be sensitive to your child's individual needs. If he has emotional dysregulation, get it mended through professional help.

m. If the child's emotional dysregulation is secondary to a primary cause like iron deficiency, ADHD (attention deficit hyperactivity disorder) or schizophrenia, get appropriate professional help.

n. Never judge, never criticize, snub, scold or hit. There is no benefit but harm only.

o. Never insult or humiliate, let them find their own limits

p. Take every negative situation as a basis for future learning.

q. Allow themselves to push hard. If he/she does not, consider it unnatural with unmet needs requiring, if necessary, specialist intervention. Never say "lazy" or other derogatory remarks.

r. Let the child have confidence to tell you everything. A child who is afraid to tell is a parental missed opportunity to help the child to learn from his/her mistakes.

s. No emotion is invalid, no opinion is silly and no behavior is bad. As an adult, it is your job to get to the bottom of it and help the child solve the crisis faced.

t. Do not do everything for your child. That is no helping. Child usually gets angry.

u. Understand what is within realistic capability of your child on par with his/her mental age and let them do it by them-

28

selves, being patient about few tentative attempts or mistakes.

v. If you cannot change yourself to become the role model you understand you should be, please understand that your child can have the same difficulties too.

w. Your child may need a shoulder to cry up on, not necessarily hands to solve problems. You need to understand that, when appropriate. Ask, if you are unsure.

x. If you have difficulties in fulfilling your role, do not assume this to be your fault. Seek professional help. These things are easily solved, if detected and acted up on early in an expert manner.

28

2. **As healthcare professional**

(*Dr Brian Stafford, Current Pediatrics, 20th edition, 2009. McGraw-Hills Publication*)

Following are the evidence based statements collated by this senior national policy level Child and Adolescent Psychiatric Consultant from the USA:

a. 50% of pediatric outpatient consultations are for EBD problems

b. 75% of the EBD problems will go to their primary care physician

c. Primary care physicians are only <20% efficient identifying EBD problems

d. Primary care physicians are gatekeepers of such problems

e. Pediatric symptom checklist enumerate 35 symptoms, starting with "complains of aches and pains" where children complains of tummyache, leg pain or headache, which often has non-organic basis, with item number 20 as "visits the doctor with doctor finding nothing wrong" as one of the valid reasons to refer to an appropriate professional [Refer to page 59 of 19th (latest) Indian Subcontinental edition of Nelson's Textbook of Pediatrics] to prevent 'downward spiralling'

f. All adult psychiatric diseases have their basis in childhood

g. Inappropriate and disjointed services results in downward spiraling.

h. Missing early interventional opportunities may etch some pathologies permanent despite appropriate intervention later on (neural plasticity), making it costlier.

i. Pediatricians are best placed as efficient gatekeepers, with adequate training, to arrest such downward spiraling.

j. Pediatrician's personal initiative and passion can make such services dramatically successful.

k. Anticipatory Guidance (trained) and Advocacy are Pediatrician's primary professional activity. For how to do so, please *vide infra*.

Recent Advances

28

Indian Academy of Pediatrics has launched a training of the trainer (ToT) module to address part of this problem through training Indian Pediatric workforce as its 5 year presidential action plan.

This is called PEICH (promoting emotional intelligence in children) Module. Level 1 workshops are being held this year, followed by Level 2 from next year, to run till end of 2017.

In this module, there is a novel concept of psychological vaccine, which was initially dreamed by Dr Jonas Salk of polio vaccine fame. He said, "if I were a young scientist, I would rather invent a psychological vaccine".

Rearing children up is no child's play. In the presence of mounting evidence, Indian Academy of Pediatrics has come up with an innovative and powerful solution, which needs to be embraced in all its splendor.

Middle school year is probably the last of the formative years, when correctional and remedial measures are still easy to implement. Once it hits the teenage years, all interventions start going egg shaped at the primary care level.

Anyone who has tried an adolescent to comply with a long term medication or a fitness regime can appreciate the developmental parenting challenges of this adolescent phase. It is therefore, immensely important that the youngsters who missed out on their opportunity in pre-school and junior school years get the benefit in their middle school years.

After all a **stitch in time, saves nine aka prevention is** *always* **better than cure.**

28

Points to remember

1. Emotional coaching parenting style is the best form of parenting.
2. Children at this age normally have their developmental stage-specific needs in growth, cognitive development, moral development, self-concept, social development, sexual development.
3. Try to become a role mode.
4. Be truthful, consistent in your approach and logical every time.
5. Never justify your weaknesses.
6. Do not give in to temptations.
7. Expose him to good and bad things of life.
8. Never judge, criticize, snub, scold or hit.
9. Don't insult or humiliate, let them find their own limits.
10. Anticipatory guidance (trained) and advocacy are paediatrician's primary professional activity.
11. Middle school year is probably the last of formative year when correctional and remedial measures are still easy to implement.

FURTHER READING

1. Nelson's Textbook of Pediatrics, 19th Edition
2. Current Pediatrics 2009, 20th Edition
3. EqiupKids; Dr. Sandip Kelkar
4. PEICH Module: Dr. Nita Jagat
5. Health for All 2004

Social Development of the Child

Shabina Ahmed

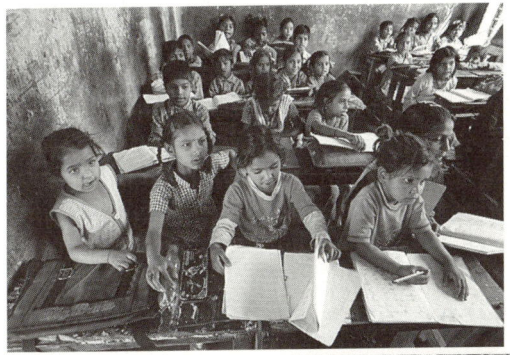

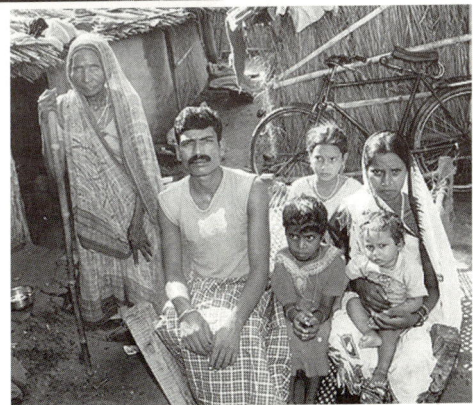

INTRODUCTION

Social development means the ability to adjust to the society outside the home environment. It is closely related to emotional development and communication development, in shaping the child's overall personality.

By its abstract nature, it presents a challenge to those in contact with the child to meet the desirable outcomes of the early years. However, knowledge of normal social behavior is helpful in understanding the child:

i. at his developmental level

ii. modulate expectations from the child

iii. helps recognise slow achievers

iv. detect deviant mannerisms

v. helps timely intervention

As children move out of infancy, their social world extends beyond their immediate family and there are marked expectations from them to conform to social norms. This leads to development of skills and capacities to achieve a reasonable degree of conformity.

As age advances there is acquisition of new skills and children begin to play social roles. However it does not develop in a smooth continuous fashion, as certain setbacks in the family, school and nursery may result in regression to an early phase. Much of the development occurs in tandem with other developments of the child and very dependent on adult–child interaction. The home environment in the early years is very important and starts playing a role when they go to school.

Parent–Child Relationship

Parenting style has a great impact on promotion or retardation of social development. Observant parents reinforce children behaviour, e.g. if a child has been thoughtful and empathetic towards others and the child is rewarded and praised, it will promote such behaviour later, more than when if it goes unnoticed. Early experiences in the formative childhood years largely determine what sort of adults children will become later.

Happy experiences motivate to seek more such experiences while unhappy experiences make them view the world and people critically. Democratic parenting helps children in social adjustments, while authoritarian parenting makes the child to be withdrawn and fearful and performs on pressure leading to maladjustment.

29

Pattern of Social Development

Social development in early years follows a steady pattern but may have variations due to health, emotional and environmental reasons.

At Birth: Babies at birth are not concerned as to who is attending to their physical needs.

At 6 weeks: The infant gives a true responsive smile to a person.

At 2–3 months: They can distinguish people from inanimate objects and develops the understanding that people supply their needs but they show no preferences.

29

At 4–5 months: The baby attracts attention by bouncing, raising, arching the body, cooing, pouting, and wants to be picked by anyone who passes by. They learn to react to a friendly versus stern face and to pleasant voices versus angry voices.

At 6–7 months: The baby by this age can differentiate friends and strangers, may befriend strangers, may briefly smile and then shows anxiety. This is the stage of"shy age".

This also is the period of development of attachment. The baby strongly attaches to the mother or caregiver and is afraid of strangers. During this period there is gaze contact with the mother and with the surrounding people, intently observing the face and looks at pictures of face and of dolls. Babies are beginning to smile at other babies.

At 8–9 months: The baby starts imitating. He tries to imitate speech, babbles monosyllables then bi syllables and initiates interaction by following gestures; vocalizes and starts playing interactive activities likes throwing objects on the floor and takes pleasure when somebody picks them up and hands over things to adults.

At 9–12 months: They now begin to manipulate toys, bangs objects and inhibits to **"No-No"**.

At 13–18 months: The child initiates interaction by pointing at objects and establishes a triangular gaze contact with the caregiver to show, share and to ask.

Negativism begins to develop, resists request and demands from adults. This manifests in physical withdrawal, hiding behind the mother or caregiver and may have angry outbursts.

At 18–24 months: Baby begins to cooperate with the caregiver in dressing, feeding and bathing. Initiates social play with ball and engages in make-belief play endowing representation and quality of real life to toys. This is when pretend play stage arises and the child enacts the activities of home and care and this is where imagination and creativity starts and the main playmates are parents and grandparents or the siblings.

29 In the first year babies can be handled easily, pleasant to be with and they are said to be in equilibrium, but around the middle of the second year the child becomes fussy and noncompliant particularly during feeding time ; they assert themselves, refuses to come to another's lap, becomes uncooperative and is said to be in a *stage of disequilibrium.* Around the second year they again exhibit pleasant nature. This is also the *ego development period*, when the child needs to be handled carefully. This is so because events like toilet-training and feeding may adversely affect the child in the long-term outcome in conflict resolution and social adjustment in later life.

Role of Play

Throughout infancy, play is mainly solitary and plays without any rules. It is mainly sensory in nature, hitting, touching, wiggling and rolling. There is no interaction with other babies and is called an *onlooker play or parallel play.* They however enjoy interactive games with adults like 'peek-a-boo', 'pat-a-cake' and 'hide- and-seek games'.

During this period there is no need to buy specific toys and play equipment. Any object that stimulates curiosity and exploration, particularly cause and effect relationship will help. As the child grows, patterns of play unfold and it becomes more varied and complex, depending on the intellectual development and motor capabilities.

Play is an integral part of development; it provides opportunities for many forms of learning particularly in areas of creativity, problem-solving, leading to imagination and internal language. It also helps the child to cooperate and respect the other person. If appropriate play does not take place, children deal with his or her environment in a restrictive stereotyped style.

CONCEPTS OF DEVELOP THROUGH SOCIAL CONTACT:

As Eskerman and Rheingold have pointed out, "It is through exploration that the infant learns about the world of people as well as things". Through play children derive joy and keep themselves amused, allay boredom and helps them to be self-sufficient. This inculcates self-confidence to cope with the various problems that they face as they grow. Play provides satisfaction and opportunities for creativity and serves as an incentive to emerge with their innovative ways of thinking and problem-solving as well as concepts.

29

Babies respond to familiar faces through pleasurable responses and regards strange people with fear. They respond to a whole situation and gradually respond to forms on the person. This is why you might often find children afraid to get into the doctor's clinic and over time fears only the doctor. As babies pass through the sensory motor stage, they fairly come to know what people are talking and begin to question who, why, what and gradually by age 2, starts generalising, but still cannot differentiate animate from inanimate objects. It is noteworthy to mention that many of the concepts needed for adjustment to life are learned at the babyhood stage, and all the social horizons will be broadened later on these foundations.

Concept of self develops by looking at the mirror and pointing at different parts of the body, and gradually the psychological self-concept develops based on people interactions and what other people think about them.

By 8 months, babies begin to respond to others emotions, play stunts, make funny faces and derive great pleasure in imitating, sustaining and causing reactions in the people around them. By two years, sex-role concepts develop as how members of the two sexes look behave.

ROLE OF FAMILY ENVIRONMENT

Baby's attitudes and behavior in social relationships is largely dependent on the early environment which is limited primarily to home environment. As the child grows and modifications take place in the environment, children learn new things but the core patterns of behavior of the early years still remain the same. This clearly explains the importance of early family relationship. It particularly affects:

a. Display of emotions

b. Attachment behavior

29 In a disturbed parent-child relationship, where adequate love and nurturance have not been provided, the children show extreme forms of temper tantrums, not responsive to social smiles and develop attention-seeking behaviours. Further, it has been seen that if the babies do not get close, warm, satisfying relationships, it affects their attachment behaviours and feel insecure, cannot develop satisfying personal relationship, and do not develop friends with peers as well as family members

Parent–child relationship is often disturbed in a large-sized family, as some of them do not get adequate attention.

The foundation stone of attitudes, behaviours, social relationships, personality structure is laid in babyhood, but events in later life also play a great role in reinforcing and modifying the person.

Common causes of disturbance of parent/child/family relationship:

- Dream child concept: If the baby is pretty, appears intelligent, then everybody is happy; but if there is any variance, it affects the relationship.
- As child becomes demanding, it becomes less appealing.
- Parental anxiety and the child react by resentment, crying and negativity.
- Parenting style: Authoritarian style and corporal punishment is very damaging to a relationship.
- Mothers are employed.
- Mothers are overworked
- Arrival of new sibling
- Preference: the child starts showing preference to certain family members who take greater care.

SOCIALISATION IN EARLY CHILDHOOD

As children move into their third and fourth years, they become aware that other people have thoughts and feelings similar to their own. This leads to greater sympathy and empathy and a greater wish to please. At the same time they develop the understanding what occurs for their own behavior, and what might arise due to others' behavior.

This is a gradual training to become a member of a 'gang' in late childhood. Early childhood is called 'pregang age'. Foundations of socialisation are laid at this age due to increasing contacts with peers.

It is at this point that the quality of social contact is more important rather than the number of friends. Those children, who get more pleasure by interacting with people than objects, fare better in life.

Through play, as it progresses from parallel play to assertive play, then cooperative play, they begin to be in a group and interact with group members. It is here they understand the rudiments of team play, conscious of others views and gradually polish the edges of social behaviour to emerge with new emergent behaviors.

Waldrop and Halverson , reported that children's sociability at 2½ years was predictive of socialisation at 7½ years. In early childhood, companions are associates and playmates and from this group they begin to have "friends" of own age and level.

In some associates they find some traits compatible, and in some they may feel amusing, but as they select their friends or playmates, they select good, honest, cooperative generous friends.

Sometimes if the companionship is not met due to isolation, or geographical reasons, pets and dolls become imaginary playmates. Early childhood is often called the "Toy stage". This is the age where symbolic operations play and rule systems, imaginations and creativity develop.

Highly intelligent children show preference for dramatic play, creative activities and for books. Socioeconomic status definitely influences the type of play. Children who are well developed involve more in motor skills and those who are weak deviate to amusements.

Creative children spend much of their time in doing something original.

With increasing intellectual abilities to explore their environment, children's ability to understand people, objects and relationships increase and new meaning being associated with meanings learned through their early years. They observe details that were missed earlier.

Children between 2 and 8 years are in the preoperational stage as defined by Piaget. The capacity to exert self-control in frustrating situations increases. They can understand the rewards of waiting. Being able to delay gratification is an essential element in social development.

Emotional expression is also gradually brought under control and temper tantrums decrease. Instead of physical outbursts they become mainly verbal, out bursts in frustrating situations.

As they enter into late childhood called, the "gang age" the children seek for a greater desire to be accepted as a member of a group. They do not like to be at home. However, children's gang differ from adolescent gang as their main purpose is to find fun not to engage in mischief. The gangs are mostly of the same sex. This is an important socialising area.

Group acceptance helps to develop ego and self-confidence. But children may be seen to be spending more time with them and this poses a friction point with their parents affecting parent-child relationship. In grouping, they may develop discrimination amongst friends by their tendency to stay with similar attitude friends. These feelings may be extended to being cruel and derogatory to others. Children who experience such events become withdrawn and depressed.

Children have a tendency to associate with similar socio-economic and racial groups. They generally change friends if they see if the other person is bossing or rude. The degree of acceptance of children in a gang is very much dependant on child rearing. Children brought up in democratic homes have better acceptance then those that come from authoritarian parenting.

At this age, play interests surround around movies, televisions and reading. They become less active and interests are diversified. The children get interested in **construction play** like drawing, painting, clay modelling and other creative work. They like to **explore** under guidance, the environment, they may be interested in mountaineering and in movements like the scouts & guides and NCC. Some **collect** stamps, birds, flowers as a hobby and this places them one up others. Some go for specific games, according to abilities.

Family relationship has a marked effect on the child's emotional stability and school performance, social adjustments. Family is the first social environment and whatever they see at home affects peer relationship. In authoritarian parenting, children are followers and confronting, while in democratic parenting, encourages leadership ability, and creativity. Aspirations and achievements are affected by parental guidance.

Family relationships deteriorate depending on parental attitudes towards their role, when children fail to meet parental expectations.

SOCIALIZATION IN ADOLESCENCE

As the child passes in to adolescence stage the most difficult task for them is to make social adjustments. Adjustments have to be made with the opposite sex and adults outside home and to the school demands. They have to preserve themselves from increasing peer influence, however most adolescents want to emerge in their own right. This is how peer group influence weakens and friendship is narrowed down.

Social activities are less important than personal friendships but social participation gives social competency and better understanding of opposite sex and helps development of poise in social situations. Childhood groups and friends gradually break up to give away to friends of similar interest, with whom they can express and are appreciated and feel secure. By end of adolescence, they begin to have preference of opposite sex as friends.

Their social interests depend upon the amount of opportunities the children have been exposed in childhood in:

- Personal interests and parties
- Drinking in parties
- Drugs
- Interest in conversations
- Helping others
- World affairs
- Criticism and references

As adolescence progresses, frictions develop in the family relationship particularly when there is rejection of restrains placed by parents in their various activities. Parents are considered old fashioned and there seems to appear a generation cultured gap between them. This is further worsened by the communication gap that takes place due to their unwillingness to sit and discuss. Parental methods of disciplining, feeling victimized, hypercritical attitude are detrimental to growth. But however as adolescence progresses, family relationship improve. Parents at this time must give them more privileges

SOCIAL BEHAVIOR PATTERN DEVELOPMENT

- **Immitation:** Children model attitude and behavior which they appreciate
- **Rivalry:** Feeling of competition and to excel emerges around 4 years
- **Cooperation:** By the 3rd year it develops in team activities and group plays
- **Sympathy:** Develops by 3rd year, enhanced by play contacts
- **Empathy:** Begins early childhood
- **Social Approval:** Starts after closure of early childhood
- **Sharing:** Sharing institutes generosity and is an important integration of social development
- **Attachment Behavior:** If part child relationship has been congenial, then the child attacks herself to people and adjust outside more satisfactorily.

Points to remember

1. Social development means the ability to adjust to the society outside the home environment and is closely related to emotional development and communication development, in shaping the child's personality.
2. Parenting style has a great impact on promotion or retardation of social development.
3. Concepts needed for adjustment to life are learned at the babyhood stage.
4. Early conducive home environment influences the baby's attitudes and behavior in social relationships.
5. Social adjustments are difficult during the adolescent stage.

29

FURTHER READING

1. Personal and social development: Hamah Mortimer, published by Scholastic Ltd.
2. Development psychology: "A life span approach" Fifth edition– Elizabeth B Hurlock a Tata McGraw-Hill edition.
3. Waldrop, MF, and C.F Halverson. Intensive and Extensive peer Behaviour; Child Development 1974; 45: 19–26.
4. Eckerman CO and H.L. Rheingold. Developmental Psychology, 1974.
5. Child psychiatry: A Developmental Approach, 3rd edition, Phillip Graham, Jeremy Turk and Frank Uerhust.
6. Developmental and Behavior Paediatrics—Lenne, Carrey, Crocher-3rd edition.

Power of 'Emotional Intelligence' in Parenting

Sandip Kelkar

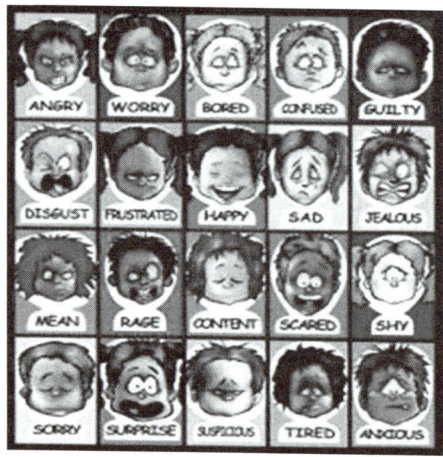

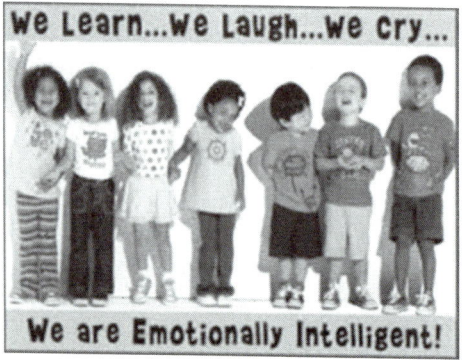

Parenting is a terrific experience, but it could be terrifying foremost. Raising kids is a daunting task by any standards. Each child is unique, so what works for one may not work for others because kids are not like mathematical equations where two plus two adds up to four. Worse still, when a child is born he/ she doesn't come out with a 'User manual' to guide you on parenting: on details of their internal structure of mind, on which buttons to press to have better working, etc. so you have to charter your own path full of challenges. You have to select better choices and do good and less harm to your child. This puts enormous pressure on parents because of the constant dangling uncertainty which lurches on their minds of 'Whether I am doing right or wrong"?

I am sure this article on *Power of 'Emotional Intelligence' In Parenting...* will take you through a journey to face many of these uncertainties in an Emotionally Intelligent way! In these challenging times we as parents will have to give a new vigor to our parenting and that's possible by utilizing this novel concept of 'Emotional Intelligence'. Time and again the research has proven that the parents who are aware of this concept of EI and practically apply it while parenting will automatically raise children with higher 'Emotional Intelligence'.

30

But why this novel idea and the exploration now? What is this concept of 'Emotional Intelligence' (EI) all about? And how do we as parents utilize power in this novel concept while parenting? This article will essentially revolve around these three points.

Why this Exploration now? And why bring EI to Parenting?

This modern world is rife with challenges facing kids and parents which have grown by leaps and bounds in recent times. The childhood has changed and parents need to learn scientific techniques and strategies to deal with children, need to know the appropriate way of having dialogue with their children and should be aware of how to give 'Quality' to the time spent with them. These challenges have essentially grown due to rapid growth of Economic and Technological innovations all around us not keeping in pace with the slower evolution of human beings. The challenges are many viz.

1. Increasing competitiveness and less of collaboration in this modern world
2. Changing family structure, from old 'Joint Family' to more nuclear families
3. Diminishing time parents are spending with their children
4. Children are exposed to various unfiltered external influences especially from media and television—the so-called "Third Parent"
5. Rising divorce rates and marital conflicts leading to 'Single Parenting'
6. Changing attitude of society which was previously "Have a nice day" to presently 'Make my day' attitude
7. Everincreasing influence of addictions (drugs, alcohol, etc.) on children
8. Enormous pressures put on the child by parents to somehow make him into a 'Super child'
9. Growing violence, aggressiveness in the society.

30

If you notice these challenges, most of them are related and have impact on 'Emotions' in children as well as parents. If we want to do parenting in a more effective way then we need to be more intelligent about how to deal with and utilize Emotions in our lives. We as parents have to nurture in ourselves certain set of skills related to Emotions better known as Emotional Intelligence. What is this novel concept of Emotional Intelligence?

What is Emotional Intelligence?

Emotional Intelligence is a set of skills and abilities (Beyond IQ) to effectively deal with and utilize emotions. Measure of Emotional Intelligence is called as Emotional Quotient (EQ).It includes abilities called as 'EI skills' or Emotional Skills the likes of:

1. Ability to recognize, understand and constructively express emotions more commonly called as Emotional Literacy (i.e.) knowing the language of emotions, Emotional self-awareness
2. Ability to handle difficult, disturbing emotions like anger, fear, disappointment, frustration, etc. and manage them effectively

3. Ability to control impulses and delay gratification
4. Ability to motivate self and others
5. Ability to use accurate, realistic, positive thoughts (optimism skills) when there are adversities in life
6. Ability to identify and tune into emotions in others (empathy skills)
7. Ability to know other person's perspective and read nonverbal cues
8. Ability to use emotional social skills and work in group with cooperation

In a nutshell "Emotional Intelligence" reflects how smart we are with our emotions

All these EI skills are learnable skills and can be developed in ourselves as parents and in our kids. Research has proven that children with these 'EI skills' developed are more assertive, less lonely, less impulsive, more focused, more responsible, more popular and outgoing, have greater academic achievement. They are better equipped to face all the life challenges and in general enjoy better emotional and physical health.

How can we use these set of EI skills while parenting? This is a key question which can be answered only if we know what is at the core of parenting?—*Our Parenting Style.*

What is at the Core of Parenting?

The parenting style

Parenting is a complex activity that includes many specific behaviors that work individually and together to influence child outcomes. It is assumed that the primary role of all parents is to support, influence, teach, facilitate and sometimes control their children.

Since last few decades developmental psychologists have been interested in knowing how parenting style influences the development of children's social and emotional competence. Parenting style captures two important elements of parenting:
1. Parental responsiveness (warmth, supportiveness) and
2. Parental demanding (control, supervision and disciplinary efforts)

As reported in the journal genetic psychology monographs in 1967, the work by Diana Baumrind was some of the earliest research that looked at the connections between different styles of parenting and children's personalities and behavior, more commonly called as 'Baumrind Typology'.

Parents according to whether they are high or low on parental control and warmth creates a typology of four parenting styles: Authoritarian, Uninvolved, and Permissive and Authoritative

One way to look at parenting is to divide it up along the lines of control and warmth. In this way, you can put parents into four very broad categories:

30

		Control	
		High	Low
Warmth	**High**	(A) High warmth, high control ("authoritative") children "self-reliant, self-controlled"	(B) High warmth, low control ("laissez-faire") children with "little self control"
	Low	(C) Low warmth, high control ("authoritarian") children "discontent"	(D) Low warmth, low control

It's time that we start reflecting for few minutes and start knowing about "where do I fit in these parenting styles?" To simplify the styles I have elaborated few characteristics of each parenting style. Take one minute and honestly reflect on which style does you fit in?

In **EI language**, the parenting styles can be classified as:
1. Dismissing (low warmth, low control)
2. Disapproving (low warmth, high control)
3. Laissez-faire (high warmth, low control)
4. Emotion coach (high warmth, high control)

Now Imagine this..'Your 3 yrs old daughter has accidentally broken her new toy, which you have bought her just a few hours back. She comes crying to you with all tears" How do you normally respond?

Which set of these underlying characteristics you showcase most of the times? Each of these parenting styles will have certain effects on children.

The Dismissing Parent (Low Warmth, Low Control)

Characteristics

1. Treats child's feelings as unimportant, trivial
2. Disengages from or ignores the child's feelings
3. Wants the child's negative emotions to disappear quickly
4. Characteristically uses distraction to shut down child's emotions
5. Does not try to solve problems with the child and believes that passage of time will resolve most of the problems
6. Focus more on how to get over emotions than on the meaning of the emotions itself
7. They often try to shrink the problem down to size, encapsulate it and put it away so it can be forgotten.

Effects of this style on children

1. They learn that their feelings are wrong, inappropriate and not valid
2. They may learn that there is something inherently wrong with them because of the way they feel
3. They may have difficulty regulating their own emotions
4. They learn to ignore their feelings and don't learn how to deal with emotions.

The Disapproving Parents (Low Warmth, High Control)

Characteristics

1. Judges and criticizes the childs emotional expressions
2. The children are reprimanded, disciplined, or punished for expressing emotions like fear, anger and sadness.

30

3. Believes expression of negative emotions should be time limited
4. Believes negative emotions need to be controlled, they reflect bad character traits
5. Believes emotions make people weak, children must be emotionally tough for survival
6. Believes negative emotions are unproductive and waste of time.

Effect of this style on children

1. In general same as for the dismissing type
2. Kids learn that emotional-intimacy or the expression of emotions is a high risk proposition; it can lead to humiliation, abandonment, pain and abuse
3. Your anger is causing embarrassment to others.

The Lassez-Faire Parent (High warmth, Low control)
Characteristics

1. Freely accepts all emotional expression from the child
2. Offers comfort to the child experiencing negative feelings
3. Offers little guidance on behavior
4. Does not teach the child about emotions
5. Does not teach problem solving methods to the child
6. Believes that managing negative emotions is a matter of physics; release the emotion and the work is done

Effects of this style on children

1. They don't learn to regulate their emotions
2. They have trouble concentrating; forming friendships and getting along with other children
3. They often lack the ability to calm themselves when they are angry, sad and upset.

Parents as Emotion Coach (High Warmth, High Control)
Characteristics

1. Values child's negative emotions as an opportunity for intimacy and an important opportunity for parenting

2. Can tolerate spending time with sad, angry or fearful child; does not become impatient with the emotion

3. Is aware of and values his or her own emotions

4. Is sensitive to child's emotional states, is not confused or anxious about the child's emotional expression and knows what needs to be done

5. Does not make fun of child's negative feelings

6. Does not say how the child should feel

Effects of this style on children

1. They learn to trust their feelings, regulate their own emotions; and solve problems constructively

30

2. This style would directly influence EQ components such as emotional self awareness, assertiveness, empathy, interpersonal relationship, flexibility, impulse control and self regard

3. Make children more responsible

4. Children can communicate their feelings with others and stay Connected.

Now you will know which Parenting style of Dealing with children is most effective to nurture Emotional Intelligence skills in children. It's off course...Emotion Coach Style. Let's now dive deeper into specific steps we can take to become 'Emotion Coach' for our children? When a problem or crisis is there in the household, when intense emotions are expressed in the family, emotionally intelligent parent is expected to follow certain steps as **Emotion coach**:

1. First acknowledge your own feelings about the situation and the child involved. Every situation or stimulus in the environment triggers stored up feelings (both negative and positive). Most times these feelings are not relevant to the present situation and so should not be a guide to the reaction to the situation.

2. Recognize the negative feelings that can potentially block good thinking and put them aside to be dealt with later.

3. Listen closely to what the child is saying, paying attention to the emotional message beneath the words or actions-what is the child trying to show? How is he hurting? Why is he hurting? What is the underlying trigger for this hurt?

4. Respond to the child's hurt, not to the words or to the behavior that results from the hurt; but rather to the need for comfort or safety to release the hurt feelings that are triggering the inappropriate behavior.

Parenting as emotion coach should be a natural way of parenting, and not only when there is crisis or problem and it includes:

1. Teaching children how to correctly identify and label their feelings. This means teaching the feeling words, not only sad, glad, and scared, but also the variations of these such as frustration, excitement, etc. and to identify the real origin of these feelings.

2. Helping children correctly perceive others' feelings and therefore appropriately responding to them. Frustration means something is hard to comply. Anger usually means that someone is trying to hurt you (even yourself as in when you berate yourself for doing something wrong)". The appropriate response to frustration is different from the response to anger.

3. Helping children deal with their feelings in appropriate ways. This includes assisting them to see and understand another's point of view. According to Child Development theorists children below age 6 or 7 have difficulty seeing another's point of view. They can only see the world form their own perspective. As they get older and their development proceeds with good guidance they get better at understanding and tolerating other people's point of view and therefore are better at cooperating and compromising.

4. Helping children build good relationships. Although human beings are born with an inherent connection to all human beings, they are not necessarily born with the skills needed to develop and nourish these connections.

30

5. Teaching constructive and creative problem solving skills. So these are few steps we can follow in the process of Emotion Coaching.

Emotion Coaching Process

1. Become aware of child's emotion

2. Recognize the emotion as an opportunity for intimacy and teaching

3. listen emphatically, validating the child's feelings

4. Help the child find words to label the emotion s/he is having

5. Set limits while exploring strategies to solve the problem at hand.

30

While Solving Problem

- Find the goal(s) of the behavior— what did you want?
- Help child verbalize actions taken towards goal(s)—What did you do to get it?
- Assess effectiveness—How did that work?
- Examine full range of possible behavioral options—What were/are all the options?
- Choose the most effective option—What is the best choice?
- Check back to see how the plan worked—Let's see how that goes?

In conclusion parenting style as **Emotion Coach** would help children grow as caring, responsible human beings, which is truly the need of the hour!!

Until now we have seen why do we need to utilize power of Emotional Intelligence in parenting? What is this concept of Emotional Intelligence and how do we become more adept at facing children's emotions by changing our parenting style to 'Emotion Coach' style? Now in this last part of the article we will see how do we raise children with higher EQ by utilizing this concept of EI in parenting by way of 'Emotionally Intelligent Parenting'

EMOTIONALLY INTELLIGENT PARENTING

Parenting is all about caring, supporting and Guiding (controlling within limits) your child. But when we talk about Emotionally Intelligent Parenting it means much more than just this. It is about demonstrating EQ skills our self and trying to instill those in our kids in a natural way. This will help in the long run in bringing up our children as caring, empathic, independent, imaginative, adaptable and responsible human beings. This will also help our children in raising their EQ. in this sense; they will be less impulsive, less anger prone, more motivated, and confident and better in academics. There are few things parents can do to raise an Emotionally Intelligent child.

30

1. Role Plays EQ Skills Yourself

Your kids are watching you very closely. They see how you respond to frustration, anger, they see how you solve problems, they see how you show resiliency when the times are tough and they see whether you're aware of your own feelings and the feelings of others. You need to model EQ skills in front of them and slowly they will imbibe those skills.

2. Its OK to Say "No" to Your Kids

Your kids will demand something or the other daily, as they see lots of stuff in their surroundings. It's OK to say no to your kids saying no will give your kids an opportunity to deal with disappointment and frustration and to learn impulse control. Kids who always get what they want typically aren't very happy.

3.'Know Yourself' when You are with Your Kids"

Many a time's parents come unglued with some issues and thoughts and feelings when they are with their kids and this reflects in their actions knowingly or unknowingly. So try to 'Know yourself' the issues which are bothering you, try to find out feelings and emotions behind those issues. Knowing your issues does not make them go away — it just makes it easier to plan for and to deal with them. This will reflect on kids in a positive way.

4. Practice and Build Emotional Literacy Skills in Your Kids

Start labeling feelings in yourself and your kids. Avoid name calling. Instead name the underlying feelings the child is having, e.g. Say, "He seems angry," rather than "What a jerk." When your kids are whiny or crying, saying things like, "You seem sad," will always be better than just asking them to stop. If your child needs to talk, stop and listen to what he has to say. He needs to know that his thoughts, feelings, desires, and opinions matter. Help him get comfortable with his emotions by labeling them. By accepting his emotions without judgment, you validate his feelings and show that you value what he has to say. If you share your own feelings, he'll gain confidence expressing his own.

30

5. Let them Face Some Problems and do not Solve all the Problems for them

When kids are beyond the toddler years, you can let them face more problems rather than solving them yourself. You can help them to be more responsible, e.g. when your child is solving a difficult math problem instead of telling him/her how to solve let him/her do it him/herself. Kids who try to solve difficult problems on their own will learn to overcome obstacles in solving them. Constantly telling your kids what to do does not help them to develop confidence and responsibility. For example, instead of asking your child to get paper and pencil for writing, you may ask "What do you need for writing"?

6. Mistake Child Makes is an Opportunity for You to Showcase Your EQ Skills

Your child is bound to make mistakes some time or the other. These are valuable lessons for your child's confidence if your child puts his plate too close to the edge of the table and it tips, encourage him to think about what he might do differently next time. That way his self-esteem won't sag and he'll understand that it's okay to make mistakes sometimes. When you goof up yourself, admit it, acknowledging and recovering from your mistakes sends a powerful message to your child—it makes it easier for your child to accept his own shortcomings. See yourself as having something to do with every problem that comes along. Most problems in families get bigger when parents respond to them in a way that exacerbates the problem. If your child makes a mistake, remember how crucial it is for you to have a calm, reasoned response. This is an opportunity for you to model calm collective response, resiliency, anger management and listening skills in your child.

30

7. Get Your Kids Involved in Household Duties at an Early Age

Research suggests that kids who are involved in household chores from an early age tend to be happier and more successful because from an early age, they're made to feel they are an important part of the family. Kids want to belong and to feel like they're valuable.

8. Limit Your Kid's Access to Television

Young kids need to play, not spend time in front of a television. To develop creativity and problem-solving skills, allow your kids time to use free play. Research strongly suggest that what your kids learn from you and from free play with others will provide the seeds for future emotional intelligence. TV viewing not more than 1–2 hours per day is acceptable according to research. According to renowned psychologist Dr. Shapiro, parents may put family on a TV Diet for not more than 1–2 hours per day which applies to everyone in the family and not just children. It will be much better if you accompany the child while TV viewing and try to use it as an opportunity to build up his/her vocabulary of feelings by asking him/her the feelings the character on TV is displaying.

9. Talk Freely about Feelings as a Family

Emotions and feelings are the most neglected and suppressed part in our communication as family members. We as parents need to talk more freely about feelings and emotions so that it becomes our natural way of communication state your emotional goals as a family. These might be no yelling, no name-calling, be respectful at all times, etc. Families that talk about their goals are more likely to be aware of them and to achieve them. As the parent, you then have to "walk the talk."

10. Give Your Kids Unconditional Love

A child's self-esteem flourishes with the kind of no-strings-attached devotion that says, "I love you, no matter who you are or what you do." Your child benefits the most when you accept him for who he/she is regardless of his strengths, difficulties, temperament, or abilities. So lavish him with love. Give him plenty of cuddles, kisses, and pats on the shoulder. And don't forget to tell him how much you love him. When you do have to correct your child, make it clear that it's his behavior—not him—that's unacceptable. For instance, if your child is pushing his friend, instead of saying, "You're a naughty boy! Why can't you be good?" say, "Pushing your friend isn't nice. It can hurt. Please don't push." There is no greater way to create emotional intelligence in your child than to see them as wonderful and capable. One law of the universe is, "What you think about expands." If you see your child and think about them as wonderful, you'll get a lot of "wonderful." If you think about your child as a problem, you'll get a lot of problems.

30

Points to remember

1. We as parents should utilize the power in this novel concept of emotional intelligence while parenting.
2. "Emotional Intelligence" reflects how smart we are with our emotions.
3. All these EI skills are learnable skills and can be developed in ourselves as parents and in our kids.
4. Children with these 'EI skills' developed are more assertive, less lonely, less impulsive, more focused, more responsible, more popular and outgoing, have greater academic achievement.

   They are better equipped to face all the life challenges and in general enjoy better emotional and physical health.
5. Parenting styles can be classified as:
   - Dismissing (low warmth, low control)
   - Disapproving (low warmth, high control)
   - Laissez-faire (high warmth, low control)
   - Emotion coach (high warmth, high control)

     These parenting styles have their own characteristics and they affect their children hence parents should become good emotional coach.
6. Parents should know when to give freedom and how to say no.
7. Parents should give their kids to unconditional love.

30

Developing Self-Esteem in Children

Amol Anndate

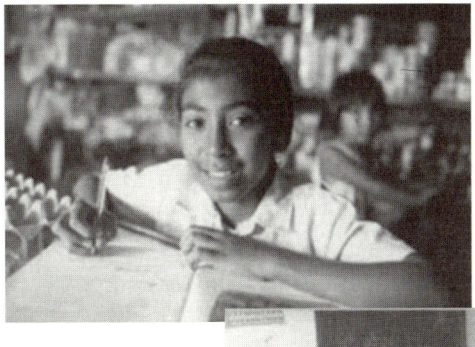

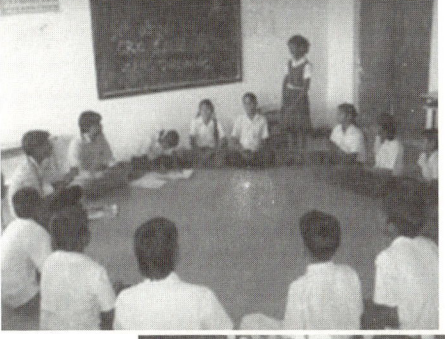

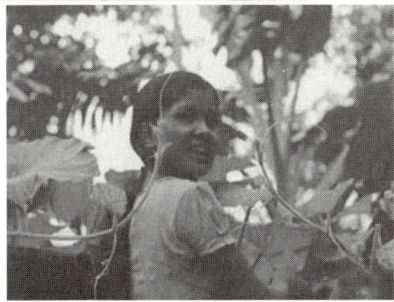

A. The Need of Self-Esteem

Many a times self-esteem is not nurtured, developed or hearted in childhood unintentionally by parents and society. This makes children to believe many negative thing about themselves. As they grow older the power of this negative image grows harder. Its roots are planted early in the children. Although the child may scale height of success as an adolescent but many a times he feels developed and disapproved as this child with low self-esteem continues to stay inside him.

Hence parents, society and pediatrician should work towards self-esteem needs of children and find ways of reversing a child budding negative self image at its early stage. This doesn't need any specialized training or counselor but it can be done on day to day basis by parents.

Self-esteem seems to be the foundation of self confidence but self-esteem doesn't mean over confidence. Child with self-esteem knows himself and accepts himself with his limitations. These children are not ashamed of their limitations but simply see them as a part of the reality .They are perhaps as a boundary they are challenged to expand keeping self-esteem alive. Self-esteem is as necessary for each child as water is for plants. Self-esteem is the daily food for emotional health of a child.

B. Role of Parents

Since children look upon parents as their biggest support and source of inspiration parents play a vital role in shaping self-esteem of child. A loving atmosphere is necessary for every child. No one can live healthily for long without loving and being loved. It is not that parents don't love their children; in fact they love them the most. But there is a constant battle between their head and heart where head wants the child to be tough and competent for surviving in this world while heart wants them to be untouched from the hardships. As a result of this battle parents start deciding for the minutest needs of the child. They want child's life to go by their mature adult conscience. This is the foundation of destroying self-esteem of the child. In this journey of shaping the future of child by the parents the child starts feeling inadequate, incompetent unlovable, unpopular and ultimately became unapproachable.

C. Stepping Stone for Developing Self-Esteem by Parents

1. **Be available to children:** In today's busy world child becomes the most neglected factor so spending quality time and making the children realized that parent's care enough for them helps to grow self-esteem.

2. **Listening without making judgments:** Parents need to be good listeners and that too without giving conclusions or opinions on what the children are saying. If at all something has to be told it should be done on some other occasion and not as continuity when the child is expressing himself on the topic.

3. **Keeping the sharing mutual and emphasizing similarities:** Many a times you can share your simple problems with the child. This makes them feel that you value them enough to share some part yourself with them. This helps to grow self-esteem in the child.

4. **Taking children to special places:** For children to accept a unique experience with an important person is to accept themselves as important and valuable.

5. **Be real and don't pretend:** Many a times false promises or commitments makes the children feel as fooled and creates a negative self image. Hence such things should be avoided and when children find you real they also will be real with you.

6. **Be nonthreatening:** While setting rules and boundaries parents should make it appoint to be nonthreatening. As compared to adults children sense of self is still fragile, vulnerable and easily knocked out.

7. **Never embarrass children:** Many a times children are made to perform in front of strangers and nonperformance leads to embarrassment and insult. Never force children for such performances. Also let them know that they don't have to prove anything to you or others.

8. **Capitalize on existing success:** It is not bad to have expectations but more important is taking advantage of what they already have going for them. Utilize the interest and success that already exist. Success builds most easily and effectively on appreciation of past success.

31

9. **Watch for growth sparks:** Sometimes child comes up with sparks of skills. Make them realize that this is really a unique and specialized skill and that the child is really blessed to have this skill.

10. **Fostering the freedom of choice:** In Indian society the importance choice of parents is so deeply rooted in childhood that it continues till choosing a life partner. Hence freedom of choice has to practice since early childhood. This will also help the children take responsibility of the results.

11. **Dealing with strong emotions and failures:** Children need to understand that academic success is not the ultimate success and that it's ok to fail. They should be given realization that they are not loved because they are successful or it is not that they will not be loved if they have failed. This helps the child to bounce back.

31

D. Role of Teachers and Schools

Many a times a child with lack of self-esteem takes a mask of bossy and aggressive behavior in the school and they are just turned down by the school as 'difficult child'. But a detailed investigation into the child's behavior will reflect the lack of self-esteem. Insulting or punishing such children or sending note to parents or threatening them of a punishing or complaining to principal furthers demoralizes the child. Hence, such child should be given tasks of their likings and interviewed in a friendly way about the emotions they are going through. More ever they should be reported to parents for support and not for complaints.

E. Role of Pediatricians

Patients coming with repeated functional complaints or hysteria can be a sign of disturbed self-esteem. Also the body language of a decreased self-esteem can be easily noted by the pediatrician during routine consultations and reported to the parents. Pediatricians can be friends to the child and extend support to such child. Remembering names of children and addressing them by name for next consultation helps a lot to boost self-esteem of the child.

Need of developing self-esteem in children for the society— not only does the social environment affect such children but the children affect their environment. An angry and frustrated child touches off anger and frustration in the family and at school. At the same time the self-esteem of people around such child diminishes as their frustration grows, they feel increasingly inadequate in dealing with the needs of such child. Situations like this often start a destructive cycle where everyone involved continues to lose self-esteem. Hence, developing self-esteem in a child is necessary not just for him but for the society at large.

31

Points to remember

1. Be available to children. Spend quality time with your children. Play with them. Take them to places.
2. Be proactive listeners and non-judgmental opinions and views can be given at appropriate times.
3. Be real and don't pretend.
4. Appreciation of past success will help him to overcome his recent failures.
5. Don't embarrass him in front of strangers.
6. Help him to understand his emotions and deal with it successfully.
7. Teachers should discuss the child's behavior and find effective solution rather than being punitive.

Sleep Problems in Children

Jaydeep Choudhari

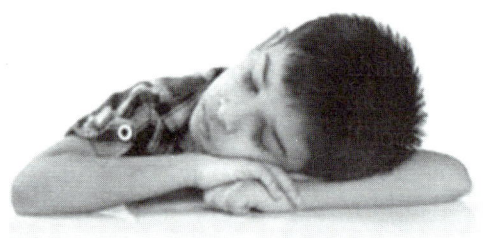

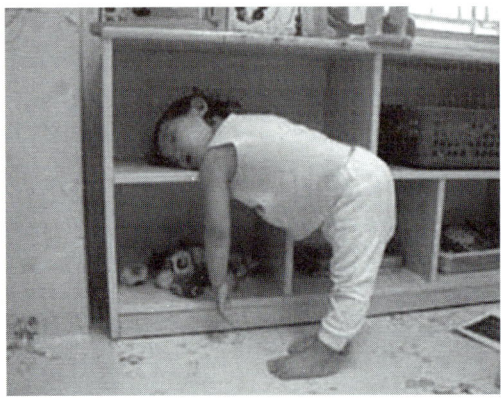

Good sleep makes the mind alert which is critical for good academic performance and learning skills. A proper sleep pattern is essential for physical and psychological wellbeing. Various factors influence children's sleep. It is affected by age of the child, day of the week (whether it is school day or weekend) and also the place where the child lives. Ideally a child should sleep in a room with optimum temperature, quiet, comfortable and well ventilated room with minimal light. Small children may be put to sleep by lullaby or bed time stories. Older children should not watch television before going to bed, for at least 1 to 2 hours prior to bedtime. Television should not be kept in the bedroom.

Sleep problem is actually a sleep pattern that is unsatisfactory or cause of concern to the parent, child or physician. The conception and interpretation of proper sleep also varies as sleep pattern is different in various families. A pattern which may be of great concern to a family may be inconsequential or trivial to another family. Most of the sleep related problems are transient and self limited. Professional help is generally sought when the child's sleep problem causes parental sleeplessness.

32

Normal Sleep Patterns

The timing, organization and structure of sleep changes and evolve during childhood years. Normal neonates sleep most of the day except when they are hungry. The 24 hour rhythm is usually established between the ages 3 and 6 months. The total sleep duration decreases from an average of 14 hours per day at 6 months of age to an average of 8 hours at 16 years of age. Increase in duration of night-time sleep occurs during the first 1 year after birth with a decreasing trend of daytime sleep. Children sleep less on school days than on weekends. Girls sleep a little more than boys. Obese children usually sleep less. Children like adults sleep more in winter than in summer.

There is no fixed duration that one should sleep. Sleep requirement varies according to sleep practices, environmental demands and probably regulated by genes. Short sleepers spend 4–5 hours per day in sleep and still feel fresh and energetic. Long sleepers sleep for 10–12 hours a day.

Poor Sleep Consequences

Regular low quality and low duration sleep are associated with a range of psychosocial and physical disturbances in children. Impaired attention, memory consolidation, creativity, learning and academic performance, increased impulsivity, aggression and hyperactivity are some of the manifestations. A sleep deprived child may have poor school performance. Short sleep duration may be associated with increased risk of overweight and obesity in children.

Types of Sleep Problems

The following are the types of sleep related problems.

i. *Dyssomnias:* Disorders of initiating and maintaining sleep.
ii. *Hypersomnias:* Excessive sleepiness.
iii. *Parasomnias:* Abnormal activity or behaviour during sleep.

32 Evaluation of a Child with Sleep Disorder

Complete sleep history is the most important guiding factor. A comprehensive sleep diary for 2 weeks helps in analysis of the child's sleep problem. A detailed medical, developmental and behavioural history should be taken. Physical examination should include assessment for tonsil or adenoid enlargement, sinusitis with post-nasal drip, bronchial asthma, gastrocolic reflux, abdominal colic and examination of central nervous system.

Common Sleep Problems in Children

Sleep terror

It is seen in children between 4 and 12 years age. It is episodic in nature. There may be history of sleep terrors in the family. It is characterized by a state of confusion and partial arousal usually during the first third of night, in the transition from NREM stage 3 or 4 to light sleep. Sleep terror usually lasts for a few minutes, occasionally for about 30 minutes. It is associated with autonomic activities like sweating, tachypnea, tachycardia, mydriasis, confusion, tremulousness and sometimes vocalization. A state of terror or intense fear is reflected in facial expression. Moaning, shouting, screaming and agitation may accompany. Some children may start walking or running during an episode. There may be associated somniloquy, night awakenings and separation anxiety. Attempts to wake up the child during an episode may exacerbate the child's disturbance.

The episodes usually end abruptly and the child rapidly returns to deep sleep. Children with sleep terror have poor recall of their dream and they are difficult to arouse.

Most children outgrow sleep terrors. Precipitating factors are fever, sleep deprivation, some drugs like antihistaminics, bronchodilators, antireflux medication, etc.

Management: It is usually a self-limiting disease, parental reassurance and guidance are essential. Proper sleep routine should be followed. Stress should be relieved. Short acting benzodiazepines li ke clobazam or lorazepam may be given for 3–6 months if there is a danger of self harm.

32

Nightmares

It occurs in the last phase of REM sleep. It is usually seen in 6 to 10 year old children and is precipitated by previous traumatic or stressful event. Nightmares are characterized by disturbing dreams and followed by post-event anxiety and refusal to go to sleep. The child remembers the dreams. Proper sleep habit is the main treatment. Violent and frightening television programs just before bed time should be avoided.

Night time fears

Childhood fears to some specific objects like ghosts, storms, darkness, cockroaches, flying insects and lizards are normal and universal. These fears may manifest in various ways, like resistance in going to sleep and even as frightening dreams. Fear of darkness may be alleviated by low night light. Other fears may be countered by parental support and good bedtime stories.

Somnambulism

Somnambulism or sleep walking is generally seen in the age group 4 to 8 years. It is an altered state of consciousness or impaired judgement. Sometimes a child walks in sleep in a dazed confused state with eyes open and reacts to external stimuli. The child does not appear to recognize surrounding person. There is no recall. Sleep deprivation or febrile illness may be the precipitating factors. Somnambulism is associated with the risk of safety concern for the child. The condition can be managed by avoidance of sleeplessness, anticipatory arousal and benzodiazepines or tricyclic antidepressants.

Somniloquy

Somniloquy or talking during sleep is a common feature in general population. It is seen in children as well as in adults. It is seen both in NREM and REM sleep. It is a benign condition and often features legible sentences with meaning and good recall. It can coexist with other parasomnias like somnambulism and night terrors.

Confusional arousals

Confusional arousals are common in children. The child suddenly wakes up, utters a few words or cry inconsolably. It appears as if the child is not able to recognize people around and again falls asleep.

Bruxism

Bruxism or forceful grinding or rhythmic clenching of teeth including rhythmic movements of mandible during sleep is seen in more than 50% of children and also in adult population. There is no confirmatory evidence of the belief of bruxism as the manifestation of worm infestation. Emotional or psychological factors may contribute to bruxism.

Delayed sleep phase disorder

There is delay in initiation of sleep beyond socially acceptable or desired bedtime which leads to difficulty in and delayed waking up. It is commonly seen in adolescent years. It is usually associated with day time sleepiness. The sleep-wake schedule is progressively delayed by two or more hours beyond scheduled bedtime and it leads to difficulty in daily activities. The treatment plan should be to gradually shift the bedtime by 15 minutes. Melatonin, 1 mg and increased up to 3 mg, when given 1 hour before the desired time of onset of sleep is effective

32

in altering the sleep phase. Proper sleep environment should also be maintained.

General Management

Sleep habit and hygiene is the most important aspect of management of sleep problems. Sleep habits are relative and varies in different families to a great extent. Proper sleep habits should be inculcated in all children from early age. Following are the main components of sleep hygiene:

i. Definite time to go to sleep and wake up,
ii. Proper environment—comfortable bed, dark, quiet room,
iii. Television, computer, mobile phones should be restricted,
iv. Avoidance of caffeine rich food and beverages in the evening and night,
v. Avoidance of play and exercise before bedtime.

32

Sleep problem is often not a disease. Many healthy children may also suffer from sleep related disorders. Parents can play a vital role in management of sleep problems in children. Sharing bed with small children or bedtime stories may solve many sleep related problems.

Other non-pharmacological therapies are extinction and graduated extinction, fading, scheduled waking, sleep restriction and light therapy.

Pharmacological therapies should be reserved as the last resort. The drugs include melatonin, short acting benzo-diazepines and anti-histaminics.

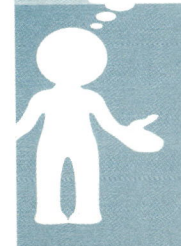

Points to remember

1. Good sleep makes the mind alert which is critical for good academic performance and learning skills.
2. The total sleep duration decreases from an average of 14 hours / day at 6 months of age to 8 hours at 16 years of age. Short sleepers

spend 4–5 hours a day and long sleepers sleep for 10–12 hours a day.

3. These are the following types of sleep related problems.

   a. *Dyssomnias:* Disorders of initiating and maintaining sleep.

   b. *Hypersomnias:* Excessive sleepiness.

   c. *Parasomnias:* Abnormal activity or behavior during sleep.

4. Common sleep problems in children are sleep terror, nightmares, somnambulism, somniloquy, bruxism, and confusional arousals.

5. Define time to go to sleep and wake up.

6. Television, computer, mobile phone should be restricted.

7. Avoid caffeine rich food and beverages.

8. Avoidance of play and exercise before bedtime.

9. Medications after consultation only.

32

FURTHER READING

1. Choudhury J. Sleep Problem. In: Choudhury J, editor. Behavioral Problems in Children and Adolescents, 1st edition. New Delhi: Jaypee Brothers; 2013.

2. Sheldon S, Ferber R, Kryger M. Principles and practices of pediatric sleep medicine. Philadelphia: Elsevier Saunders; 2005.

3. Chhangani B, Greydanus D E, Patel D R, Feucht C. Pharmacology of sleep disorders in children and adolescents. Pediatr Clin North Am 2011; 58: 273–91.

4. Owens J A, Moturi S. Pharmacologic treatment of pediatric insomnia. Child Adolesc Clin North Am 2009; 18: 1001–16.

5. Bharti B, Mehta A, Malhi P. Sleep problems in children: a guide for primary care physicians. Indian J Pediatr 2013; 80: 492–8.

6. Petit D, Touchette E, Tremblay R E, Boivin M, Montplaisir J. Dyssomnias and parasomnias in early childhood. Pediatr 2007; 119: 1016–25.

7. Bhatia M S, Gupta R. Common sleep disorders. In: Gupte S, editor. Recent Advances in Pediatrics – 19, Hot Topics. New Delhi: Jaypee Brothers; 2010.

Bedwetting (Enuresis)

Jaydeb Ray

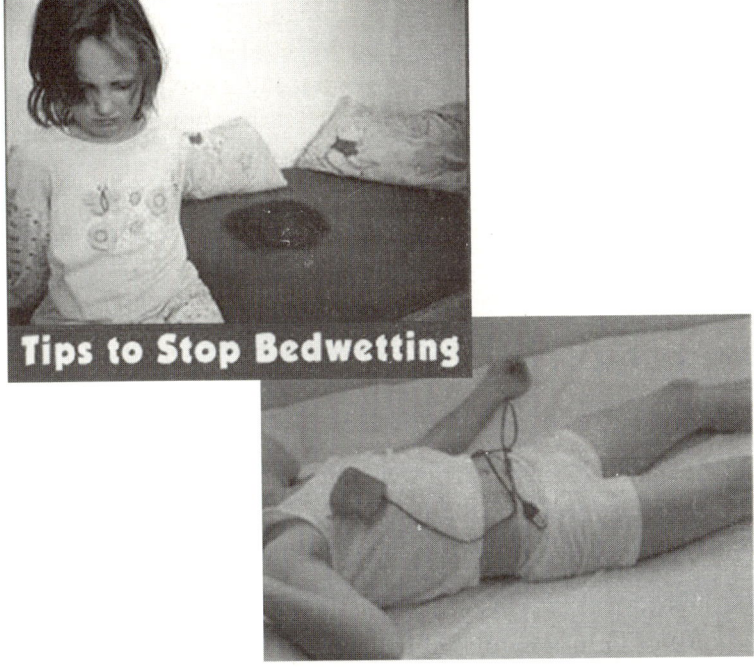

Bedwetting (enuresis) is a common childhood problem. Children learn to control daytime urination as they become aware of their bladder filling. Once this occurs, the child then learns to consciously control and coordinate his or her bladder. This generally occurs by four years of age. Nighttime bladder control usually takes longer and is not expected until a child is between five and seven years old. Repeated (twice a week for 3 consecutive months) discharge of urine into clothes or bed after a developmental age when bladder control should be established is known as enuresis.

A FEW FACTS REGARDING BED WETTING

Agewise Problems

The number of children with bedwetting varies by age;
- At five years of age, 16 percent of children have some difficulty staying dry at night.
- By 15 years of age, only 1 to 2 percent continues to wet the bed.

33

Sex: Boys are twice as likely as girls to wet the bed.

Genetic link: If one parent was a bed wetter the probability of having enuresis in the child is 45%;

If both parents were bed wetter's the probability increases to 77%.

On the other hand only 15% will be affected if neither parent had enuresis
- **Bedwetting goes away on its own in most children.**

Causes of Bedwetting

Although not all of the causes of bedwetting are fully understood, the following are some that are possible:
- Your child is a deep sleeper and does not awaken to the signal of a full bladder.
- Your child has not yet learned how to hold and empty urine well. (Communication between the brain and bladder may take time to develop.)
- Your child's body makes too much urine at night.
- Your child is constipated. Full bowels can put pressure on the bladder and lead to problems with holding and emptying urine well.
- Your child has a minor illness, is overly tired, or is responding to changes or stresses going on at home.
- There is a family history of bedwetting. Most children who wet the bed have at least one parent who had the same problem as a child.

- Your child's bladder is small or not developed enough to hold urine for a full night.
- Your child has an underlying medical problem.

WHEN ONE SHOULD TAKE CHILD TO DOCTOR?

- **Child is older than 5 years and still wets the bed:** If children reach school age and still have problems wetting the bed; it most likely means they have never developed nighttime bladder control.
- **Child was once dry at night and then began wetting the bed again:** A parent who had enuresis as a child may not be concerned about his or her six-year-old with enuresis. Parents of a four-year-old with enuresis may worry because their older child was dry at age three. If this happens to your child, simply go back to training pants at night and try again another time. The problem usually disappears as children get older
- **Bed wetting upsets your child or you:** For most children, enuresis is a problem when it interferes with their ability to socialize with friends.
- **Wets or soils his or her pants during the day:** If you are concerned about your child's bedwetting or your child expresses concern, talk with your child's doctor. You may be asked the following questions about your child's bedwetting:
- Is there a family history of bedwetting?
- How often and when does your child urinate during the day?
- Have there been any changes in your child's home life such as a new baby, divorce, or new house?
- Does your child drink carbonated beverages, caffeine, citrus juices, or a lot of water before bed?
- Is there anything unusual about how your child urinates or the way the urine looks?

Myths and Misconceptions

Myth: Wetting the bed is unusual

Reality: Up to 16% of five-year-old have yet to achieve nighttime dryness, and many school-age children suffer from the problem as well. Bedwetting in young children **is** *common*.

Myth: Wetting the bed is caused by laziness or a failure to pay attention to body signals.

Reality: Bedwetting occurs during sleep, and research suggests that kids who wet the bed are.

Physiologically different: They may be harder to awaken at night. These traits may have a genetic basis, which would explain why nocturnal enuresis seems to run in families.

Myth: Wetting the bed is sign of psychological maladjustment or antisocial tendencies.

33

Reality: It's true that bedwetting is sometimes associated with stress. But does a child's failure to awaken before urinating indicate that he is psychologically disturbed? **No.**

Myth: There's no point trying to cure bedwetting if a child is depressed or anxious. You must treat the psychological symptoms first.

Reality: Some kids who wet the bed are also distressed. But their psychological problems aren't necessarily preventing them from getting dry, and successful treatment of their bed wetting symptoms may improve their psychological problems.

Myth: Parents can ignore the problem. Kids will eventually grow out it.

Reality: Nocturnal enuresis is sometimes caused by medical conditions like constipation, urinary tract infections, obstructive sleep apnea, and diabetes. So if your child is wetting bed, it's wise to have him screened for underlying medical problems. This is particularly important if your child has suddenly become incontinent after going for at least 6 months without wetting the bed.

Signs of a Medical Problem

However, most medical problems that cause bedwetting to recur suddenly have other signs, including:

- Changes in how much and how often your child urinates during the day

- Pain, burning, or straining while urinating
- A very small or narrow stream of urine or dribbling that is constant or happens just after urination
- Cloudy or pink urine or bloodstains on underpants
- Daytime and nighttime wetting
- Sudden change in personality or mood
- Poor bowel control
- Urinating after stress (coughing, running, or lifting)
- Certain gait disturbances (problems with walking that may mean an underlying neurologic problem)
- Continuous dampness

If your child has any of these signs, your child's doctor may want to take a closer look at the kidneys or bladder. If necessary, your child's doctor will refer you to a pediatric urologist, a doctor who is specially trained to treat children's urinary problems.

Managing Bedwetting

Initial treatment of bedwetting includes education and motivational therapy. Behavioral alarms or medication may be tried if enuresis does not improve with these interventions.

Punishments, humiliation (the child is not doing it on purpose), teaching the child to "hold it till morning", keeping the child thirsty, diapers—they give the wrong message.

Keep the following tips in mind when dealing with bedwetting

- **Do not blame your child:** Remember that it is not your child's fault. children should not be punished for bed-wetting
- **Be honest with your child about what is going on:** Let your child know it's not his or her fault and that most children outgrow bedwetting.
- **Be sensitive to your child's feelings:** If you don't make a big issue out of bedwetting, chances are your child won't either. Also remind your child that other children wet the bed.
- **Protect the bed:** A plastic cover under the sheets protects the mattress from getting wet and smelling like urine.

- **Let your child help:** Encourage your child to help change the wet sheets and covers. This teaches responsibility. It can also keep your child from feeling embarrassed if the rest of the family knows. However, if your child sees this as punishment, it is not recommended.

- **Child drinks** most of his or her fluids in the morning and early afternoon to prevent overfilling of the bladder during the night. Before trying this, keep a diary of the amount of fluids your child drinks in a 24-hour period .Based on the total, you can create a schedule to spread fluids through the morning, afternoon, and evening. One recommendation is to offer 40 percent of fluids in the morning, 40 percent in the afternoon, and only 20 percent in the evening. For example, if a child generally consumes 32 ounces (approximately 1 liter) in 24 hours, the parent should offer 13 ounces (approximately 400 milliliters)—about 40 percent—in the morning, 13 ounces (approximately 400 milliliters) in the afternoon, and 6 ounces (approximately 200 milliliters)—about 20 percent—in the evening.

- **Encourage** the child to urinate regularly during the day and just before going to bed (a total of four to seven times). Also remind the child to empty his or her bladder immediately before bedtime.

- **Take steps before bedtime:** Have your child use the toilet and avoid drinking large amounts of fluid just before bedtime. Avoid sugary and caffeine-containing drinks, especially in the evening

- **Try to wake your child up to use the toilet** 55 min after going to sleep to help your child stay dry through the night. If the child wakes at night, take him/her to the toilet. Remind the child every night to get out of bed and use the toilet when she/he needs to urinate.

- **Help the child locate the toilet** easily by using night lights in the bathroom and hallway. Consider placing a portable potty seat in the child's room if the toilet is far from the child's bedroom

- **Protect the child's mattress** with a waterproof sheet to avoid urine odor

33

- **Stop using diapers**, training pants, or pull-up pants at home since these may prevent a child from wanting to get out of bed, especially if the child is older than eight years. They may be used for special occasions, such as overnight visits with family or friends
- **After wetting accidents during the night**, encourage the child to go to the bathroom before changing into dry pajamas. You can place a dry towel over the wet part of the bed, or you can make the bed in several layers, alternating a fitted sheet with a waterproof pad; this allows you and/or the child to quickly and easily remove the wet items and avoids the need to re-make the bed. Leave dry pajamas and towels out so that a child can find them easily.
- Ask the child to help with morning bed clean-up, including removing and washing bed sheets. Also ensure that the child showers or bathes daily to avoid urine odor on the skin.
- **Set a no-teasing rule in your family:** Do not let family members, especially siblings, tease your child? Let them know that it's not your child's fault
- **Be positive:** Reward your child for dry nights. Offer support, not punishment, for wet nights.

33

Motivational therapy: Motivational therapy involves keeping a record of progress, with bigger rewards for longer periods of dryness. You and the child should agree about the reward in advance and might progress from a sticker on a calendar for each dry night to a favorite book for seven consecutive dry nights.

Bedwetting alarms: If your child is still not able to stay dry during the night after using these steps for 1 to 3 months, a bedwetting alarm may be recommended. When a bedwetting alarm senses urine, it sets off an alarm so the child can wake up to use the toilet. When used correctly, it will detect wetness right away and sound the alarm. Be sure your child resets the alarm before going back to sleep.

Bedwetting alarms are successful 50% to 75% of the time. They tend to be most helpful for children who are deep sleepers and have some bladder control on their own. Ask your child's doctor which type of alarm would be best for your child.

Keep a diary of wet and dry nights. Give positive reinforcement for dry nights and for successful use of the alarm sequence

MEDICINES

Medicines are available to treat bedwetting for children 6 years and older. Though medicines rarely cure bedwetting, they may be helpful, especially when children begin attending sleepovers or overnight camps. Your child's doctor can tell you more about these medicines and if they are right for your child. Remember to ask about possible side effects.

Complementary and alternative therapies: Several complementary and alternative therapies have been tried in children with nocturnal enuresis, including acupuncture, chiropractic maneuvers, and hypnosis. However, there are not enough data from scientific studies to know if these therapies are effective. Complementary and alternative treatments are not currently recommended for children with bedwetting.

33

Points to remember

1. The child learns to consciously control and coordinate his or her bladder by four years of age. Nighttime bladder control usually takes longer and is not expected until a child is between five and seven years old.
2. Bedwetting goes away on its own in most children.
3. Parents should know causes of bedwetting and when to consult the doctor.
4. Parents should know myths and misconception about nocturnal enuresis.
5. Managing bedwetting requires motivational therapy, bedwetting alarm, star calendar and medicines.

Anxiety, Fears, Phobias and Panic Attacks

Anjan Bhattacharya

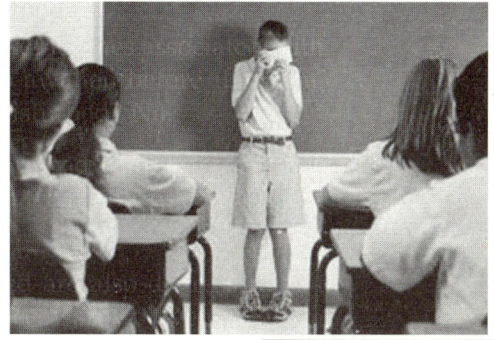

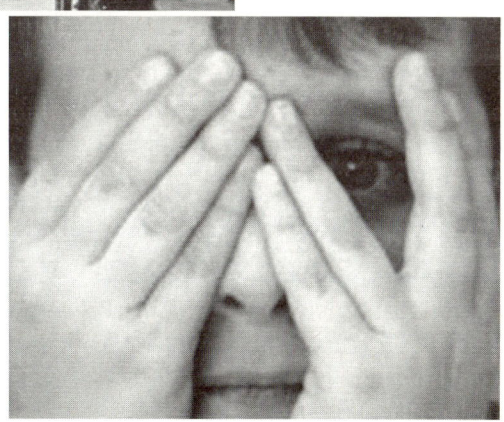

Every human being feels anxiety or fear at some stage in their life. It is understandably uncomfortable. But for children, such feelings are not only normal, they are also necessary. Facing these feelings help them prepare for greater challenges of adult life.

What is Normal?

Anxiety, by definition, is "apprehension without apparent cause." In reality, there is no clear and present danger, but the imaginary mood feels real enough.

Anxiety provokes "fight or flight" reaction instantly. The pulse speeds up, beads of sweat start showing, and "butterflies" in the stomach soon follow. But, a little bit of anxiety can actually help people remain alert and focused.

Having fears or anxieties about certain things survival benefits as it makes children behave in a safe way. For example, a child with a fear of injection would avoid playing with needles.

34 But the nature of anxieties and fears change through phases of development:

- In babies stranger anxiety is manifested predominantly, that is why they go through their 'clingy phase' of holding on to their parents and familiar adults.
- For toddlers the predominant expression is separation anxiety. They become emotionally distressed if either parents leave. This phase is typically between 9–18 months of age
- Four to six year olds show anxiety about things that are not present, such as fears of monsters and ghosts.
- Older children aged 7 to 12 often experiences fears that mimic real life situations like war or natural disaster.

When children grow, one fear may disappear or replace another. For example, a child who could not come near uncle's pet dog at age of 5 becomes an animal lover, some years later. Similarly, some fears may extend only to one particular kind of stimulus, for example, a child may want to become a soldier in later life but currently cannot brave the doctor's chamber!

Features of Anxiety

Anxiety and fear in children change with age. Usually encountered are fear of strangers, heights, darkness, animals, blood, insects, and being left alone. Children often learn to be afraid of a specific object or situation after having an unpleasant experience, such as a finger burnt or trapped in the door.

Separation anxiety is common during life's transitions, e.g. when young children are starting school, admitted to hostel or later during puberty.

If anxieties persist, the child's sense of wellbeing may be jeopardised. The anxiety associated with social avoidance can have long-term consequences e.g. a child with fear of rejection can fail to learn important social skills, leading to disabling social isolation.

Adults are often tortured by fears that originate from their childhood experiences. A common example is an adult's fear of public speaking originating as a result of embarrassment in peer group many years before. That is why parents and adults have such great responsibility to identify the early features so that appropriate low level input can avoid development of pathological states life phobia or panic attacks in later life. Early detection can lead to early intervention with its consequent benefits, if we know these early signs well, at the community level.

34

Some of such symptoms are as follows:

- becoming too clingy, impulsive, or distracted
- nervous movements, such as temporary twitches, rapid eye blinking
- sleeping problems
  - i. getting to sleep (poor sleep induction)
  - ii. staying asleep longer than usual (poor sleep duration)
  - iii. falling asleep at day time (daytime somnolence)
  - iv. Disturbed sleep (poor sleep architecture)
  - v. Often wakes up in sleep (fragmented sleep maintenance phase)
- Sweaty hands, palm, brow, body, armpits, etc.
- accelerated heart rate and breathing
- nausea, occasional retching, e.g. seeing food or before going to school
- headaches; stomach aches, leg pains, "growing pains" (aches and pains)
- deep sighing breathing (in full consciousness)

Please note that the above signs can also be features of other clinical states, e.g. ensure that the deep sighing breathing is not a missed "Kussmaul's breathing" of diabetic ketoacidosis or daytime somnolence of obstructive sleep apnea, and therefore, need to be ruled out with due diligence!

One other very important lessons of Pediatric practice is that, parents can usually tell when their child is feeling excessively uneasy about something. Doctors, especially Pediatricians have an overarching duty to sympathetically listen to the concerns raised by parents. In Pediatric practice, it is also an essential skill to be able to talk to the child according to their developmentally age-appropriate way. More often than not, a sympathetic listening can help a child get over his/her anxiety or fear and move on with his/her life.

34

What is a Phobia? Why Children get Panic Attacks?

It is the unusual persistence of anxieties and fears that lead to problems. Contrary to a parent's hope that the child will outgrow it, sometimes the opposite happens and the cause of the anxiety, when not alleviated, becomes more prevalent.

The anxiety or the fear becomes a phobia, or a fear that is extreme, severe, out of proportion and persistent.

Panic disorder is a common and treatable disorder. Children and adolescents with panic disorder have unexpected and repeated periods of intense fear or discomfort, along with other symptoms such as a racing heartbeat or feeling short of breath. These periods are called "panic attacks" and last minutes to hours. Panic attacks frequently develop without warning.

Symptoms of a panic attack include
- Intense fearfulness (a sense that something terrible is happening)
- Racing or pounding heartbeat
- Dizziness or light-headedness
- Shortness of breath or a feeling of being smothered
- Trembling or shaking
- Sense of unreality
- Fear of dying, losing control, or losing your mind

A phobia or panic attack can be very difficult to tolerate, for the child as well as those around them, especially if the anxiety-producing stimulus (anxiety trigger) is hard to avoid (*e.g.* lizzards). Parents and the child may be helpless in this situation without professional help.

It is however; important to emphasize that, unless an anxiety, fear or even phobia is hindering day to day functioning of a child, referral to a professional may not be warranted. Local management of subclinical and subthreshhold by family, teachers and early start professionals at the community level may suffice.

It may therefore, be helpful here to have some general guideline about when to escalade:

34

Parenting Guidelines on Anxieties, Fears, Phobias and Panic Attacks

Honest answer to the following questions may hold the key for early detection:

Is your child's fear and behavior related to it typical for your child's age? If the answer to this question is yes, it is a good bet that your child's fears will resolve before they become a serious cause for concern. This is not to say that the anxiety should be discounted or ignored; rather, it should be considered as a factor in your child's normal development.

Many children experience age-appropriate fears, such as being afraid of the dark. Most, with some reassurance and perhaps a night-light, will overcome or outgrow it. However, if they continue to have trouble or there is anxiety about other things, the intervention may have to be more intensive.

What are the symptoms of the fear, and how do they affect your child's personal, social, and academic functioning? If symptoms can be identified and considered in light of your child's everyday activities, adjustments can be made to alleviate some of the stress factors.

Does the fear seem unreasonable in relation to the reality of the situation; and could it be a sign of a more serious problem? If your child's fear seems out of proportion to the cause of the stress, this may signal the need to seek outside help, such as a

Pediatrician, child and adolescent Psychiatrist or a Developmental Pediatrician.

Is there a family history? These can run in the families. Therefore, genetic links are discovered. Neurobiological associations are understood with increased association with such conditions with other diagnoses like hypochondriasis or psoriasis, etc.

Parents should look for patterns. If an isolated incident is resolved, making it more significant than it is would be harmful. But if a pattern emerges that is persistent or pervasive, parents should take action. If they do not, the phobia is likely to continue to affect their child.

Parents ought to contact their doctor and/or a mental health professional who has expertise in working with children and adolescents. Remember, honest answers to the above questions are needed. In the Indian context, barriers to such honesty may be:

- current level of parental understanding,
- denials,
- fears,
- prejudices,
- cultural beliefs,
- habits of "normalization", etc.

Helping the Child

Parents, family members, teachers and health professionals can help children develop the skills and confidence to overcome fears so that they do not evolve into phobic or panic reactions.

To help the child deal with fears and anxieties:

- Recognize that the fear is real. As trivial as a fear may seem, it feels real to your child and it is causing him or her to feel anxious and afraid.
- Being able to talk about fears helps—words often take some of the power out of the negative feeling. If you talk about it, it can become less powerful.
- Never belittle the fear as a way of forcing your child to overcome it. Saying, "Don't be ridiculous! There are no

34

monsters in your closet!" may get your child to go to bed, but it will not make the fear go away.

- Do not cater to fears. If your child does not like dogs, please do not cross the street deliberately to avoid one. This will just reinforce that dogs should be feared and avoided. Provide support and gentle care as you approach the feared object or situation with your child.

- Teach kids how to rate fear. A child who can visualize the intensity of the fear on a scale of 1 to 10, with 10 being the strongest, may be able to "see" the fear as less intense than first imagined. Younger kids can think about how "full of fear" they are, with being full "up to my knees" as not so scared, "up to my stomach" as more frightened, and "up to my head" as truly petrified.

34

- Teach coping strategies. Try these easy-to-implement techniques. Using you as "home base," the child can venture out toward the feared object and then can return to you for safety before venturing out again. Please do not expect him/her to succeed fully, the first time around.

- The child can also learn some positive self-statements, such as "I can do this" and "I will be okay" to say to himself or herself when feeling anxious.

- Relaxation techniques are helpful, including visualization (of floating on a cloud or lying on a beach, for example) and deep breathing (imagining that the lungs are balloons and letting them slowly deflate).

The key to resolving fears and anxieties is to overcome them. Using these suggestions, you can help your child better cope with life's situations.

RECENT ADVANCES

A. Classification

Consistent with the previous version of the Diagnostic and Statistical Manual of Mental Disorders (DSM-IV), DSM-5 includes the fol lowing anxiety disorders:

　i. Specific phobia, e.g. arachnophobia (fear of creepy crawlies/insects)

ii. Generalized anxiety disorder (e.g. anxiety in common life situations)

iii. Social anxiety disorder (formerly social phobia)

iv. Panic disorder (e.g. claustrophobic panic reactions)

v. Agoraphobia (i.e. the irrational fear of open spaces)

Key Changes in DSM–5 include

i. Agoraphobia has been classified as a stand-alone diagnosis (i.e. no longer linked to the presence or absence of panic disorder)

ii. Separation anxiety disorder and selective mutism have been re-classified as anxiety disorders (rather than in a section for 'disorders usually first diagnosed in infancy, childhood or adolescence') and

iii. Obsessive compulsive disorder (OCD), post-traumatic stress disorder (PTSD) and acute stress disorder are, respectively, grouped under OCD and related disorders and trauma-related and stressor-related disorders (i.e. no longer included within the anxiety disorder category).

34

While core features of each anxiety disorder are broadly considered with DSM-IV, in order to minimize the over-diagnosis of transient features of Agoraphobia, specific phobia and social anxiety disorder, those under the age of 18 are now required to have had symptoms for *at least* six months.

B. Assessment

Young people with anxiety disorders are unlikely to present for help independently with parents commonly raising their concerns to general practitioners. In the dearth of standardized screening tools for children and young people and in view of very good assessment tools, the National Institute of Clinical Excellence (NICE), UK highlights the need for a comprehensive assessment by an appropriate healthcare professional.

Since there is a high level of comorbidity in children and young people with anxiety disorders, it is **essential** to assess for possible co-existing neurodevelopmental problems, substance misuse, social and mental health matters and speech and language problems rather comprehensively in competent hands.

C. Management

The most commonly evaluated treatments for anxiety disorders in children and adolescents are Cognitive Behavioral Therapy (CBT). Kendall's 'Coping Cat' is modelled in many CBT based programs. Recent Advances focused heavily on Low Intensity Interventional models of CBT in anxiety disorders in under 18s.

Two such approaches that are subjected to systematic evaluation are:

  i. Bibliotherapy: Brief treatments in which parents are guided to work through a book that instructs them on how to help their child overcome their difficulties with anxiety, and

  ii. E-therapies: Treatment delivered via computerized platforms.

34

Where bibliotherapy or E-therapy proves to be subnormal, the need for full use of CBT, medication and other multidisciplinary input cannot be overemphasized.

Future Directions

There is now irrefutable evidence that with early detection and competent early intervention, even with low intensity but standardized input, children and young people with anxiety disorders show favourable outcomes. Little is known however, about why sometimes treatment is ineffective!

Recently, several independent predictors of treatment outcomes from CBT have been identified: gender, primary anxiety severity, comorbid mood and externalizing disorders and the genetic factors 5HTTLPR, NGF rs6330. The clinical utility of these predictors remain to be determined.

Use of anxiety management in autism spectrum disorder along with current available treatments like the applied behavior analysis (ABA) found significant anxiety reduction with improved final outcome with the standardized available tools. These studies are encouraging in demonstrating that, with appropriate adaptation, existing treatments can be effectively applied to broader population that those typically included in these recent treatment trials.

SUMMARY AND CONCLUSIONS

- Anxiety and fear are normal experiences for children and young people
- These feelings have evolutionary advantages to prepare a child for adult life
- If these persists for a prolonged period, especially when of irrational proportion, they fall under pathological group
- Pathological group also includes Phobias and Panic reactions
- All these pathological states need to be addressed in children
- Unless these pathological states interfere with healthy living, these can be effectively managed locally
- If local management proves ineffectual over a period of six months, prompt escalation is warranted
- With the advent of modern low-intensity intervention, primary, secondary and tertiary care pathways can be followed
- Professional management of anxiety, fear, phobias and panic attacks must be managed by professionals competent in it
- Comorbidities are norm and must be managed together efficiently

34

Points to remember

1. Anxiety and Fear are normal experience for children and young people.
2. Phobia's which are in irrational proportions needs prompt investigations and management.
3. Relaxation techniques and deep breathing exercises are helpful.
4. Auto-suggestive positive statements can alleviate anxiety.

FURTHER READING

1. Nelsons Textbook of Pediatrics, 19th Edition
2. Kids Health: Reviewed by: D'Arcy Lyness, PhD. Date reviewed: October 2010
3. Creswell C, Waite P, Cooper PJ. Assessment and Management of Anxiety Disorders in Children and Adolescents. *Arc. Dis. Child* 2014;**99**:674-678
4. NICE. Social anxiety disorder: recognition, assessment and treatment (CG159). http://www.nice.org.uk/CG159: [NICE guideline]; 2013
5. American Psychiatric Association. *Diagnostic and statistical manual of mental disorders*. 5thedn.Arlington, VA. American Psychiatric Publishing, 2013

34

35

School Refusal or Avoidance

Suchit Tamboli, Zafar Meenai

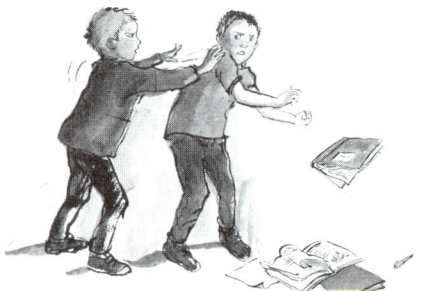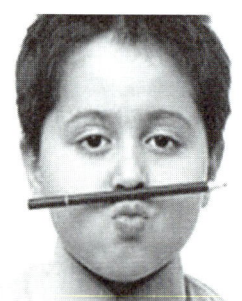

School refusal or avoidance is an extreme reluctance to attend school for a sustained period of time school is a theatre in which many developmental and behavioral issues are on **stages** students judgment about themselves are moulded by constant feedback from peers and teachers, giving them clear input regarding their personal assets and short comings in the social, emotional and academic domains mal-adaptation to school can occur as a result of broad range of negative influences. In many children mal-adaptation leads to school disinterest, disengagement and subsequent school attendance problems school absence or refusal is found to be associated with psychiatric disorders especially conduct disorder or depression.

SOURCES THAT LEAD TO MAL-ADAPTION OF SCHOOL

1. Psychotic and emotional disturbance: Either generalized anxiety or separations are associated with conduct disorder.

A behavioral history looking at causes and timing of anxiety as well as signs and symptoms of depression helps identify these difficulties. Careful family and social history is also very important.

2. **Temperament:** Many children have temperaments that make the school experience difficult and frustrating. An affected child feels that his or her success in school is determined solely by external forces, which can after lead to reactive depression and anxiety disturbances.

3. **Social imbalances:** Rejection by their peers perceived conflict and lack of personal support in friendships is associated with multiple forms of school mal-adaptation including loneliness and avoidance. During family interview specific question about student's friendships and activities help to identify problems.

4. **Neurodevelopmental dysfunctions:** Learning disorders, attention or motor deficits can make school experiences un pleasurable . Specific tests need to apply for identification.

5. **Social cultural influences:** Many children do not have academic role models at home or in community. They may have difficulty in identifying with education as it relates to providing opportunities for a more productive and stable future.

6. **Family/Environmental stresses:** A child may feel guilty for going to school in the morning, anxious and fearful of going home at the end of the day. We must rule out possibility of Neglect/Abuse. In some cases family therapy, marital counseling is necessary.

7. **Chronic diseases and physical challenges:** Diseases like leukemia, rheumatic can lead to absenteeism.

Management of School Refusal

The goal of management of school refusal is prevention of further disengagement, which can lead to school dropout.

- **Behavioral intervention:** For disruptive students behavioral contract between teachers, parents and students can be effective. Positive reinforcement and consistency are essential for success. Children who are too disruptive to other students

35

35

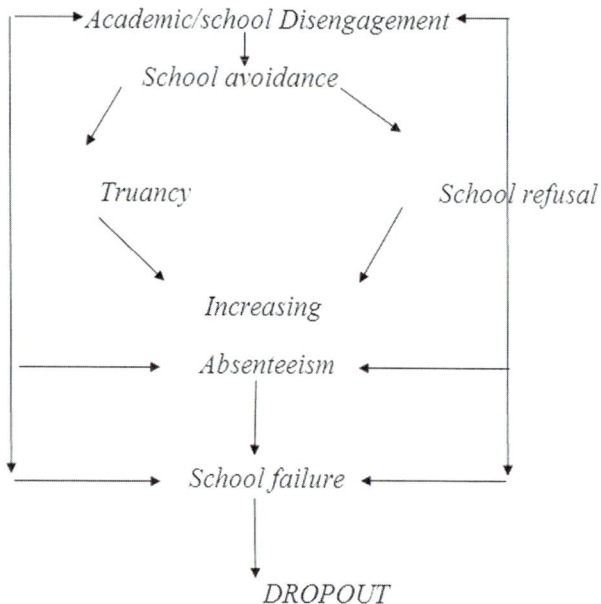

often must be placed in special classroom with more structure background. If impulsivity is the cause of behavior, trial of stimulant mediation is appropriate.

- **Developing strengths:** Children with learning problems can suffer with self esteem problem. They are disengaged from school. They should be developed in their area of interest and to improve their confidence.

- **Neurodevelopment intervention:** Special education focused on skill development and bypass strategies is important once the breakdowns in learning are indentified. Language, occupational and physiotherapy may be indicated.

- **Counseling:** Childs emotional difficulties and behavior should be focused in counseling as well as follow-up is necessary to observe the positive changes in behavior.

- **Social skills training:** Because of lack of social skills. Children are withdrawn. Some schools have social skills groups.

Children with low IQ/below average IQ and should be educated separately according to their needs. Special tutors giving special guidelines are helpful. Children with learning disability should be educated knowing the progress in each area/subject. They may complete the syllabus of different standards at the same time.

Children with school phobia should be assessed for diagnosing the type of phobia. It may be of teachers, failure in subject, bullying, being teased by classmates.

Discussing with parent and teachers and giving assurance is important.

Many children have mental health problems such as depression and conduct disorder which may suppress the school activity. Finding out the causes of depression it may be familial educational or genetic and treating with medicine may be necessary.

35

Other health problem may be anemia and fatigue after illness, abdominal complaints, frequent urination and frequent passing the stools may cause school refusal. Myopia or difficulty in hearing may cause disturbances in learning. Frequent attacks of asthma which are aggravated by exam stress should be identified and treated.

Points to remember

1. School refusal or avoidance is an extreme reluctance to attend school for a sustained period of time.
2. The sources that cause mal-adaptation of school are generalised or separation anxiety, temperamental personality traits, peer problems, learning disorders, attention or motor deficits, as well as family/environmental stresses.
3. Behavioral modification intervention, positive reinforcement and consistency are essential for success.
4. Remedial teaching, special education, speech, occupational and physiotherapy may be indicated.

Scholastic Problems in My Child

Samir Dalwai, Sandhya Kulkarni

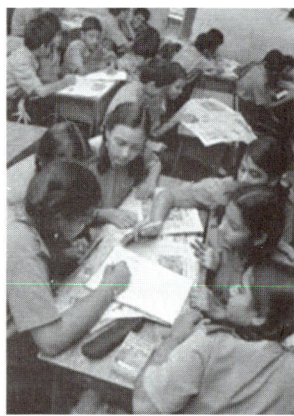
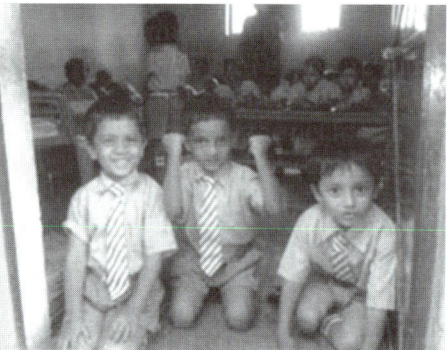

The word 'school' evokes such happy feelings and fond memories—little wonder that it leads to a smile on the face of every person—young or old—at any time of our life! Any phase of our childhood somehow is always connected to school, teachers, friends, pranks, laughter, and a lot of mischief!

Parents practically relive their childhood during their children' primary school years. A family that consulted us had made a decision to shift their children to a better school; one which had a big playground and laid a lot of emphasis on outdoor activities. The parents had spoken to the children about this and they were quite aware of the change. They were also eager and excited to go to a new school.

Initial days were full of excitement as they seemed to like the new place a lot! They seemed to gel well with the new classroom, friends, teachers and the environment! The parents heaved a sigh of relief and got involved with their busy schedules. The mother was however not very sure about the daughter Sera, who had become very quiet as days passed and would narrate in the evening some incident that had happened in the class and disturbed her.

Soon enough, her day began with—'Can I not go to school only for today? I promise that I will definitely go tomorrow. I have a headache, tummy ache, aches in my legs, feel like vomiting", basically a lot of vague complaints. Initially, the mother gave in but later there was no end to the excuses. Something was amiss as such behaviour had never occurred earlier. The parents went to the school and spoke with her class teacher. She literally opened a Pandora's Box and mentioned so many more observations about Sera.

36

According to her, Sera had become very lonely in the class, never spoke to or mixed with anyone and mostly kept to herself. She did not copy anything from the board.

Due to this interactive response from the school teacher, the parents became aware of Sera's concerns. With further help from the school counsellor and the class teacher, they could handle this situation much better and slowly Sera started getting back to her old self.

Sometimes, a seemingly insignificant factor, like a change in the residence or in the school, may influence the child adversely because children are tuned into their specific environment and may resist change. If the child does not like his/her class teacher for any reason ("she seems too strict" or, she may have severely punished your child sometime for some reason in the past), the child demonstrates rebellion by refusing to focus on studies.

Scholastic problems may also present through **behavior** such as inattention, lack of interest in studies, physical complaints particularly in the school hours or absolute reluctance and refusal to attend the school. As with Sera, the child may complain of a stomachache or headache in the mornings and refuse to go to school.

Scholastic problems may also be of the nature where child is unable to exhibit his skills in reading, writing or math, but may be well versed conceptually and can answer well orally. This could be a sign of a **learning disability**.

On the other hand, there could be concerns such as inability to grasp content, poor retention of studied matter and a general underdeveloped conceptual understanding. This could reflect some level of **intellectual sub normality**.

Other concerns such as **hyperactivity, inattention and easy distractibility** could also affect academic performance.

Children can never express with ease what is going on within their mind. In a large number of cases, a school going child undergoing emotional trauma is picked up only when she fails in the examination. That acts as a warning sign for the child's parent or caregiver to look into the matter and do something about it before the problem gets out of hand and the studies begin to get negatively affected. Hence, the focus must always be the child first and after that, the academic performance.

Parents need to understand that often the child is reprimanded and even threatened to study without exact awareness or the severity of their concerns, which torments the child from within. **Academic performance merely acts as a symptom.** Treating the symptom is not possible without handling the underlying problem. Slowly but surely, the problem resurfaces, with symptoms that get worse each time. It is necessary for parents as well as teachers to pick up their cues; it is imperative that those in contact with the child always notice their cry and rush for their help to prevent matters from getting out of hand.

Academic difficulties may be a reflection of an underlying cognitive/neuropsychological/emotional or behavioral problem, which negatively influences the child's development. Thus, many reasons may coexist contributing to the poor performance of a school-going child. The solution is two fold:

- to alleviate the primary cause wherever possible and
- To work on the academic functioning through scientific intervention programs.

For parents, it may be difficult to always identify the root cause. They would only see the outcome and try to deal with "the outcome" (and not the cause) insensitively at times. In such a scenario, it is necessary to seek professional support to identify the cause and use remedial measures to solve the problem before it gets too late. The school lays the foundation of a child's intellectual, social and emotional domain. Timely help provided when they subtly ask for it is the duty of parents. This will assist to fulfil their academic and socio-emotional development in school.

Points to remember

36

1. Change in residence or school can adversely affect behaviour and aversion for the school and academics.
2. Learning disability could be the reason why your child is not performing well despite good intelligence.
3. Hyperactivity, in attention and easy distractibility could also affect academic performance.
4. General underdeveloped conceptual understanding or intellectual sub normality could be reason for scholastic under achievement.
5. Alleviate the primary cause.
6. Remedial teaching, individualised education program and behavioural modification therapy helps child perform well in schools.

37

Electronic Media and Children Behavior

Suchit Tamboli

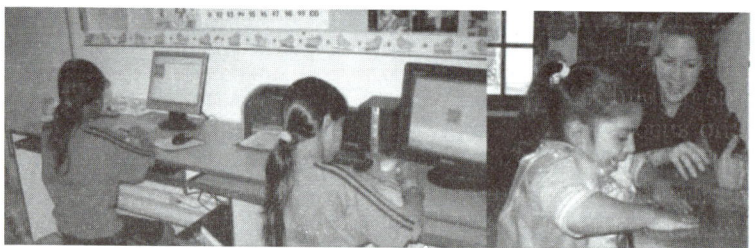

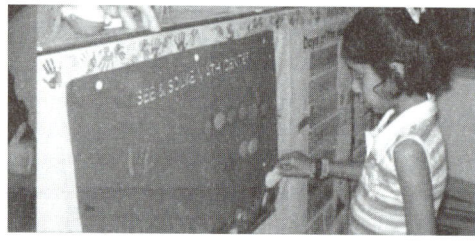
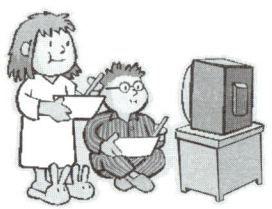

INTRODUCTION

We are all the product of mass media culture. We live in a sea of mediated communication. Less in global village than a vast bazaar of messages, we are more in contact with the thoughts and intentions of others than at any other time in history.

The world of electronic media is changing dramatically. Television dominated the media world through 1990–2000, now competes in an arena crowded with cell phones, I pods, video games, instant messaging, interactive multiplayer video games, virtual reality sites, web social networks and email. In India 30 crores people directly use media. More than 17,000 crores rupees are collected through advertisements. There are 2130 dailies and more than 100 channels. In 1980 first serial with Hum log, Rajani had been started and now multiple options like fear factor, big boss, voice of India, etc. are available.

The vast majority of children have access to multiple media. A teen can watch a television show on a computer long after its aired on. They have almost constant access to media often at times and in places where adult supervision is absent.

A typical child watches 15,000 to 18,000 hours of television by age of 18 years compared with attending 12,000 hours of school. They spend more time using media than do engaging in any single activity other than sleeping. Television viewing has become the Indian drug of choice.

37

MEDIA HISTORY

Taking media history should be important part of history taking by pediatrician. It should include how many hours to which media and under what conditions, content of program, selection criterion, and supervision by adult, v chip, other leisure time activities, inference discussion, and nutritional history. The most important is supervision by parents and content. Media is used as a third parent or servant is very important as both parents are working mother in kitchen and father in reading or out for his work and he is having remote in his hand and does not know to select the programs and watch movies or cartoons. Hence, the remote control is in which hand is very important.

Our own survey of 1263 students from different socio-economic class and different educational background of parents shows: 79% of parents and children perceived TV as a media for entertainment while 84% children and parents watch TV for 2 hours. Remote control of TV is family discussion (49%) and father (34%). Rule for viewing TV is after studies by 45% of the parents. 78% of parents and 85% of children did not watch TV after 10 pm. Parents blamed TV (51%) for the behavioral problems important being stubborn (21%) sleep 20% and imitating stars 16%. The programs blamed for behavioral problems are movie 29%; Horror shows 20%, and songs 20%. 50% parents have more than two cell phones in their house.

Sending sms or email jokes contribute 36% while creative messages 41%. Majority children take breakfast in front of TV (45%) while 22% eats fast food and potato chips. Favorite media of the parents (40%) is TV and internet was preferred media of Children (35%). The best alternatives for electronic media are sports 31%, parental interaction and story book 20 %.

We also noted difference in English and Marathi medium students' attitude. Perception of television as entertainment is more with English than Marathi medium. Habit of taking meal is independent of medium. In English medium as age advances instead of sports serial and movies were preferred. In both medium duration of child watching TV is same as parents hence parents must be careful about that. As an alternative to media English medium students preferred sports while Marathi medium students preferred parental interaction.

The conclusion of studies shows that the electronic media has great effect on children's behavior.

Trends in media use: It is important to distinguish between media use and media exposure. Media use Refers to the amount of time young people devote to all media.

Media exposure: Refers to media content encountered by young people expressed in units of time that is hours of TV exposure.

Total media exposure, media multitasking has been increased but total use remained relatively constant and there is little evidence that any medium especially television is being displaced. Children's simultaneous use of different media or media multitasking is very common. Television in a background child uses computer or cell phone for instant messages. Computer is "Media multi-tasking station". Cell phones can be a television and internet portal and radio all in one. Both opportunity and environment plays an important role in concurrent media use. Girls report more concurrent media exposure than boys.

Neurodevelopment and learning: There is growing literature about impact of electronic media exposure on attention, memory, executive functions, language and communications, visual-spatial processing, reasoning and social and emotional functioning. Impact depends on age and content of the media. The impact of television on visual processing and language appears to be neutral.

Media technology can be used effectively as a teaching tool in school but the results depend on how teachers use the technology and their own comfort level with the media. Unlike the phonologic code of written language visual mass media do not require training in a formal notational system. Children with learning disability watch more television then peers, have more difficulty in distinguishing fiction from reality and have difficulty with drawing inferences and narrative continuity.

Transfer of learning from TV is possible if

37

1. Must understand content
2. Must create an abstract
3. Must remember the content and see its relation to new problem
4. Must apply the remember content to the new problem.

Addiction of Television

It can be identified as follows

1. Using TV as a sedative
2. Indiscriminate viewing
3. Loss of control while viewing
4. Feeling angry with one self for watching too much
5. In ability to stop watching.
6. Feeling miserable when kept away from watching.

Age Related Media

Children learn through observation .Infants and toddlers needs direct experience and more interaction with real people to develop cognitively hence they do not learn by electronic media. By the age of 3 years electronic media with educational content that uses repeating an idea presenting images and sounds that capture attention. 5 yrs children learn more words than 3 yrs children from media.

Background TV interferes with toddler's ability to focus on play they do not begin to discriminate between TV and real life events until preschool years. Socio demographic factors like income, education may not affect children's viewing until late in childhood.

Children's ability to attend to television increases until about 9 years, when is reaches about 70 % of viewing time, attention to television appears to be closely related to the child's understanding of the content. **Content if designed correctly can enhance learning.**

Teenagars spend their lives immersed in electronic media. While doing homework on internet they do instant messaging to their friends and television on background or they are listening to music on ipod.

Media and Behavior

Electronic media can positively influence social behavior, knowledge and understanding. It can be accused of increasing aggression and having negative effects on learning. It is endless source advertising, portrayals of violence and opportunities for dangerous encounters with strangers and possible exposures to pornography.

Family TV diary, maternal employment, education, older sibling in the family influence educational programs. Heavy media use becomes recognized as a possible symptom of personal maladjustment.

Attention, Cognition and School Achievement

More is not necessarily better. An academic achievement of children peaks at 1–2 hours of educational programming and declines with heavier use (more than 4 hours). There is significant negative link between grades media exposure. Playing video games can have positive effects in developing visual spatial skills such as visual tracking, mental rotation and target localization. Gaming may also improve problem solving skills. There is inconsistent evidence of link between heavy electronic media use and ADHD. High doses of entertainment before 3 years of age give rise to attention problems 5 years later. The children learn the things we teach them.

37

Children cannot learn from educational messages to which they do not pay attention. For maximizing attention to program cuts between shots, camera, sound effects child's voice etc. are the technique used by producer. It also depends on comprehension, repetition, viewer characteristics and transfer of learning.

Edutainment seek to instruct its audience by embedding lessons in some familiar form of entertainment like TV programs, computer and video games, films, music, website, multimedia, etc. Objective can be in one of following domains physical, cognitive, emotional, social skills, esthetic, moral etc. parents to talk "early and often" to preadolescent and adolescent children.

37

Sleep

The presence of a television set in the child's bedroom may be a relatively under recognized, but important, contributor to sleep problems in school children. Why parents have bedroom TV for children because it frees them up, they can watch own shows, it keeps children occupied but such watching becomes an isolated experience and that is harmful for developmental at risk for sleep disorders. The children having television set in bedroom watches one hour more than average. Bedroom television is linked to number of poor outcomes including academic, social and physical activity. Teenagers' use of Cell phones after bedtime contributes to poor sleep. The American Academy of Sleep Medicine (AASM), Experts recommend that adolescents should get about 8–9 hours of sleep each night for good health and optimum performance.

Media and Emotional Development

Screen media plays crucial role in children's emotional development. They learn ability to recognize emotions in others feel empathy or share emotions with others.

Aggression, Fear, Violence

Content of some entertainment and news can instill fear and anxiety in children. Children between ages 3–8 years are frightened by fantasy characters. Older children are affected by realistic scenes of injury of violence.

Media violence exposure has a larger effect on later violent behavior than does substance use, abusive parents, poverty, living in a broken home or having low IQ. Media have a powerful influence on health and behavior. Girls experience more fear from media than boys as they get older.

Media violence is a risk factor for aggressive behavior but is not related to crime.

Risky Behavior and Sexual Problems

37 Society's traditional adolescent issues intimacy, sexuality and identity have all been transformed by electronic media. Transformations is also due to greater teen autonomy, decrease face communication, increase peer group relations in expense of family relations and greater teen choice. Five critical types of adolescent health risk behavior identified, obesity, smoking, drinking, sexual risk taking and violence.

Exposure to sexual content in music, movies, television, and magazines accelerates adolescents' sexual activity and increases their risk of engaging in early sexual intercourse. The media should be encouraged to provide more sexually healthy content, and youth service providers and physicians should be aware that earlier maturing girls may be interested in sexual information.

Willingness model for risky behavior as to pathways one that is reasoned and the other is spontaneous and opportunistic. Reaction to favorable social circumstances rather than planned are seen.

Nutrition and Obesity

Television consumption has clear relationship to obesity. A couch Potato by definition expands very little energy .Even doing nothing uses up more calories than watching television. The second mechanism that links is the change in eating habits. The role model actors endorsing high calorie products cannot be under estimated. An increased consumption of sweets, salted snacks and artificially sweetened drinks, bhajias and chiwadas and less in take of vegetables and fruits. Obesity is also related with amount of time spent in front of television and eating meals in front of television.

Eating right and being healthy is as easy as **5-4-3-2-1 go**

5. Or more fruits and vegetables

4. Servings of water

3. Servings of low fat dairy

2. Spend no more than 2 hours per days on watching TV or similar activity

1. At least one hour of physical activity a day.

Social Marketing and Campaign

37

Campaigns to present and control tobacco use, increase physical activity, improve nutrition and promote condom use are example of successful social marketing.

Social marketing has also been used to promote better parent–child communication and improved family health. It can provide children and adolescent with reason and opportunities to engage and in healthful alternatives by demonstrating behavioral alternatives that tap into their wants and needs.

Social marketing's 5 new strategies

1. improved audience segmentation (use research data) to identity behavioral predictors

2. to develop tailored messages for specific groups

3. co branding

4. to make full use of technology

5. social networking

Child as a Consumer

Advertising and product placement for cigarettes and alcohol as well as exposure to movie character smoking and drinking has increased under age drinking and initiation of smoking.

4Ps of Marketing

Product, Place, Price and Promotions. They use public presentations to influence consumer's attention. Stealth advertising in which marketers attempt to conceal the internet of advertisement for effective marketing repetition, attention, getting product features, branded characters and premiums, product placement, viral marketing, recognition and retention, product request and purchase are the technique used.

Negative outcome of advertisement—parent–child conflict, cynicism, obesity and materialistic attitudes. To reduce children request using power assertion (restrictive mediations) and reasoning (active mediation), no information (co viewing) is necessary.

37 Media Policy, Role of Media Literacy

Children spend with media, parents and policy makers needs to focus on what is being offered to children on the various media platforms. Rating of programs for all media, regulation of advertisements is necessary. The programs should be more pro social. Media policy should contribute to positive role in developing in child's life.

Media literacy training involves school based efforts to teach children to understand media conventions, such as advertisement technique. (1) Transition between advertisement and program content must be distinct, (2) hot selling is not allowed, (3) product being sold cannot be integrated into program content.

Marketing practices such as repetition, branded environment and free prizes are effective in attracting children attention.

AAP Recommendation

1. Be alert to the shows your children see.

2. Avoid using television, videos, or video games as a baby-sitter. Simply turning the sets off is not nearly as effective as planning some other fun activity with the family.

3. Limit the use of media. Television use must be limited to no more than 1 or 2 quality hours per day. Set situation limits too: no television or video games before school, during daytime hours, during meals, or before homework is done.

4. Keep television and video player machines out of your children's bedrooms.

5. Turn the television off during mealtimes.

6. Turn television on only when there is something specific you have decided is worth watching. Don't turn the TV on "to see if there's something on."

7. Don't make the TV the focal point of the house.

8. Be active: talk and make connections with your children while the program is on.

9. Be especially careful of viewing just before bedtime. Emotion-invoking images may linger and intrude into sleep.

10. Be explicit with children about your guidelines for appropriate movie viewing and review proposed movie choices in advances.

11. Become "Media literate."

12. Limit your own television viewing. Set a good example. Be careful when children are around and may observe material from "your" program.

13. Let your voice be heard to insist on better programming for our children.

37

Points to remember

1. Children spend more time using media than do engaging in any single activity other than sleeping.

2. Taking media history and identify the addiction should be important part of history taking by pediatrician.

3. Children's simultaneous use of different media or media multitasking is very common. Computer and cell phone is "Media multi tasking station".

4. Television use must be limited to no more than 1 or 2 quality hours per day. The most important is supervision by parents and content. The medium is the message. Content matters.

5. Media technology can be used effectively as a teaching tool in school. Playing video games can have positive effects in developing visual spatial skills.

6. Avoid using television, videos, or video games as a baby-sitter, use it as a third parent.

7. Media violence is a risk factor for aggressive behavior but is not related to crime.

8. Media use: its cool but don't let it rule (your life)

9. Television consumption has clear relationship to obesity.

10. To control tobacco use, increase physical activity, improve nutrition and promote condom use are examples of successful social marketing.

11. Media policy should contribute to positive role in developing in child's life.

12. Work ahead is to discover what is beneficial, for whom it is beneficial, and when it is beneficial.

37

Section

6

Special Child

Special Needs Child—
Help Me Doctor

Samir Dalwai, Santosh Nimbalkar, Deepti Kanade-Modak

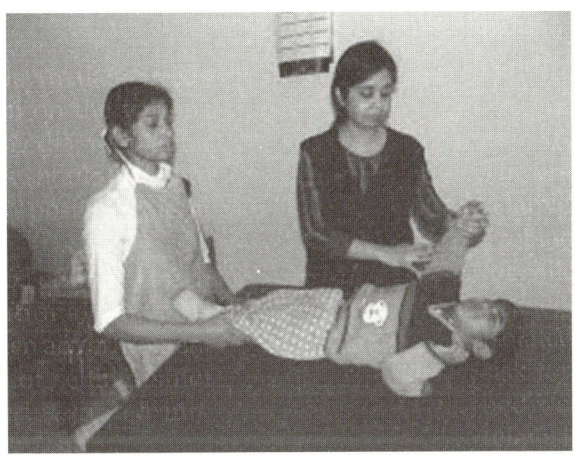

Growth and development are the most important aspects of child health. Every child has a unique growth and development pattern. However, some children develop a pattern of development which differs from the normal. Such patterns of development vary on a spectrum of mild deviance or delay to profound deviance or delay. Parental anxiety about child's weight gain and health is valid but it's imperative that parents should be aware about developmental milestones.

Child development occurs in 4 areas
- Motor (Sitting, Standing, Walking, Running, Climbing)
- Language (Vocabulary and Communication)
- Social (Interaction and Play)
- Adaptive (Day-to-day living)

Within each of these areas, there is a normal range within which the child should be able to achieve her/his milestones. Children whose development varies from the normal spectrum, either in terms of delay or deviancy or both, need to be evaluated by a qualified developmental pediatrician. **Developmental Pediatricians** help to identify the child's concerns and guide the parent towards the process of intervention.

Identification and thorough professional assessment for developmental concerns should be done as early as possible in order to decrease the impact upon life. Delayed identification and hence, delayed intervention leads to secondary problems creeping in, and often these are more difficult to manage later on than the primary ones. Parents and school teachers have a key role in this vital process of early identification and correct remedial action.

In general, most parents are unaware of the facilities available to their differently abled child, and further lack the required information to access them. Parents need to enquire and approach qualified rehabilitation personnel for scientific guidance.

When parents realize about child's developmental concerns, they may go through a series of adjustment phases as follows:

- Awareness of the problem
- Recognition of the problem
- Search for a cause
- Search for a cure, and
- Acceptance of the child.

Acceptance is the key to training and supporting differently abled children. Parents who accept that they need to take perseverant measures to work with the child and that there is a solution, are the Parents who are able to give the maximum benefit of the intervention to the child.

Parents need to remember the **4 core areas of rehabilitation**:

1. **Scientific and documented individualized intervention.** This will include therapeutic services such as occupational therapy, speech therapy, remedial education, physiotherapy, nutrition and counseling. Every child requires a **combination** of any of these depending on his

or her specific developmental concerns. Since areas to be worked on and goals to be achieved are many and since the process is spread over months, it is vital to have a written document called individualized therapy plan (ITP) or individualized education plan (IEP) for the same.

2. **Education:** Mainstream education should be the goal of the parent to help the child explore his best potential within the milieu of typically developing children. Inclusion benefits all the children in the classroom and not merely the special child. However, since most schools lack the facilities for individualized programs for a special child, the parents may need to avail of the same outside the ambit of the school; otherwise the school may find itself helpless to do anything much for the child. The Courts have ruled in favor of allowing Shadow Teachers inside the classroom, if that is in the best interest of the child (the author was the Chairman of the Committee formed to look into this aspect of the matter of Arvind Shetty *Vs* Jamnabai Narsee School, http://archive.indianexpress.com/news/autistic-child-fit-to-attend-regular-school-panels-final-report/1164231)

38

3. **Rights, provisions and facilities:** Availing the necessary provisions and exercising the rights for differently abled children. The Nation Trust set up by the Government of India in this regard offers significant information and details of the same. Different State Governments have their own provisions in place.

4. **Community support:** Parents are the best advocates of their child's concerns. Parents' need to elicit support of significant members of the extended family, community and society. The Community as a whole needs to work towards reducing stigma and discrimination towards the differently abled child and support the child in the process of 'Inclusion'.

Finally, parents should bear the following in mind

- All children have strengths and challenges, and these strengths must be identified and reinforced and challenges should be given the necessary support and intervention wherever required.

- Identification and Intervention require the assistance of a qualified, multidisciplinary team working in close coordination with each other, and working according to a Documented Program that is shared with the parents.
- Foster feelings of self-esteem in your child.
- Do not compare the performance of the differently abled child with other siblings
- Parents who convey hope provide a major force in helping children overcome challenges and become resilient.
- Parents can help differently abled children develop a sense of responsibility and contribution to their family and society.

38

Points to remember

1. Parents should know that child development occurs in 4 areas—motor, language, social and adaptive.
2. Parents should know that early identification and interventions done by qualified multidisciplinary professionals minimizes secondary and tertiary problems.
3. Acceptance of the differently abled child is key to success in management of these children.
4. Rights, provision and facilities of such children should be known to parents.

The 'Only Child'

Anil Mokashi

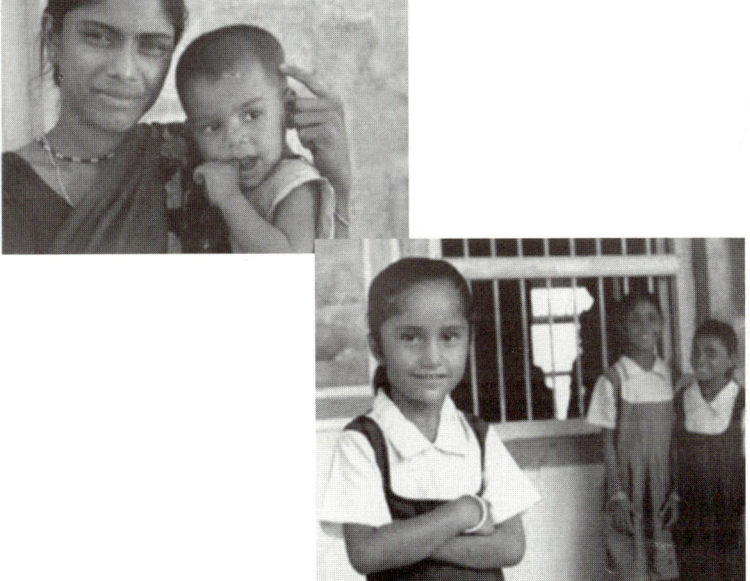

People say the 'only child' is a 'lonely child'. They say it is harmful for the child to remain single. Is it true? Is it really bad to have a single child? The answer is 'No'. Hundreds of studies have proved that only children are no different from their peers.

The families buzzing with 5–6 children, 5–6 aunts and uncles all growing together less than one roof is a history. 'We two our two' brand square families were common in previous generation. Now the trend is of a 'single child'. That is the new generation 'traditional family'.

Being single and having no siblings, is a question of family environment that child grows in. Many couples prefer to have a single child. China has a 'one child policy'. First born child is a 'temporary only child' till the second child is born. A child with a much older sibling also has a similar family environment.

It costs to bear and rear children. It costs money, time energy and everything. Family stress, marital disharmony, career, bad obstetric history, fear over next pregnancy, advanced age, infertility or death of a sibling are some of the causes of having single child. The decision to 'stop at one' is difficult. There are advantages and disadvantages of a single child. There are dos and don'ts in raising a single child.

39

Disadvantages of a Single Child

'Little emperors'

He is the boss of the house. He commands. He demands. He gets everything he wants. People say only children are spoiled, selfish, aggressive and what not! They say only children do not develop normally as they do not get opportunity to interact with brothers and sisters. But research proves that it is not true.

'One-Two-Four' Problem

When the only child grows to become an adult, he has to support six elderly. His two parents and four grandparents. With increasing life span, the number of elderly family members is increasing fast. Many self employed elderly do not have retirement benefits. And the problem is not of economic provisions only. Day-to-day living support and emotional support is also a need. Without support the elderly become destitute or resource less.

The Single Girl Child

In Indian culture, a single girl child becomes a 'sandwich generation'. She is sandwiched with responsibilities of three generations. She finds it difficult to get married if she is the only or an important earning member of the maternal family. She may land in despair and become pessimistic. If she gets married, she has to care for her own aging parents, her husband, children and in-laws. She is needed by everybody.

Advantages of a Single Child

You can give more of everything to a single child. More attention, more quality time, more educational facilities and more developmental facilities. Eventually a single child achieves better. He is more likely to make outside friends and become extremely independent. By limiting the number of members, the family can raise its socio-economic status, per capita income, offer better heath care. As there is no option, the family is bound together and is likely to have better interpersonal relationships.

39

Parenting a Single Child

Do not feel guilty

You have not done any injustice to him. You need not be apologetic. Do not try to overcompensate for keeping him alone. Opting for a single child is your personal decision taken for his better future. You have every right to have your opinion.

Give more attention, but don't overdo

View your single child as an advantage. Give your quality time to make him a responsible adult. Responsible for his thoughts and actions. A housewife mother should have some interest other than raring her only child. Otherwise she will try to live his life for him. A working mother should not try to force all her childcare in her available and convenient time. Feeding, cleaning, education, play, hobbies, extra curricular, discipline, everything can not be packed (zipped) in the available hour or two. The bud has to blossom; don't try to force open the petals! A balance is very important. He needs his space and independence for his development.

Do not shower gifts, shower time and words

Do not try to fulfill all his wishes. He will learn to emotionally blackmail you. Along with money, time, attention, love and care are also important resources. Costly gifts and excessive pocket money are not necessary. Affluence gives a wrong signal. He will not be able to face life in the true spirit.

In a nuclear double income family, the child might crave for company. In your absence, he may get involved with wrong company, or suffer alone. You have to play multiple roles. You have to be his brother, sister, friend as well as a mother. Do not praise him for everything, whether it's well done or not. Maintain discipline. Otherwise he may become self-centered or pampered.

Keep him Busy

39 Engage him in activities like painting, drawing, craft (fine arts) music, dance, sports, indoor games, etc. Consider his aptitude. Give him exposure to many activities and let him select one to pursue. Books can be long lasting friends. Let him watch TV and surf the net for a limited time. Excessive TV and net removes emotions and makes the mindset mechanical. Activities make him creative.

Expand Your Family and Family Friends

Socialization can prevent loneliness of the only child. Encourage him to have his own friend circle. Teach him the need of family friends. Teach him how to develop friendship. Teach him the significance of lasting friendship.

Grandparents provide a wonderful bonding. If he is not lucky enough to live with his own grand parent, search for an elderly couple without grandchild in the neighborhood. You will certainly find one. Develop relationship. Open the windows of communication. It will be mutually beneficial. He should have cousins, a ton of cousins! Assumed brother or assumed sister is a suitable concept. Find out one in the vicinity. Nurture the relations on rakhi, bhaubeej, tilgul and other similar occasions. Adoption of the second child is also an available option, practiced by innumerable couples nowadays. This step may teach him caring and sharing. Expose him to social gatherings, ceremonies, music concerts, clubs and like minded groups. He should know how to organize 'birds of same feather'. Give him an opportunity to socialize with strangers. Make him independent while maintaining strong family ties. Family gives him roots and stability. Independence without family ties is like a 'kite without string'.

Reorganize Your Family at Appropriate Time

Only 'diamonds are for ever'. Time changes everything else. Time changes the way family lives, eats, thinks. Time changes relationships. The change is inevitable. You can not stop the time clock. You have to change with times. Any change is difficult. But you have to change for better. You have to teach him to accept change. You have to teach him how to change. Reorganize your family at an appropriate time.

Marriage, career, death, disease and aging are the times that force families to change. The changes should be predicted and appropriate actions planned. Changes in the family should be a smooth transition rather than a jerky catastrophe. Career and marriage of only child needs special consideration. Parent should shift to the place where child works or the child should work where parents stay. A neighborhood flat is the ideal solution in present day context.

Ultimately

Don't lose your heart if your only child misbehaves. All children misbehave some time or other. The grass is always greener. They say "a friend is better than a brother. Brother takes a share, friend gives one! It all boils down to parenting, pure and simple. Positive parenting is the bottomline

You can spoil one child or a group of them.......
Doesn't matter about the 'only child' thing.

Points to remember

1. There are advantages and disadvantages of a single child.
2. A single child can be given more attention, more quality time, more educational facilities

39

and have better interpersonal relationship. They score higher in self esteem and achievement and are emotionally secure.

3.· Single child's parents should be authoritative in nature to give maximum opportunity to develop.

4.· Single child's responsibility of taking care of his parents, grandparents increases as he is the only dependent member of the family.

5.· Give time to your child. Give unconditional love and make him feel secure.

6.· Socialization will help him to develop good interpersonal relationship, excellent communicative skills and improve his emotional and social intelligence.

Cerebral Palsy: Parent's Perspective

Ashok Rai

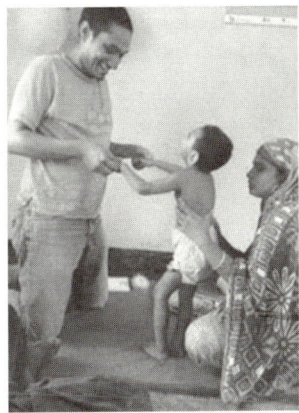 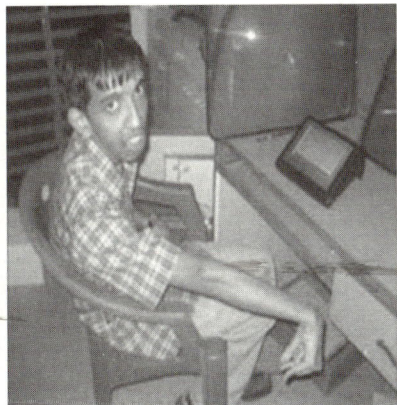

CEREBRAL PALSY

Developmental disabilities are one of the common causes of morbidity seen in children, affecting as much as 5% of the children. The numbers are likely to increase in future as more and higher risk infants survive and graduate from the neonatal intensive care units. The condition is more common in lower socioeconomic groups. The child with special needs or medical/ psychological conditions brings with him a host of problems and demands for their parents that become additional source of stress apart from parenting stress.

Cerebral palsy is the most common physical disability in childhood. Children with cerebral Palsy usually survive into adulthood and the condition is often poorly understood in adulthood. Recognising and managing cerebral palsy's many important comorbidities are as important as treating the motor disabilities.

It is a common developmental disability first described by **William Little** in the 1840s. It is one of the three most common life long developmental disabilities. The other two being autism and mental retardation causing considerable hardship to affected individual and their families.

DEFINITION

Cerebral Palsy is "an umbrella term covering a group of non-progressive but often changing, motor impairment syndromes secondary to lesions or anomalies of the brain arising in the early stages of development. It may be stated as a static encephalopathy in which, even though the primary lesion, anomaly or injury is static, the clinical pattern of presentation may change with time due to growth and developmental plasticity and maturation of the central nervous system.

Incidence

CP is a common problem, the worldwide incidence being 2 to 2.5 per 1000 live births. Incidence is higher in premature infants and in twin births.

Ascertaining the Cause of Cerebral Palsy

CP in developing countries is most often attributed to birth asphyxia and birth trauma and indeed birth asphyxia is still a leading cause in India. However, the other important causes include developmental abnormalities, intrauterine and postnatal infections, and iodine deficiency disorders, prematurity and metabolic disorders. Identifying the actual cause is important, since it avoids needless blame on obstetric management and the feeling of guilt in parents.

It may be difficult to pin point the exact cause when the child presents in infancy with CP. In patients delivered in hospital, the intrapartum events would have been recorded and help in ascertaining the cause. In patients delivered at home, it may be very difficult to ascertain the exact cause. However, it may be noted that neonates with significant birth asphyxia are likely to have abnormal behavior in the first 24 hrs following birth and are unlikely to accept breastfeed.

Clinical Presentation

Cerebral palsy, except in its mildest forms, can be seen in the first 12 to 18 months of life. The condition presents when children fail to reach their milestones and when they show qualitative differences in motor development, such as asymmetric gross motor function or unusual muscle stiffness or floppiness. Cerebral palsy is usually characterised clinically by the parts of the body affected although conventional terminology used to describe cerebral palsy is less precise. Descriptions of the predominant motor disorder refer to spastic, dystonic, athetotic and ataxic features.

40

The Gross Motor Function Classification System (GMFCS)

This is a recently developed system which has been found to be a reliable and valid system that classifies children with cerebral palsy by their age specific gross motor activity. The GMFCS describes the functional Characteristics in five levels, form I to V. Level I being the mildest and level III usually require orthoses and assisting mobility devices, while children in level II do not require assisting mobility devices after age 4. Children in level III sit independently, have independent floor mobility and walk with assisting mobility devices. In level IV, affected children function in supported sitting but independent mobility is very limited. Children in level V lack independence even in basic antigravity postural control and need power mobility.

Associated Deficits

Mental retardation is common in CP in upto 60% of the case. **Singhi et al., 2003** in a study in India report MR in 72.5% of affected children. Children with spastic quadriplegia have greater degree of cognitive impairment than children with spastic hemiplegia.

Visual impairment and disorders of ocular motility are common (28%) in children with CP. There is an increased presence of strabismus, amblyopia, nystagmus, optic atrophy and refractive errors. Children whose CP is due to periventricular leukomalacia are also more likely to have visual perceptual problems.

Hearing impairment occurs in approximately 12% of children with CP. This occurs more commonly if the etiology of CP is related to very low birth weight, kernicterus, and neonatal meningitis or sever hypoxic ischemic insults.

Epilepsy is common in children with CP. Children with spastic quadriplegia or hemiplegia has a higher incidence of epilepsy than patients with diplegia or ataxic CP. In an Indian study, it was found that 35% had epilepsy. 66% of children with spastic hemiplegia, 43% of spastic quadriplegia and 16% of children with spastic diplegia had seizures as an associated feature.

Apart from these, orthopedic problems like scoliosis, dislocation of hips and medical problems like neurogenic bladder, feeding difficulties, urinary tract infection and constipation are also seen especially in severe cases and spastic quadriplegia.

Speech and Language Disorders

Speech is affected in CP due to bilateral corticobulbar and oromotor dysfunctions. Both receptive and expressive language deficits are common and go hand in hand with mental retardation. Articulation disorders and impaired speech are present in 38% children with CP.

Diagnosis

The diagnosis of CP is essentially clinical and involves a detailed prenatal, natal and postnatal history along with careful physical and neurodevelopmental examinations. As in all medical conditions, a systematic approach focusing on maternal, obstetric and perinatal histories, review of developmental milestones, and a thorough neurological examination and observation of the child in various positions such as supine, prone, sitting standing, walking and running is essential in the diagnosis of cerebral palsy.

It is very difficult to diagnose CP in infants less than 6 months except in very severe cases. Early diagnosis is very important for providing early intervention to CP children. It depends upon the clinical acumen and experience of developmental pediatrician.

Be Cautious while Labeling Cerebral Palsy

Undue significance is attributed to delay crying in diagnosis of Cerebral palsy.

Neurodegenerative disorders and other genetic causes of developmental delay should always be excluded before labeling Cerebral palsy. Many disorders presenting with muscle tone abnormalities, seizures and developmental delay are metabolic disorders with autosomal recessive inheritance. Such disorders should be investigated thoroughly before labelling Cerebral palsy.

40

Clusters of Signs Useful for Early Identification of CP

Warning signs
- Lack of alertness
- Decreased spontaneous motility.
- Stereotyped abnormal movements.

Abnormal signs
- Reduced head circumference/fall off in growth
- Constant fisting with adduction of thumb beyond 2 months
- Delayed social smile
- Primitive reflexes persisting beyond 6 months
- Obligatory ATNR
- Delayed appearance of postural reflexes and developmental milestones
- Persistent tone abnormalities
- Persistent asymmetry in posture, movement and reflexes

Investigation

Investigations are not needed to confirm the diagnosis of CP. They should be used to find out the cause and exclude other illnesses:

A. **Neuroimaging:** Neuroimaging studies are carried out to know the etiology of cerebral palsy. MRI studies are preferred to CT scans.

B. **EEG:** EEG in required in children with epilepsy or seizures.

C. **Genetic and metabolic tests:** These tests are required in diagnosis of genetic and metabolic disorders causing such type of diseases and if there is family history of childhood neurological disorder associated with CP.

Parents First Question About Cerebral Palsy

40

Patient's first question to Doctor is: "is it curable? How bad this condition is? and whether child will sit, walk and talk". These questions are very difficult to answer for a pediatrician. Evidence based information should be provided to parents and their families. Pediatrician should try to alleviate parental stress as much as possible. Honest and open communication should be done with mother, father and no blame should be given to any parent.

Management

Cerebral palsy cannot be cured. The World Health Organization's model of health and disease focused on function and is an important framework to guide modern thinking about treatment of children with cerebral palsy. The goals of management should be to use appropriate combinations of interventions (including developmental, physical, medical, surgical, chemical and technical modalities) to promote function, to prevent secondary impairments and, above all, to increase a child's developmental capabilities.

A multidisciplinary team of health care professionals develops an individualized treatment plan based on the patient's need and problems. It is imperative to involve patients, families, teachers, and caregivers in all phases of planning, decision making and treatment.

Our aim in management should be

A. Classify different type of CP

B. Care for spasticity management

C. Rehabilitation of child by physiotherapy, occupational therapy speech therapy

D. Orthotic and orthopedic management

Management of Spasticity

Reduction of spasticity is only one of many facets of the overall management of motor disorders of cerebral palsy. While in some children, spasticity may interfere with motor function, in others, it may in fact be useful to maintain posture and capacity to ambulate. Different pharmacological agents, e.g. Baclofen, benzodiazepines, dantrolene are used for the reduction of spasticity in selected patients.

Botulinum toxin injection is used in very few patients. It causes a focal, dose dependent, reversible chemodenervation of muscle. The most benefitted patients are one who is hypertonic either spastic or dystonic, whose abnormal muscle tone is interfering with function or who is expected to develop joint contracture with growth because of hypertonia.

40

Habilitation

While there is no cure for the basic lesion that leads to CP, there is a lot that can be done to help the child achieve his potential. The main aim is to access the functional capacity of the child in various domains and to plan as intervention programmes to maximize it. Physiotherapy, occupational therapies are mainstay of therapy for rehabilitation of these patients.

a. **Physiotherapy:** Physiotherapy should be started as soon as diagnosis of CP is established. Early intervention helps in prevention of contractures and deformities in these patients. Neurodevelopmental therapy essentially involves training of the child through normal sequence of motor development, abolition of primitive and abnormal reflexes, reinforcement of normal postural reflexes and facilitation of normal movements.

b. **Occupational therapy:** Occupational therapy focuses on the development of skills necessary for the performance of activities of daily living. These include play, self care activities such as dressing, grooming, feeding and fine motor tasks such as drawing and writing.

Besides PT/OT, play therapy, hippotherapy (horseback riding therapy) are also being used in some centres.

Speech therapy, behavioural therapy and education are the mainstay of therapy is later phases.

Counseling

Parental involvement is pivotal for the success of any intervention programme. Guidance and counseling is a continuous endeavour to ensure parental acceptance of the problem and their participation in prolonged treatment programmes.

40 Avoidance of consanguinity, routine immunization especially MMR, good pre and perinatal care are most essential for prevention of this type of illness.

Points to remember

1. Cerebral palsy is commonest preventable neuro developmental disability.
2. Recognition of early markers / warning signs is importance
3. High risk neonatal follow up with detailed visual assessment including (retinal) and newborn hearing screening can present tertiary morbidities and permanent blindness and hearing impairment.
4. Early intervention in the form of hearing, visual, tactile kinaesthetic stimulation therapy is mandatory.

FURTHER READING

1. Emery AEH. Muscular Dystrophy : The facts, Oxford, Oxford University Press, 2000.
2. Rosen MG, Dickinson JC. The incidence of cerebral Palsy. Am J Obstet Gynecol 1992; 167:417–423.

3. Nelson KB, Ellenberg JH. Childhood neurological disorders in twins. Paediatr Perinat Epidemiol 1995; 9:135–145.
4. Anjeja S. Evaluation of a child with cerebral palsy. Indian J Pediatr 2004;71(7):627–634.
5. Cans C. Surveillance of Cerebral Palsy in Europe: a collaboration of cerebral palsy surveys and registers. Dev Med Child Neurol 2000; 42:816–824.
6. Palisano RJ, Rosenbaum PL, Walter SD, Russell DJ, Wood EP, Galuppi BE. Development and reliability of a system to classify gross motor function in children with cerebral palsy. Dev Med Child Neurol 1997; 39:214–223.
7. Singhi PD, Jagirdar S, Malhi P. Epilepsy in children with Cerebral Palsy. J Child Neurology 2003; 18:174–179.
8. Sankar C, Mundkur N. Cerebral Palsy: Definition, Classification, Etiology and Early Diagnosis. Indian J Pediatr 2005; 72(10): 865–868.
9. Rosenbloom L. Diagnosis and management of Cerebral palsy. Arch Dis child 1995; 72:350–354.

40

The Dancing Letters and LD

Samir Dalwai, Nita Mehta

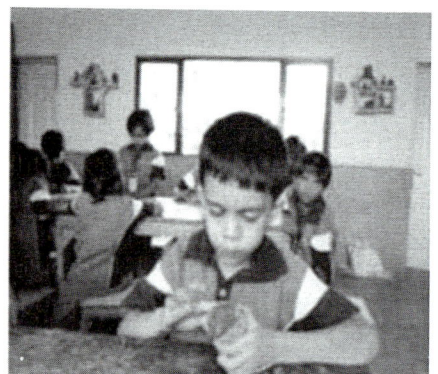

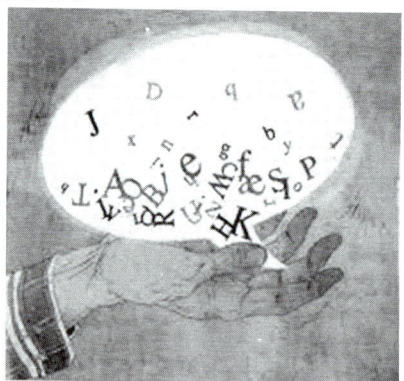

When Ananya, 7 years, got a silver star in one of the formative tests in her second grade, she was very happy to have scored at least the minimum necessary marks her class teacher had announced before the test and promised herself to continue studying sincerely to get more silver stars. The class teacher however expressed concerns to Ananya's mother about several 'silly' mistakes made by the child. She pointed out omission of letters in many words such as "pace" for "place"; addition of letters like "bill" for "bill". Ananya's mother is worried how her child will cope with studies as she moves to higher grades. Arpit, 10 years old boy, is an excellent football player and enjoys Math. He squirms at the idea of attending English Literature classes and often finds a way to engage in an alternate activity in school. When asked by a friend, he said that he often finds reading very confusing. Words on paper fail to remind him of how they sound and 'reading 'the 'spelling' of every word in every sentence seems like a waste of time. To add to despair, Arpit, like other students, is often asked to read a paragraph or two aloud to the class. "Why don't they just drop Literature subject!" laments Arpit.

41

There are numerous other *Ananyas* and *Arpits* across India, whose **sincere, hardworking efforts often are not seen translated to their academic performance.** Many students face challenges in performing tasks that come easily to others, such as reading with desired fluency and change of intonation at punctuations, writing spellings of words, recalling and applying rules of arithmetic.

BASIC CONSIDERATIONS ABOUT LEARNING

Learning is defined as 'acquisition of knowledge or skills' through observation, study, practice, experience, or being taught. Learning to use language for reading, writing, expressing ideas and thoughts, applying mathematical operations on numbers are skills acquired by children through formal and informal ways (at home, in school).

Learning most often occurs when children are exposed to such information (stimulus), given opportunity to practice and apply (response) resulting in appreciation and/or feedback on application (consequence) (Joseph, 2008). Some factors that are at play and have crucial requirement in the process of learning are:

A. Ability to observe details (*ability of a child to receive sensory input and transmit information to the brain for processing*)

B. Understand and analyse details (*exert cognitive processes of comprehension of details, thinking and reasoning*)

C. Retain details and analysis of details with easy access in memory to recall the details (*memory to store information in appropriate location and ability to access it with ease and speed when required*)

D. Analyse and apply to new situation (*reasoning and problem solving*)

Thus, learning requires age-appropriate development of neurological connections and transmissions for each of the above skills to be functional for the child to learn the skills of reading, writing, and other academic activities.

41

LEARNING DIFFERENTLY

Many children like Ananya and Arpit find it difficult to learn and apply these skills to new situations and have different patterns of learning.

Learning differences arise from neurological differences in brain structure and function and affect a child's ability to receive, store, process, retrieve or communicate information (Cortiella, C. & Horowitz, SH, 2014).

The Diagnostic and Statistical Manual-V (2013) uses the term "Specific Learning Disorder" (SLD) to explain the concerns where an individual faces persistent difficulties in reading, writing, arithmetic, or mathematical reasoning skills during formal years of schooling. Symptoms may include:

- Inaccurate or slow and effortful reading (**Dyslexia**: difficulties in reading and spelling)
- Poor written expression that lacks clarity (**Dysgraphia**: difficulties with sizes and shapes of alphabets, spacing between words, usage of punctuations and case of alphabets)
- Difficulties remembering number facts, or inaccurate mathematical reasoning (**Dyscalculia**: Difficulty with calculations, arithmetic, mathematics, solving word problems)

The most important fact is that children's difficulties are **not** accounted by any sensory deficits, developmental, neurological or motor concerns. Children will demonstrate normal levels of intellectual functioning **as measured by appropriate assessments**. Children may have difficulties in only one 'specific' learning area or more than one area.

Epidemiology researches suggest 8–10 percent of children face one or more type of learning difficulties in reading, writing or math (Sadock, 2003).

Signs of differences in learning and performing in these areas are noticeable from pre-school years such as:

1. Preschool history of some indicator of slower language milestones (first words, first sentences) (Berninger, 2006)
2. Difficulties in pronunciation and rhyming of words
3. Slow growth in learning new vocabulary
4. Difficulties in making connections between sounds and alphabets
5. Difficulties in learning numbers, colours, shapes
6. Difficulties in counting, sequencing of numbers
7. Under-developed pencil grip

41

The child's performance gives strong indications towards significant discrepancy between the child's 'actual efforts' versus 'actual level of learning achieved'. **In spite of best efforts**, the child is unable to perform as per her/his potential.

When these concerns are not identified at an early stage and often go unnoticed without adequate support offered to the child, it causes repeated failure, poor self-concept and self-esteem, and anxiety about all events with performance expectations. There are other disturbing experiences when children face ridicule from peers and adults, are considered misfits and excluded from peer circles. When these children are unfairly criticized, it damages their self-respect and leads to behavioral concerns.

RAY OF 'SCOPE'

Neurological researches suggest that SLD is a way in which brain processes information. It is not an illness to be cured but a training program to be engaged in to offer the neurological processes better ways to perform on tasks of reading, writing and math. With right support and intervention, children with SLD can succeed in school and go on to successful, often distinguished careers later in life.

Parents can help children with SLD achieve such success by encouraging their strengths, knowing their challenges, understanding the educational system, working with professionals and learning about strategies for dealing with specific difficulties. Some important points to be aware to start training/interventions are:

41

- **Observe** for difficulties in academic performance faced by the child which do not improve with support.

- Refer to a **developmental pediatrician, psychiatrist or a psychologist** who is trained to deal with this matter, as early during school life as possible. Appropriate testing like an IQ test along with specific psycho-educational tests will establish the diagnosis.

- **Remedial education**, in addition to their regular schooling, will enable these children to cope with their academic challenges and they will learn how to read and spell correctly.

- **Occupational therapy** will help with attention, task-planning, fine motor and visual-motor coordination.

- Above all, **parental counselling and behaviour modi-fication** will go a long way in improving the home environ-ment and improving everyone's self esteem; and most important, keeping the parents focused and determined to succeed with the task at hand.

- The **participation of the school**, especially the classroom, teacher is extremely important in terms of remediation as well as inclusion, and making the child feel wanted and respected and a part of the class.

- The government of Maharashtra and now many other State governments offer **special provisions** during exami-nations. Parents need to speak with the school personnel to have necessary arrangements for the child.

Points to remember

1. Learning is defined as 'acquisition of knowledge or skills'. Through observation, study, practice, experience or being taught.

2. Learning requires age-appropriate development of neurological connections and transmissions for sensory inputs, storage, processing, comprehension and retrieval of information.

3. Child with learning disability has difficulties and spelling (Dyslexia). Poor written expression that lacks clarity (Dysgraphia) and difficulties in calculation, arithmetic and mathematics (Dyscalculia).

4. Management of Learning disability includes remedial education, occupational therapy, parental counselling and behaviour modification.

5. Inclusive education of these children by schools and special provisions during examinations will help such children gain highest academic potentials.

41

FURTHER READING

1. Berninger, VW (2006). A developmental approach to learning disabilities. *Handbook of child psychology, 4,* 420–452.

2. Cortiella, C & Horowitz, SH (2014). The state of learning disabilities: Facts, trends and emerging issues. *New York: National Center for Learning Disabilities.*

3. Joseph, L. M. (2008). Best practices on interventions for students with reading problems. *Best practices in school psychology, 4,* 1163–1180.

4. Sadock, BJ & Sadock, VA (2003). Synopsis of psychiatry.) *Classification in Psychiatry and Psychiatry Rating Scales (9e) Philadelphia: Lippincot, Williams and Wilkins,* 288–318.

Child Abuse and Safety

Anjana Thadani

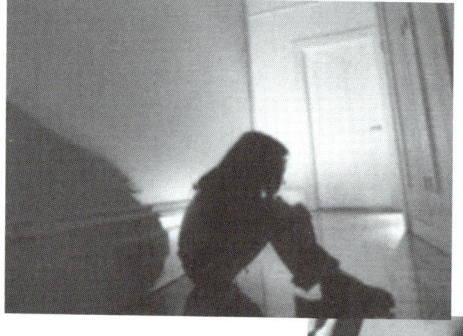

Rekha, a 13-year-old girl was referred for breathlessness, fever and mild drowsiness since past few days, on examination and subsequent investigations she was diagnosed to have Right sided lower lobe pneumonia. She also suffered from a Neurodegenerative condition and was bedridden since one year. Another disturbing finding was the presence of genital warts and a lax vagina. I took a gynecological reference who confirmed my suspicion of chronic ongoing sexual abuse. When I discussed my fears with the mother of the child, she immediately dismissed the matter and avoided any conversation with me thereafter. Rekha went home after the completion of the treatment.

Karan came for a routine consultation for mild fever and during the examination, his knuckles were burnt. I asked the child about what caused the wound when his father went out to attend an urgent call. The child told me that he fell. After the consultation I confronted the father about the wounds and the father told me that those were burn marks given by the mother for the child's bad behavior.

Sonia was refusing to go to school since past 15 days and was brought by the parents for counseling. She on further inquiry told that she was touched inappropriately by a school peon in the washroom after school. This peon apparently is a very old employee and has been indulging in such behavior regularly. What was more shocking was the attitude of the principal who chose to believe the peon and not a 6 year old student of her school. The parents retracted the child from the school. The risk of abuse continues for all the other children of this reputed school.

As medical professionals we all have come across numerous similar incidents and also the unwillingness of the parents to report these cases to appropriate authorities. Hence, it is important for us to get empowered to deal with this alarmingly increasing menace in the society.

42

INTRODUCTION

Child abuse is increasingly discussed in context of numerous cases which are constantly surfacing in the media and also cases of child abuse happening around us. Child abuse happens almost anywhere and everywhere. The abuser could be a Parent, Caregiver, Teacher, Neighbor, Family member, frequent visitor to the household, or a Stranger…almost anyone.

Similarly, no place can be considered safe from abuse and cases are reported from Homes, Schools, Streets, Institutions, Public places, etc. There is also a rise in such cases seen by medical professionals in their daily practice.

The pediatrician traditionally assumes the responsibility of looking after the well being of children, which in a holistic sense also extends to their safety concerns. The pediatrician also comes across numerous concerned parents and their queries regarding child abuse and behavior. Schools and teachers are also concerned about the safety issues. This definitely calls for a collaborative effort from all segments of society to ensure a safe and healthy environment for our children.

DEFINITION

Child abuse is a misuse of power by adults over children that endangers or impairs a child's physical, mental, sexual, emotional health and development. It refers to the intended, unintended and perceived maltreatment, whether habitual or not, of the child including any of the following:

- Psychological and physical abuse, neglect, cruelty, sexual and emotional maltreatment.
- Any act, deed or word which debases, degrades or demeans the intrinsic worth and dignity of a child.
- Unreasonable deprivation of the basic needs for survival such as food and shelter; or failure to give timely medical treatment to an injured child resulting in serious impairment of growth and development or permanent incapacity or death.

FORMS OF CHILD ABUSE

Physical Abuse

Physical abuse is inflicting of physical injury upon a child, including burning, hitting, punching, shaking, kicking, beating or otherwise harming a child. It may be the result of over-discipline or physical punishment inappropriate to the child's age. Most offenders are parents or caretakers using extreme and bizarre forms of punishment such as confinement in a closet or dark room or tied to a chair for long periods of time. Battered Baby Syndrome and Shaken or Whiplash head injuries are extreme form of physical abuse seen in infants.

Physical abuse has significant long-term medical and mental health morbidity. Children with abusive head or abdominal injuries are more likely to die or become more severely incapacitated than are children with head or abdominal injuries caused by accidents. Victims of physical abuse in childhood are

42

more likely to develop a variety of behavioral and functional problems including conduct disorders, physically aggressive behaviors, poor academic performance, and decreased cognitive functioning.

Sexual Abuse

Child sexual abuse (CSA) is a form of child abuse in which an adult or older adolescent who is in a relationship of responsibility, trust or power, uses a child for sexual stimulation. CSA means contacts or interactions between a child and an older or more knowledgeable child or adult (stranger, sibling, parent, or caretaker), when the child is being used as an object of gratification for the older child's or adult's needs. Such contacts or interaction are carried out against the child using force, trickery, bribes, threats or pressure.

Different forms of sexual abuse are:

A. Severe forms
- Assault, including rape and sodomy
- Touching or fondling a child
- Exhibitionism: Forcing a child to exhibit his/her private body parts
- Photographing a child in nude

B. Other forms
- Forcible kissing
- Sexual advances towards a child during travel
- Sexual advances towards a child during marriage situations
- Exhibitionism: Exhibiting before a child
- Exposing a child to pornographic materials

Child sexual abuse is committed by a person responsible for the care of a child or related to the child. If a stranger commits these acts, it would be considered sexual assault

Sexual abuse is also described as Touching and Non-Touching Behaviors.

Touching behaviors include fondling a child's body for sexual pleasure, kissing a child with sexual undertones, inclinations, rubbing genitals against a child's body, sexually touching a child's body, and specifically private parts (breasts and genitals) including encouraging or forcing a child to do likewise, making a child touch someone else's genitals, or playing sexual ("pants-down") games, encouraging or forcing a child to masturbate, with the child as either a participant or observer, encouraging or forcing a child to perform oral sex (mouth-to-genital contact on or by the child), inserting objects or body parts (like fingers, tongue or penis) inside the vagina, mouth, or anus of a child; includes attempts of these acts.

Non-touching behaviors include encouraging a child to watch or hear sexual acts either in person or lowering the bars of privacy, looking at a child sexually, exposing one's private body parts to a child (exhibitionism), watching a child in a state of nudity, such as while undressing, using the bathroom, with or without the child's knowledge (voyeurism), an adult making suggestive comments to the child that are sexual in nature, commenting on the sexual development of a child, encouraging or forcing a child to read or watch pornography, giving pornographic material or using the child in pornography, etc.

42

EMOTIONAL ABUSE (Syn: Verbal Abuse, Mental Abuse, Psychological Maltreatment)

Verbal abuse constitutes threatening or terrorizing a child, belittling or rejecting the child, using derogatory terms, habitual tendency to blame the child, constant criticism, constantly ignoring a child, punishing normal social behaviors, exposure to domestic violence, withholding praise and affection, constant comparison, etc. Psychological maltreatment refers to a repeated pattern of parental behavior that is likely to be interpreted by a child that he or she is unloved, unwanted, or serves only instrumental purposes and or that severely undermines the child's development and socialization. Psychological or emotional maltreatment of children and adolescents may be the most challenging and prevalent form of child abuse and neglect, but has received relatively little attention.

Psychological maltreatment encompasses both the cognitive and affective components of maltreatment. Exposure to psychological maltreatment is considered when acts of omission (ignoring the need for social interaction) or commission (spurning, terrorizing); may be verbal or nonverbal, active or passive, and with or without intent to harm; and negatively affect the child's cognitive, social, emotional, and/or physical development.

Psychological maltreatment is quite often difficult to identify because such maltreatment could pass off as bad parenting and is repetitive and difficult to intervene.

Neglect

It is the failure to provide for the child's basic needs including Physical, educational, or emotional. Abandonment is an extreme form of neglect. Physical neglect includes not providing adequate food or clothing, appropriate medical care, supervision, proper weather protection, abandonment, shelter, safety, hygiene, etc. Educational neglect includes not providing appropriate schooling, special educational needs or allowing excessive truancies. Psychological neglect is the lack of any emotional support and love, never attending to the child, allowing substance abuse in the child, etc.

Pediatricians are sometimes confronted in practice by children whose medical needs are being neglected. In the United States, medical neglect accounts for 2.3% of all substantiated cases of child maltreatment. This represents the "tip of the iceberg," because only the most egregious and intractable cases are likely to be reported to authorities.

Medical neglect usually takes 1 of 2 forms: failure to heed obvious signs of serious illness or failure to follow a physician's instructions once medical advice has been sought. Either of these situations can be fatal in some cases or can lead to chronic disability.

Several factors are considered necessary for the diagnosis of medical neglect:

1. A child is harmed or is at risk of harm because of lack of health care;
2. The recommended health care offers significant net benefit to the child;

3. The anticipated benefit of the treatment is significantly greater than its morbidity, so that reasonable caregivers would choose treatment over non treatment;

4. It can be demonstrated that access to health care is available and not used; and

5. The caregiver understands the medical advice given.

INCIDENCE

Reliable estimates are hard to come since this is a furtive form of abuse, often causing victims to suffer in dark and claustrophobic silence. However to find out the extent of child abuse in India, the first ever National Study on Child Abuse was conducted by the Ministry of Women and Child Development, covering 12447 children, 2324 young adults and 2449 stakeholders across 13 states. In 2007, it published the report as "Study on Child Abuse: India, 2007". The survey, covered different forms of child abuse i.e. physical, sexual and emotional as well as female child neglect, in five evidence groups, namely, children in a family environment, children in school, children at work, children on the street and children in institutions.

Major Findings

1. Across different forms of abuse and across different evidence groups, the younger children (5–12 years of age) have reported higher levels of abuse than the other two age groups boys, as compared to girls, are equally at risk of abuse.

2. Persons in trust and authority are major abusers.

3. 70% of abused child respondents never reported the matter to anyone.

Physical Abuse

1. Two out of every three children are physically abused.

2. Out of 69% children physically abused in 13 sample states, 54.68% were boys.

3. Over 50% children in all the 13 sample states were being subjected to one or the other form of physical abuse.

42

4. Out of those children physically abused in family situations, 88.6% were physically abused by parents.
5. 65% of school going children reported facing corporal punishment, i.e. two out of three children were victims of corporal punishment.
6. The State of Andhra Pradesh, Assam, Bihar and Delhi have almost consistently reported higher rates of abuse in all forms as compared to other states.
7. Most children did not report the matter to anyone.
8. 50.2% children worked seven days a week.

Sexual Abuse

42

1. 53.22% children reported having faced one or more forms of sexual abuse.
2. Andhra Pradesh, Assam, Bihar and Delhi reported the highest percentage of sexual abuse among both boys and girls.
3. 21.90% child respondents reported facing severe forms of sexual abuse and 50.76% other forms of sexual abuse.
4. Out of the child respondents, 5.69% reported being sexually assaulted.
5. Children in Assam, Andhra Pradesh, Bihar and Delhi reported the highest incidence of sexual assault.
6. Children on street, children at work and children in institutional care reported the highest incidence of sexual assault.
7. 50% abuses are persons known to the child or in a position of trust and responsibility.
8. Most children did not report the matter to anyone.

Emotional Abuse and Girl Child Neglect

1. Every second child reported facing emotional abuse
2. Equal percentage of both girls and boys reported facing emotional abuse
3. In 83% of the cases parents were the abusers
4. 48.4% of girls wished they were boys

According to WHO, one in every four girls and one in every seven boys in the world are sexually abused. Virani (2000) states, the WHO found that at any given time, one of ten Indian children is the victim of sexual abuse. In another study, a large number of children (40.4%) have been abused or assaulted in the offender's house. The most vulnerable age is between 3–7 years and then between 11–15 years. In 35% of the cases, the child was sexually assaulted or abused in public places like urinals, buses, local trains, etc. unfortunately only serious cases are reported to the police and more than 50% of the accused arrested are granted bail.

Another study on child abuse in Kolkata, Elaan, an NGO, found that four out of 10 boys faced sexual harassment in school. Generally the age of maximum abuse is between 9 to 12 years. The national study found that the abuse gained momentum at the age of 10 and peaked between 12 to 15. This shows that the teenagers are most vulnerable. The Study also acknowledges that child sex abuse takes place in schools. One out of two children in schools has faced sexual abuse. And overall, more boys than girls face various forms of sexual abuse ranging from inappropriate touch, exposure to pornography or violent sexual assault. The abuser could be from the peer group or an older student. Senior students often bring pornographic material to school and may force a younger boy to look at it to titillate them.

CPHCSA's study in 2006, conducted among 2211 school going children in Chennai, indicates CSA prevalence rate of 42%. Children of all socioeconomic groups were found to be equally vulnerable. While 48% of boys reported having been abused, the prevalence rate among girls was 39%. 15% of both boys and girls had been severely abused.

In a survey by Sakshi (1997) in New Delhi with 350 school-girls, 63% had experienced CSA at the hands of family members; and 25% of the girls had either been raped, made to masturbate the perpetrator or engage in oral sex.

Another study by RAHI (1997) on middle and upper class women from Chennai, Mumbai, Delhi, Kolkata and Goa revealed that 76% of respondents had been sexually abused as children, with 71% been abused either by relatives or by someone they knew and trusted.

42

In 1996, Samvada in Bangalore found that 83% if girls had been subject to eve-teasing, with 13% of these under age ten. 47% had been molested, and 15% had been seriously sexually abused as children. Nearly a third was under age ten, and had been raped, forced into oral sex, or penetrated with foreign objects. This study also states that 47% of the respondents had been sexually abused; 62% of whom had been raped once and 38% of whom had suffered repeated violations. Though often considered an act against lower-classes, CSA affects the upper classes as well. A study by RAHI in five major cities in India looked at the experiences of English-speaking middle- and upper-class adults. A whopping 76% reported sexual abuse as children of which 40% were survivors of incest. 35% of the attacks took place between the ages of twelve and sixteen, while 19% took place under age eight. Incest is by far the most common but least discussed form of sexual abuse that young girls suffer in India today.

42

(Rahi,1997), In a study of a 1000 girls from 5 different states in India, 50% of the girls had been abused when under 12 years of age, 35% between the ages of 12 and 16 years. Further adding to these startling numbers are the reported "disappearances" of rape victims in Delhi found that almost 70% of Delhi's rape victims (those who reported the crime to the police), 51% of which were minors, simply disappeared. It has been suggested that "rebuke from parents, relatives, and friends; insecurity and threats from the rapist; a lengthy trial and a little hope of conviction, and the fear of harassment if the rapist goes free" may be some of the reasons that girls simply leave home, or are even thrown out by parents when news of the rape comes out in the open.

A cross-sectional survey was conducted to examine the prevalence, type and intensity of abuse in 200 street children in Jaipur city, India. Larger numbers of children (61.8%) scored in the "moderate" category of abuse while 36.6% children indicated abuse in "severe" and "very severe" categories on the intensity of abuse. Highest mean scores were obtained on the "verbal" and "psychological" area of abuse. Gender differences were significant in health and overall abuse, indicating boys to be significantly more abused than girls.

Some self-report studies in the United Kingdom and United States found that approximately 8–9% of women and 4% of men reported exposure to severe psychological abuse during childhood.

Children with disabilities are approximately 3 times more likely to be maltreated than are children without disabilities.

RISK FACTORS

In almost 60–70% of cases the abuser is a direct family member. He may be a relative, neighbor, member of household or a stranger. History of being abused as a child, record of sexual offence, and alcoholism are risk factors to be an abuser.

It is difficult to ascertain risk factors related to children which predisposes them to abuse, but children at higher risk are Destitute children, Orphans, Abandoned children, Street children, HIV/AIDS affected children, Substance/drug abuse, etc. However, even normal children from so-called regular families are equally prone to abuse.

Parental risk factors include young immature parents with poor parenting skills, personality disorders, mental health problems, social pressures, domestic violence, single parent, alcohol/substance abuse, etc.

Certain parental conditions may also predispose their children for abuse and these include parents with terminal illness, single parent, children of refugees or migrant construction workers, children of prostitutes.

For example, some parental mental health problems are associated with unpredictable and frightening behaviors, and others (particularly depression) are linked with parental withdrawal and neglect. Similarly, in terms of family conflict, attacks on a parent almost always frighten a child, even if the child is not the direct target. Threats or actual violence as part of a pattern of aggression against one parent will sometimes exploit the other parent's or child's fears.

RESPONSE TO CHILD ABUSE

The most important role of the pediatrician is the recognition of child abuse. As discussed earlier the clinical presentation

42

would vary depending on various factors. In physical abuse it may present as head injury, fractures or bruising, while in sexual abuse it could be severe bleeding with perineal tears and may be an acute emergency. The verbal abuse and neglect are usually more frequent and chronic but difficult to identify in a busy office practice.

42

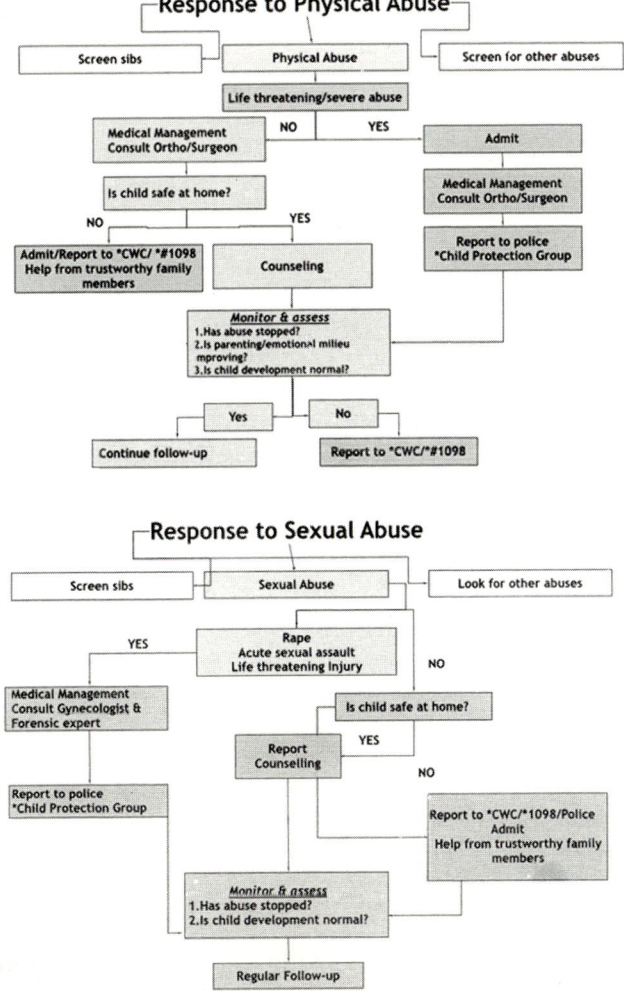

History Taking

The presence of a nurse, social worker or a counselor is a must during the assessment. The assessment should be recorded in a special Performa.

Eliciting history is very important and may be the key to reach to the core of the problem. It is important to know that in 70–85% of documented sexual abuse the physical examination is normal.

It is usually helpful to document history separately from the child and the parent or caretaker. The pediatrician should listen carefully and have a sensitive, empathic and nonjudgmental attitude.

42

Non verbal cues as 'watchful frozenness', sad mood, avoids eye contact etc should be recorded. Exact question and answers need to be recorded verbatim.

However, after the initial emergency care, a detailed medical and social history including presenting symptoms is mandatory. Points to be covered in history include place, time, witness, present and past history, noticeable behavior change, developmental and immunization history. Family history, pedigree chart and social history are extremely important.

A high index of suspicion should be maintained at all times in cases with history of fall, fracture, injury including head injury, unexplained bruises and bleeding.

In case of chronic abuse and neglect the child may present as poor growth and stunting, recurrent UTIs, abdominal pain, pain at the genitals or anus or mouth, genital sores or discharge in genital area, etc.

Inconsistency in history with poor corroboration with physical findings, psychosomatic symptomatology, previous or repeated similar injuries, delay in seeking medical help and circumstantial evidence should be noted. If the treating doctor has noticed some abnormalities and poor correlation then these have to be brought to the notice of the higher authorities or police personals and also properly documented on the patient's papers.

Fabricated illnesses include repeated presentations or persistent symptoms, unusual symptoms, family history of similar but unusual patterns, sudden death etc. It is usually seen in families with medical knowledge or training.

A psychosocial history known by the acronym HEEADDSS can be taken directly from an adolescent patient. This includes details regarding home, education, eating behavior, activities and peers, drugs, depression and suicide, sexual history and sleep pattern. Behavioral history is very important and may give specific clues regarding the abuse. This can be elicited by a trained counselor or social worker through direct interview or indirect projective techniques or questionnaires.

MEDICAL EXAMINATION

42

Parental and (preferably) the child's consent are essential for a medical examination. The child may prefer to get examined by a doctor of the same sex. He may also choose to have a trustworthy adult along with him during the procedure. The pediatrician may seek the expertise of a forensic physician and a gynecologist while examining a case of sexual abuse. The following should be recorded:

- Resistance to examination especially in a case of sexual abuse and dissociation (going to sleep during examination)
- General demeanour (like unkempt appearance in neglect)
- Vitals and tip to toe general physical examination especially noting pallor, bruises, vitamin deficiencies
- Height, weight and head circumference to be plotted on growth chart
- Sexual maturity rating for adolescents
- All injuries are to be marked on anatomical diagrams. Special sites to look for injuries include ears, inside the mouth, soles, genitalia and anus
- Systemic examination is done especially to look for injuries
- Examination of genitalia in girls should be done in supine frog leg, knee chest prone and left lateral position. Details of hymen and injuries are to be noted. Anal dilatation on a rectal examination indicates sodomy. Presence of discharge, genital ulcers, warts and inguinal lymphadenopathy are to be noted.

Detailed general and systemic examination of the child with local examination for determining size, shape, site and nature of injury should be carried out. Differential diagnosis includes bleeding disorder, hemangioma, urticaria, skin lesions, meningococcal disease, birthmarks, etc. and these conditions should be ruled out. Maculopapular lesion, bruises, bites, cuts / lacerations, thermal injuries/Burns, fractures, head injuries, Intra-abdominal injuries, petechiae/ecchymosis, etc. suggest physical abuse.

INVESTIGATIONS

Investigations as per the type of abuse and physical findings should be obtained. Multiple cross references should be obtained as required from gynecologist, psychiatrist, counselor, ortho-pedic surgeon, etc.

- Basic blood profile and parameters to ascertain nutritional status and deficiencies
- X-rays and skeletal survey is done in a case of multiple injuries or fractures and in all cases if a child is below 2 years.
- Multiple bruising entails a detailed hematological profile including bleeding and coagulation profile.

    Neuro-imaging and ultrasonography of abdomen are indicated in a case of head and abdominal injury respectively

    - Forensic samples maintaining the chain of evidence include skin, hair, clothing, saliva, oral and genitourinary secretions in acute sexual assault

    - STD screening including low and high vaginal (in post-pubertal girls) swabs and urethral swabs in boys and serology for HIV, hepatitis B and syphilis are done in case of acute sexual assault, penetrative abuse or vaginal/urethral discharge

- Pregnancy test in an adolescent girl.

MANAGEMENT

The following form important goals of a pediatrician's response:

1. Immediate goal is to ensure safety and provide emergency care if needed.
2. Comprehensive medical assessment includes history taking, examination and investigations. All should be documented.

42

3. Short-term goals include providing immediate emotional (counseling) and social support to the child and family and treating physical problems like injuries, providing immunization, STD prophylaxis and emergency contraception.

4. Long-term goals include complete physical and psychosocial well being of the child. They also ensure his reintegration into the family and social system.

Immediate response in an acute presentation is needed if the child is brought serious or with a life-threatening injury or with acute sexual assault and has to be reported within 24–72 hours of the abuse. The child will need emergency care and the police would require immediate forensic samples to book a strong case against the abuser. Such cases are best managed in a government hospital setting. However, the following steps need to be taken:

• Immediate hospitalization in an intensive care setting.
• Brief history with stabilization of vital parameters.
• A written complaint to the local police station or appropriate authority in the hospital as per the protocol.
• Definitive treatment with proper documentation of injuries and swabs in case of sexual assault
• Referrals to gynecologist and orthopedics and general surgeon.

It is mandatory to report the abuse to the Police and other Social Service agencies like Child Welfare Committee (CWC) and Child Helpline (#1098) or local NGOs may be contacted if the parents refuse to follow the treatment plan or if there is an immediate threat to safety of other sibs. CWC and child helpline can also be contacted in any case where child rights are violated like neglect, child labor, corporal punishment at school, child marriage, etc.

The definitive medical management would depend on the general condition of the child and the extent of injury. After the initial management it is important for pediatricians to refer families for additional assessment and treatment if psychological abuse or neglect is suspected.

The pediatrician should network and form a local child protection group to respond appropriately to child abuse. Such a group could easily be formed in the local medical college, as all the health personnel are available under one roof. Social worker should lead the networking between different professionals as well as parents. The team members should include:

- Social worker
- Police
- Lawyer
- Pediatrician
- Psychologist and psychiatrist
- General and orthopedic surgeons
  Gynecologists
  Forensic experts

42

Counseling of parents and informed consent becomes the responsibility of pediatricians after evaluation. Relevant authorities must be notified. Treatment and rehabilitation of these children is of utmost importance and all care should be taken to prevent ongoing abuse.

Hence, all pediatricians should assess suspected harm with the same thoroughness and attention as they would do with a life threatening condition. Poor management after disclosure can increase psychological damage. Pediatrician should believe, support, reassure, treat and ensure rehabilitation of victims of child abuse.

ROLE OF A COUNSELOR

It is important to observe the child's mood and affect during the entire examination period. A series of immediate emotional reactions may be observed as a result of abuse and would include denial, shock, anger, frustration, guilt, blame, shame, sadness and horror.

Counseling of the child and family forms the corner stone of the management. The immediate counseling of the child that can be done by the pediatrician should focus on the following:

- Believe the child, reassure and absolve feelings of guilt/blame
- Explain about the existence of a medical, family and social support system.

- Listen carefully to all fears and concerns associated with disclosure.
- Teach coping and assertive skills.

Counselor should develop approaches for asking children about their relationships with caregivers, experiences of discipline and feelings of self-worth, safety, and being loved. This might include an assessment of parent–child interactions through the use of interviews or consultation with other clinicians, such as mental health providers, to assess the child's feelings and understanding about the situation.

Children showing signs of behavioral and psychological problems should be assessed to identify specific conditions, such as depression or post-traumatic stress disorder for which specific age appropriate therapies should be administered on a long-term follow-up.

42

Consequences

Long term medical consequences of acute abuse could be head injury, severe bleeding, shock and death in severe cases.

However persistent child abuse may lead to failure to thrive, developmental delay, permanent physical disability, pregnancy and transmission of STDs/HIV along with psychological disorders.

Late behavioral manifestations include externalizing and internalizing behavior patterns. The child may show disgust, revenge or desire for punishment, self blame and post-traumatic stress disorder. Personal and social adjustment problems include weak inter-personal relations, poor social interactions, criminal behavioral tendencies and unconventional sexual behavior.

PREVENTION OF CHILD ABUSE

Role of Pediatrician

- Pediatricians need to consider child abuse as one of the differential diagnosis in case of assault, unexplained injury, etc.
- They have an important role in prevention, treatment and rehabilitation of cases of child abuse.

- Regular screening for abuse can be done during routine immunization visits or during other follow up medical visits. These visits can also be used for sensitizing parents for identifying early signs of child abuse.
- Regular seminars and workshops can be organized for the parental groups over the weekends to explain the parents the concepts of positive parenting.
- The parents can also be taught the effective disciplining methods with the help of behavior modification techniques.
- It is important for Pediatrician to network with counselors and teachers for creating community support and awareness.
- Pediatricians should encourage schools to implement effective and supportive interventions to prevent child abuse in any form.
- Pediatrician should also report suspected cases of maltreatment and abuse to the appropriate authorities.

ROLE OF PARENTS

Most of the parents complain about the challenges of bringing up children in today's world. Most parents teach their child walking, eating, alphabets and numbers, but fail to teach the basic safety rules. Parents need to be aware of the normal development and behaviors of the children at different ages. This would empower them to strategize their responses.

Awareness among Parents

This should include building awareness among parents about the following issues:
- Age appropriate child behavior and development
- Non abusive discipline strategies
- Effective communication skills with children and rapport building
- To accept an assertive 'no' from children
- To avoid enforced physical contact of children with relatives or friends for 'social purposes'
- To build self esteem of the child
  Studies have conclusively revealed that the abuser is most often from family or a known person in the home or familiar

Good Touch, Bad Touch

Use simple animated images of a boy and girl with bathing suits on to teach parts of the body:

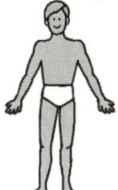 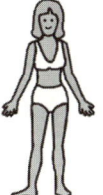

Good Bad touch

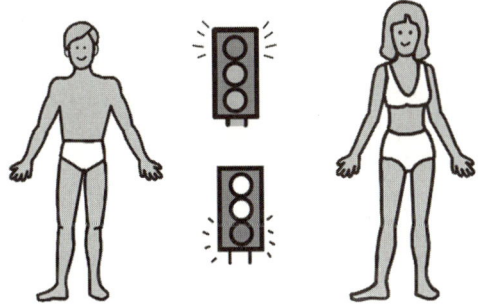

There are parts of our bodies which are good for people to touch.

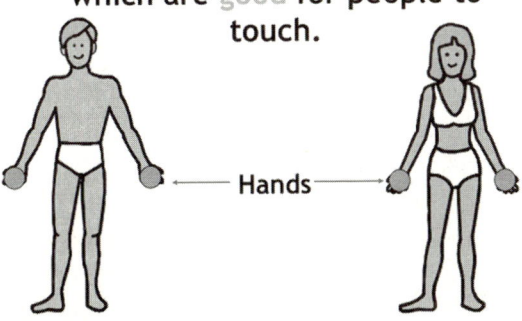

Hands

42

There are parts of our bodies which we might not like **people to touch.**

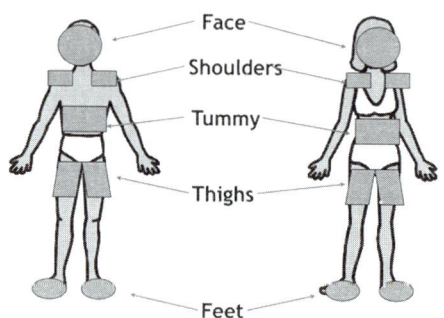

42

There are some parts of our bodies which are bad to touch. These are private parts and we should not touch anybody there or have them touch us there.

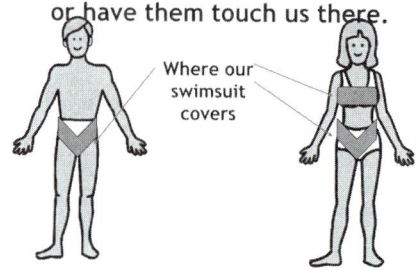

Where our swimsuit covers

Do you remember all the good, ok and bad **touches?**

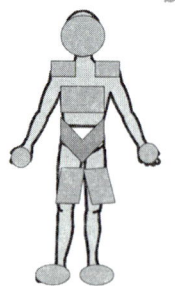 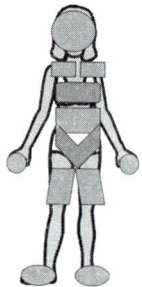

environment yet parents chose to instruct the children about the potential harm a stranger could cause them. The parents need to teach the children about understanding their bodies and how to respect them. A clear guide about appropriate behavior with regards to self and others is a must.

These concepts and behaviors' have to be taught with proper age appropriate play methods or stories to the children. The concept of good touch and bad touch is helpful and can be taught in a very non-threatening manner. Many videos are available online and can be viewed with the child along with meaningful discussion. Also it is very important that the children are taught the proper response when they encounter any threatening situation. The parents need to be available to respond and help the child. Also the rapport building is needed so that your child can share all the secrets with you.

42

Parental preparedness is the key in prevention as well as identification of child abuse. Daily conversation with the children with reference to their whereabouts is helpful. Parents with teenager's children are usually more anxious and need to be more vigilant. It is helpful to track their friends and the places they hang around. Some children may not voice any protest verbally but may show some subtle changes in the behavior which can be taken as RED FLAG SIGNS.

The significant behavioral changes could be

- Changes in diet pattern, loss of appetite, or trouble eating or swallowing or sudden changes in eating habits
- Poor school performance
- Sudden mood swings: rage, fear, anger, insecurity or withdrawal includes fear of certain people or places, nightmares, trouble sleeping, or other extreme fears without an obvious explanation,
- Stomach illness all of the time with no identifiable reason,
- Sudden appearance of bed-wetting or thumb sucking,
- Adult-like sexual activities with toys or other children, new words for private body parts, resistance to bathing, toiling, or removing clothes,
- Talking about a new older friend,
- Suddenly having money, toys or other gifts for no apparent reason,

- Cutting, burning or otherwise intentionally harming herself or himself, i.e. drug use, alcohol abuse, sexual promiscuity,
- Running away from home,
- Depressive symptoms and negative self image.

INTERNET AND CHILD ABUSE

Internet along with the availability of unsupervised content is a double edged sword. It is the responsibility of the parents that they should be able to unveil the mysteries of Adolescence in a healthy manner. Internet should not be the answer to their numerous dilemmas. It simply distorts the facts and adds confusion to their young minds. Addictions to easily available pornography sites are common but dangerous for a healthy sexual development. The parents need to be watchful and limit the access to the kids.

42

With the growing use of smart phones among teenagers, the awareness and perception of the real life dangers has sharply reduced. Parents need to talk about the potential dangers at different situations and help them judge situations and people.

CHILD HELPLINE 1098

In 1996 Childline India Foundation has launched the country's first toll-free tele-helpline for street children in distress. We need to make children and community aware of these services and encourage them to use them in case the child finds himself in a dangerous situation and also to use them for other children in distress.

ROLE OF SCHOOL AND TEACHERS

What seems to be hugely missing today is the lack of sensitivity with which the child abuse cases are handled by school authorities as seen in the widely reported 2014 case of sexual abuse in the Bengaluru School. The school authorities, Teachers and other staff members cannot brush off the responsibility for the complete well being of the child in the School campus and during transit.

While working with a case of suspected abuse by a senior teacher in a Government school, I gained some insights. The students of secondary section were interviewed separately while the teachers also had to fill in a questionnaire regarding the suspected Teacher's behavior. Most of the children reported the objectionable behavior of the teacher, while all teachers except one young and brave lady said nothing had happened. Later, after the case was concluded it was found the teacher has gotten away with his abusive behavior for last 15 years and no one had ever complained.

Another case of severe abuse which I witnessed way back during my residency and have left a long lasting impact. Jasmine was brought to the casualty of the busy municipal hospital with severe swelling and bleeding of the face and subconjunctival hemorrhage. The reason for this injury was physical abuse by the math teacher. Jasmine had an underlying bleeding disorder.

42

WHAT SCHOOLS CAN DO

- Conducting workshops for students with age-appropriate content right from pre-primary level unto secondary level.
- Life skills especially self-esteem, assertive and communication skills need to be taught to all adolescents and children.
- Training of teaching and non teaching staff should be mandatory with regards to identifying child abuse and reporting the same.
- Child abuse cell to be constituted with PTA participation and school counselor and few senior teachers.
- Background check during staff recruitment and also for other associated services.

Role of pediatricians is very important as they are involved with care of the child from birth to adulthood. There is a need to increase awareness and sensitization among pediatricians for child abuse. High index of suspicion should be maintained while evaluating a child with suspected abuse or where some pointers of abuse are found.

Empowering the children and their parents with the knowledge about child protection and personal safety is the need of the hour and is in fact the 'key' to eradicate the menace of child abuse from the world.

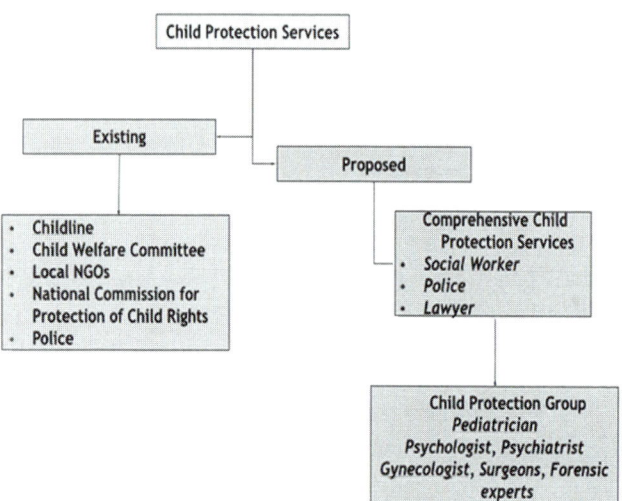

42

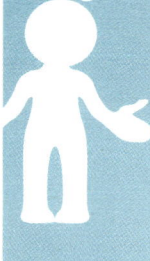

Points to remember

1. Child abuse is a misuse of power by adults over children that endangers or impairs a child's physical, mental, sexual, emotional health and development.
2. In most cases the abuser is known to the child.
3. Child abuse and sexual abuse can have devastating long term, physical and psychological consequences on the child.
4. Education and awareness about child abuse, neglect and sexual abuse should be given to parents, teachers.
5. Parents should implement non abusive discipline strategies, effective communication skills and rapport building.
6. Concept of Good Touch and Bad Touch should be taught to children.

FURTHER READING

1. Jyotsna Tiwari. Child abuse and Human Rights Vol 1: Current trends in child abuse

2. CK Parikh. Textbook of Medical Jurisprudence, Forensic Medicine and Toxicology

3. Asha Bajpai. Child Rights in India: Law, policy and practice

4. D SM-V-TR: Diagnostic and Statistical Manual of Mental Disorders 5th edition

5. Ministry of Women and Child Development, Government of India Study on Child Abuse: India 2007

6. Diane E. Papalia Human Development 5th Edition

7. Indian Academy of Pediatrics Child Rights and Protection Program manual 2007—Training of Trainers

8. Recommendations on recognition and response to child abuse and neglect in the Indian setting. Kiran Aggarwal, Samir Dalwai, Preeti Galagali, Devendra Mishra, Chhaya Prasad, Anjana Thadhani and Child Rights and Protection Program (CRPP) of Indian Academy of Pediatrics (IAP) Indian Pediatr 47(6):493-504 (2010)

9. Incidence, type and intensity of abuse in street children in India. Mathur M1, Rathore P, Mathur M. Child Abuse Negl.2009 Dec; 33(12):907-13. doi: 10.1016/j.chiabu.2009.01.003. Epub 2009 Nov 7.

10. Psychological MaltreatmentRoberta Hibbard, MD, Jane Barlow, DPhil, Harriet MacMillan, MD, and the Committee on Child Abuse and Neglect and AMERICAN ACADEMY OF CHILD AND ADOLESCENT PSYCHIATRY, Child Maltreatment and Violence Committee

11. The Pediatrician's Role in Child Maltreatment Prevention Emalee G. Flaherty, MD, John Stirling Jr, MD, The Committee on Child Abuse and Neglect

12. Recognizing and Responding to Medical Neglect Carole Jenny, MD, MBA, and the Committee on Child Abuse and Neglect

13. Clinical Report—The Evaluation of Sexual Behaviors in Children Nancy D. Kellogg, MD, Committee on Child Abuse and Neglect

14. Evaluation of Suspected Child Physical Abuse Nancy D. Kellogg, MD, and the Committee on Child Abuse and Neglect

15. Maltreatment of Children With Disabilities Roberta A. Hibbard, MD, Larry W. Desch, MD, and the Committee on Child Abuse and Neglect, and Council on Children With Disabilities

16. The Problem of Child Sexual Abuse in India, Laws, Legal Lacuna and the Bill – PCSOB-2011, J Indian Acad Forensic Med. April-June 2012, Vol. 34, No. 2 ISSN 0971-0973, Review Research Paper Alok Kumar, Asha Pathak, Sandeep Kumar, Pooja Rastogi, Prateek Rastogi

42

17. Prevalence of Violence against Children in Families in Tripura and Its Relationship with Socio-economic Factors, Sibnath Deb, Subhasis Modak, J Inj Violence Res. Jan 2010; 2(1): 5–18.,doi: 10.5249/jivr.v2i1.31

18. Child abuse,Neha Gupta, N.K. Aggarwal, Delhi Psychiatry Journal Vol. 15 No.2 October 2012

19. http://www.tulircphcsa.org

20. www.prevent-abuse-now.com

21. www.stopitnow.com

22. www.protectkids.com

23. www.childlineindia.org.in

42

43 Parenting of An Adopted Child and Selection of Day Care Centre

Shrikant Chorghade

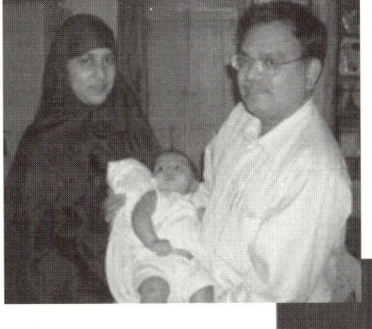

A couple, who is having a genetically transmittable disorder or parents who are infertile and eagerly want a family, turn to adopting a child. Many times couples having their own biological child, volunteer to adopt a child as a social responsibility. All such parents must be aware that parenting an adopted child is a difficult task. In India, normally no parents feel it necessary to know about their task of parenting, or to approach a counselor before becoming biological parents. It is never thought of. But in my opinion every couple must approach a counselor before taking a decision of becoming a biological parent or before adopting a child.

The decision of adopting should always be well thought of process. There are some aspects which adopting parents should be aware before they finally decide on adoption. They must think of following probabilities which are as follows:

1. It has been found that adopted children are likely to have more emotional problems and learning difficulties than biological children. This is not to scare the adopting parents but to make them aware that adopting children need systematic thoughtful parenting and adoptees must feel loved and secure with adopting parents, if they desire a favorable outcome.

2. Adopted children being genetically unrelated are likely to be different in looks, intelligence and personality. This may invite derogatory comments from known people or strangers. Adopting parents must be aware of these facts so that these things should not come to them as surprise.

3. By the time adopted children reach adolescence they start thinking and may become curious to know about their roots. This curiosity to know their biological parents may cause them stress and they may be keen to try to meet them. When the adopting parents come to know of this situation they are likely to be stressful and irritated. Inability to trace the biological parents may also be stressful to the adoptee and result into behavioral aberrations. Parents should not become anxious, on the contrary should help the adoptees in tracing their heritage if possible. Ideally if the adoptees come to know about the adoption between the edges of three to four years they easily assimilate the fact without emotional turmoil. In spite of such a gesture if during adolescence adoptee is keen to find out its root the adopting parents need not be resentful or feel insecure. They must accept and understand that it is natural for the adoptee to have curiosity about their roots. The adopting parents need not volunteer but should try to help in tracing the roots if the adoptee desires so; without being panicky, anxious or resentful about it.

4. A biological sibling in a joint family or a small family may be favored more than an adoptic if adoptee lacks in

43

performance or if biological siblings have a better performance. The parents of adoptee are likely to get disturbed. They may regret their decision of adoption. Adopting parents must always remember that putting undue stress on performances or grades or marks in schools is unnecessary. It is never a permanent affair. Ups and downs, successes and failures are a part of life. They need not blame themselves for the failures or underperformance of adoptee. On the other hand they should accept the adoptee in spite of his or her performance and always try to encourage and motivate the child to do better. Parental emotional stress is likely to be reflected in their approach toward adoptee and may make the adoptee anxious or depressed.

43

5. The attitude of the biological siblings in the family of an adoptee may cause friction amongst children and may disturb the emotional harmony in the family. The adopting parents need not get disturbed. They should accept the friction as a normal behavior of children. Even biological siblings do have differences, friction and fights.

6. The rejecting attitude of relatives and outsiders towards adoptee may emotionally disturb the adoptee and the adopting parents. Such disturbance in emotional harmony should be accepted in a proper stride and the adoptee is to be given assurance of being loved .This will help the adoptee to accept and digest the insults.

7. Senior generation in a joint family is likely to have traditional thinking which makes them believe that adoption is a family disgrace .Some grandparent, relatives, neighbors and outsiders may demean, criticize, insult or reject the adopted child and adopting parents. Such occasions should be treated as a litmus test for the adopting parents. These are the occasions to console the adoptee and offer love and affection more intensely.

All the Adopting parents must anticipate these matters and think over how to maintain their confidence and grit while facing such occasions. They must strongly believe in their decision to adopt. Adopting parents must convey to the adoptee from time to time that they selected him or her willingly only because they liked him or her. Loving an adoptee and conveying unconditional love and affection is important part of parenting an adopted child. The love and affection should frequently be conveyed to the adopted child in words and action. Parents must anticipate disturbing moments, insults and experiences and be ready to face them firmly. Every child has to go through negative experiences. The frequency may be more for an adopted child as compared to biological children. Assurance of parental love and affection of adopting parents will give emotional strength to the adoptee. Adopting parents must know and execute authoritarian style of parenting, which will help them in experiencing parenting as a pleasant job.

43

Selecting A Day Care Centre

With industrialization the size of families is gradually shrinking. A couple with one or two children has become a universal family structure. India is no exception. In urban India nuclear families is the order of the day. When both parents are working, the child in the family needs somebody to care and nurture. Presence of grandparents will give tender loving care to the child at home. In absence of grand parents, a caretaker is assigned the job. Availability of a trained care giver is rarity. Uneducated women untrained in childcare may be available for the job. If they are not available option for the parents is a day care centre. Such centers are mushrooming in many cities. The care taker looks after the feeding and recreation of the children under care, in absence of parents. The owners or proprietors of such centers are not trained in child care. In such cases the child is likely to be neglected, undernourished and emotionally deprived. The parents must be selective in choosing a day care centre to ensure best care of their child in their absence.

Child care has become a developed science. A child grows very fast in first 3 years after birth. What every child needs is fulfillment of it's needs, viz. food, shelter, love, security and opportunities to learn fulfillment of these needs will ensure child's optimum growth and development. The child also needs extra care and medication during illnesses. All these parental responsibilities should be satisfactorily shouldered by the day care centre as long as the child is in their custody.

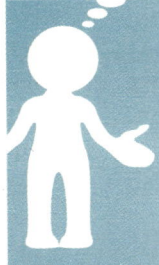

Points to remember

1. Every couple must approach a counsellor before taking the decision of adopting a child.
2. Adopted child may differ in looks, intelligence and personality which can invite unwanted or derogatory comments which the parents should know.
3. Curiosity of the adoptee to find the roots of biological parents can create tension, anxiety in the parents but instead they should help the child to find the biological parents.
4. Giving unconditional love and sense of security to the adoptee as much as to the biological sibling is equally important.
5. Parental responsibilities should be satisfactorily shouldered by the day care centre as long as the child is in their custody.

43

44

Single Parenting

Santosh Nimbalkar, Zafar Meenai

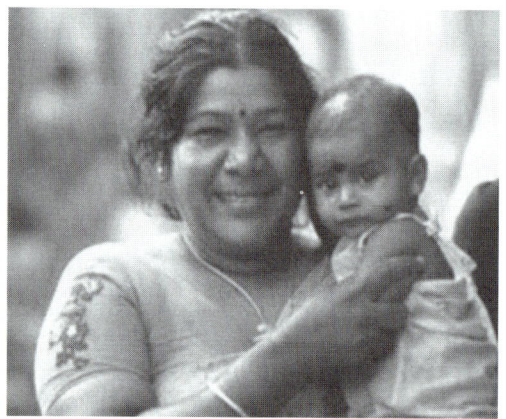

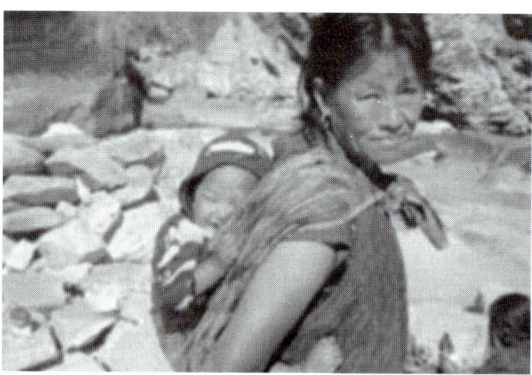

INTRODUCTION

A single parent is a parent, not living with a spouse or partner, who has most of the day-to-day responsibilities in raising the child or children. A single parent is usually considered the primary caregiver, if the parents are separated or divorced; children live with their custodial parent and have visitation or secondary residence with their non custodial parent.

Historically, death of a partner was a major cause of single parenting. Single parenting can result from separation, death or divorce of the couple with children. A mother is typically the primary caregiver in a single parent family structure because of divorce or unplanned pregnancy.

Fathers have been the less common primary caregiver in the past, presumably due to the father working most of the day resulting in less bonding with the children, or possibly a young child needing to still nurse, or if childcare was necessary while the father works, the mother would be seen to be better suited while father work. This scenario has shifted in the recent years as many fathers are taking a pivotal role as a stay-at-home dad as more mothers are in the workforce and being the sole provider to the family, resulting in fathers bonding and connecting more to their children.

DEMOGRAPHICS

In the United States, since the 1960s, there has been a marked increase in the number of children living with a single parent. The 1960 United State census reported that 97 of children were dependent on a single parent, a number that has increased to 25% by the 2000 US census. In 2000, 11% of children were living with parents who had never been married, 15.6% of children lived with a divorced parent, and 1.2% lived with a parent who was widowed. In 2010, 40.7% of births in the US were to unmarried women.

About 16% of the children worldwide live in a single parent household. In the UK, about 1 out 4 families with dependent children are single parent families, 8 to 11% of which have a male single-parent.

PRIMARY CAREGIVER

In the United States, 80.6% of single parents are mothers. Among this percentage of single mothers, 45% of single mothers are currently divorced or separated, 1.7% is widowed, and 34% of single mothers never have been married.

Cultural definition of a mother's role also contributes to the preference of mother as primary caregiver. Children will lean more towards mothers because of their protective nurturing characteristics, from a long established mother child relationship from early on attachment beginning at birth and continuing as the child grows up. In addition to their traditional protective and nurturing role, single mothers have to play the role of family providers as well, since men are the breadwinners of the traditional family, in the absence of the father the mother must fulfill this role while also providing adequate parentage. Because of this dual role, in the united states, 80% of single mother are employed of which 50 % are full time workers and 30% are part time workers.

Father as Primary Caregiver

In the United States today, there are nearly 13.6 million single parents raising over 21 million children. Single fathers are far less common from single mothers, constituting 16% of single parent families.

The number of single father has increased by 60% in the last ten years and is one of the latest growing family situations in the United States. 60% of single fathers are divorced, by for the most common cause of this family situation. In addition, there is an increasing trend of men having children through surrogate mothers and raising them alone. While fathers are not normally seen as primary caregivers, statistics shows that 90% of single fathers are employed, and 72% have a full time job.

A father must take time to be a dad as well as a friend, disciplinarian, a shoulder to cry on, dance partner, coach, audience, adviser, listener and so much more. In addition to there qualities, the single father must take on the role of the mother, a role that extends deep into morality, devotion and the ability to set up an educational yet nurturing environment. Thus it is the father's role to be a source of both residence and strength, and love and compassion.

Causes of Single Parenting

- **Death of a partner**: Historically death of a partner was a common cause of single parenting. Diseases and maternal death not infrequently resulted in a widower or widow responsible for children. At certain times wars might also deprive significant numbers of families of a parent.

- **Divorce:** In 2009, the overall divorce rate was around 9/1000 in the United States. Along with this, it has been shown that for the past 10 years or so, first marriages have a 50% chance of ending in divorce. And, for other marriages after a first divorce, the chance of another divorce increases. In 2003, a study showed that about 69% of children in America living in a household that was a different structure that's the typical nuclear family. This was broken down into about 30% living with a step parent, 23% living with a biological mother, 6% with grandparents as care givers, 4% with a biological father, 4% with someone who was not a direct relative and a small 1% living with a foster family.

44

Although all agree that divorce affects children, there is a controversy whether this is positive or negative.

Children undoubtedly need a family structure to develop into mature and productive adults. However there is much debate as to what equals a complete family. Some define a complete family as that which "Consists of a father, mother and their children living in a state of greater geographical, economic and social independence from other relatives and kin. Under this definition, a single parent home would not be categorized as a family. Not only is there the absence of one parent, but also members are often geographically separated from their primary family and because of this detachment are limited in their social interactions. Further more single parent families have trouble providing financial independence for themselves.

However, many challenge this definition of the traditional family, claiming that a family is made up of people who love and emotionally support each other. Those who defend this definition, argue that it is the affection and feelings of the people and not the structures of the family that is significant.

Since many single parent families work very well, lovingly nurturing children full capable of happiness and success, there are parent households which undoubtedly qualify as a family while a household headed by two indifferent and uncaring parents does not necessarily form a family.

There is further debate on the action of divorce itself. The advocates down that happy parents equal happy children. Their argument is that children are perceptive and sense the tension in their parent's marriage. This turmoil in turn makes the children unhappy. They further argue that happy parents are more patient and have more time for their children. Thus there are many who believe that the parents should stay together for the well-being of the children for emotional support adamantly arguing that children are important, that they don't grow up well unless we bring them up, that our needs can't shoulder theirs aside, that commitments and responsibilities to others have to take precedence over personal gratification, that nothing is more important than to see children flourish.

Some people believe that the effects of divorce on children are neither always positive nor negative but depend on the individual situation. One study showed a relation between how the child perceives the divorce and the child's behavior. Kids with a negative perception of the divorce showed larger incidents of behavior and self - esteem problems. On the other hand, children with positive allusions demonstrated less anger aggression. Thus, there are no absolute answers as to the effects of divorce on children.

- **Unintended pregnancy**: Some out of wed lock birth are intended, but many are unintentional. Where out of wed lock births are accepted by society, they may result in single parenting. A partner may also leave as he or she may want to shirk responsibility of bringing up the child. This may result in a negative impact on the child. Where they are not acceptable, they some times result in forced marriage, however such marriages fail more often than others.

In the United States, the rate of unintended pregnancy in higher among unmarried couples than among married ones. In

1990, 73 % of births to unmarried women were unintended of the time of conception, composed to about 44% of births overall.

Mothers with unintended pregnancies and their children are subject to numerous adverse health effects, including increased risk of violence and death, and the children are less likely to succeed in school and are more likely to live in poverty and involved in crime.

Single Parent Adoptions

Single parent adoptions are controversial. They are, however, still preferred over divorces, as divorced parent are considered an unnecessary stress on the child. In one study, the interviewer asked children questions about their new lifestyle in a single parent home. The interviewer found out that when asked about fears, a high proportion of children feared illness or injury to the parent. When asked about happiness, half of the children talked abut outings with their single adoptive parent. A single person wanting to adopt a child has to be mindful of the challenges they may face, and there are certain agencies that will not work with single adoptive parents at all.

Single parents will typically only have their own income to live off and thus might not have a back up plan for potential children in case something happens to them. Traveling is also made more complex, as the child must either be left in some one else's care, or taken along.

SINGLE PARENT ADOPTION IN INDIA AND ITS LAW

According to Juvenile Justice Act that was amended in 2006, adoption means, "The process through which the adopted child is permanently separated from his biological parents and becomes the legitimate child of his adoptive parents with all the rights, privileges and responsibilities that are attached with the relationship.

- In India all adoption issues are handled by the Central Adoption Resource Authority (CARA), an autonomous body governed by the Ministry of Women and child Development.
- A minimum age difference of 21 years between the single mother and the adopted child is required if they are of opposite sexes.

- A single parent should be between 30 and 45 years in age if she wishes to adopt a child in the group of 0–3 years.
- The upper limit of the child older than 3 years is 50.
- In single parent should have an additional family support.
- According to the rules the adoptive parent has to be both medically fit and financially settled.
- According to the Hindu Adoption and Maintenance Act of 1956 Indian citizens who are Hindus, Jains, Sikhs, or Buddhists are allowed to adopt not more than one child of a particular sex.
- For foreigner, NRIs and those Indian nationals who are Muslims, Parsis, Christians or Jews, according to the Guardian and Wards Act of 1890, the parent only acts as a guardian till the child atains the age of 18.

Problems Faced by Single Indian Women who want to Adopt

1. **Adoption Agencies:** Despite these being low wherein single women in India are allowed to adopt, there are still many agencies across the country that make it tough for single women.

2. **Family:** A practicing child psychiatrist, with an adopted child of her own, went on to tell me that she knows of a few divorced single mothers who "Faced the greatest obstacle from their own parents who said that they were being selfish for not providing a father to the adopted child and that they should re-marry soon." As the idea of two parents raising a child has been so ingrained in our minds, it's tough for anyone to accept single motherhood very easily.

3. **Society:** Society's views are very narrow minded and everyone wants know about the where abouts of the father. Unfortunate but true. Thus, begins the battle for respect by most single mothers in India.

4. **Schools:** A few institutions have mandatorily implemented the use of the mother's middle or maiden name during admission. But there are still many who refuse admission when the child does not have a birth certificate and a father's name.

44

5. **Work-age:** The transition from being an independent "freedom enjoying" woman to one who begins to share her life with another life is not easy. Motherhood is a demanding role even in homes where a partner might be available to pitch in with the household chores. While co-parenting has its own challenges, single parenting can also cause a lot of stress to the single mother. After a hectic day of work when single mothers might long for moments of solitude, they find themselves often burdened by guilt.

Support for Single Women Considering Adoption in India

1. **NGO:** Many NGOs help single women in India to cope with this change in their lives—joining one might help to form support group of other like minded women who could share their experiences and advice.

2. **Read:** Book's on adoption can act as good guides.

3. **Internet:** The constant availability of chats and information sharing on various groups globally on the web help a lot. For example PEOPLE'S GROUP FOR CHILD ADOPTION IN INDIA" has over 700 online members who offer mentoring to those planning to adopt.

4. **Prepare well:** The sceptism of adoptive agencies as well as the doubts raised by others will reduce when they see how well prepared, committed and confident you are in adopting a child. Evaluate your financial status minutely so that you are able to show the agency exactly how you plan to provide for your child in the future. Prepare yourself mentally to welcome a new person in your life.

To all those women who have embraced motherhood through adoption, a huge round of applause. Your choice is heart warming indeed.

44

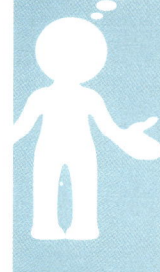

Points to remember

1. Single parenting can result from separation, death or divorce of the couple with children.
2. Unintended pregnancy may result in single parenting.
3. Single mothers are more common than single fathers.
4. Single parent has to play the dual role to meet the demands for the child's overall development.
5. Non-fulfilment of expectations of the child of single parent can have adverse behavioural problems and he/she may become non-social or antisocial.
6. Single parent adopting the child faces problems from adoption agencies, family, society and schools.
7. Juvenile Justice Act, 2006, Hindu Adoption and Maintenance Act, 1956 are laws concerned with adoption in India.
8. Central Adoption Resource Authority (CARA) of the Ministry of Women and Child Development handles adoption cases.

FURTHER READING

1. Divorce and its effects on children—stacy snow don.
2. Single parent, around the world—The New York Times.
3. "One parent families"—Australian social trends.
4. "About Single Parent". Single Parenting, April 23, 2011
5. Integrated child protection scheme.
6. Adoption laws in India.
7. Central Adoption Resource Authority.

Section

7

Adolescent

Adolescent Parenting in India Issue Based

JS Tuteja

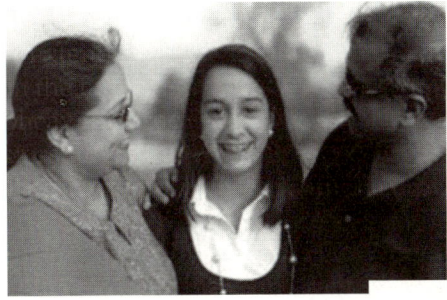

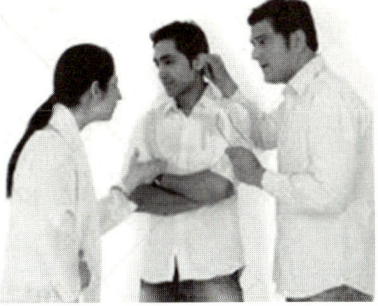

In adolescence various biological, cognitive, emotional, and social changes take place, affecting the parent–child relationship. Therefore, it seems necessary to clarify which factors influence attachment in this particular period of life. Changes in parent child relations during adolescence may differ cross-culturally due to different developmental pathways which may be characterized by the culture-specific concepts of independence or interdependence in our country. It is widely held that the development of autonomy is an important task in adolescence.

Adolescents become more independent from their parents, while peers gain in importance. Separation of adolescents from their parents, today individuation is seen as a dual process of separation and connectedness: Parents grant more independence and at the same time they remain an important source of support and advice for their adolescent children.

The traditional Indian parenting is shaped by the cultural and religious values of the country, generational wisdom, and life experiences. The goal of parenting is comprehensive development of children and it integrates the cognitive, emotional, and spiritual components of an individual's growth. It includes both the personal and social dimensions of human growth and development.

45

In Indian parenting children are brought up in an atmosphere of emphatic richness. The supportive environment of the joint family system provides support and encouragement to parents. The parent-child bond is established from breastfeeding that provides not only nutrition to the baby, but also allows increasing physical contact between the mother and the child which is remembered for the whole life. Cuddling adds physical contact between the mother and the child and also provides a sense of security for the child. The strong emotional bond established between Indian parent and child during early childhood is said to be everlasting.

Indian parenting is a value-based system. Deference for authority in social relationships is an expected behavioral norm. People are bound up by their duty to family, to parents, to children, and to society. The authoritarian type of Indian parenting limits individual autonomy and growth at various levels. Overprotection by Indian families inhibits assertiveness and prevents to develop their own identity in society. Physical punishment, tolerated in traditional Indian parenting, is said to have long lasting emotional scars on children.

India is a land of diverse traditions, all rooted in the same value system. With the trend of joint families still prevalent in India, a child is brought up in an environment where child learns to value people and relations. More than taking care of the physical growth of the child during her younger years, a grandmother in the house plays a vital role in instilling the moral values in the child.

The Indian parenting style builds the respect for other people, their values and customs. Indian parents believe strongly that their child is part of a family and a community and that it is of prime importance that the child realizes that every decision.

1. School Base Problem

Adolescents often have a hard time adjusting to new situations in schools due to unfamiliar teachers, rigid schedule of the school for which they are usually not familiar. When feeling overwhelmed, teens may express their emotions by becoming argumentative, fighting in family with other children in family or with classmates, or withdrawing into themselves. Parents can find it difficult to keep calm in such situation but they should not lose themselves in anger when things don't go right.

Let us think about proper goals that parents can work to improve situation in school for the teens. They can plan to strive to help their teens and to feel to be more successful.

Approach of Parents

A) Keep eyes open

Sometimes parents notice that something is not right with a teen and they get distracted. Parents are usually very busy, it's fact and near to the truth. They have great pressures and responsibilities pulling themselves to too many directions. The teen who seems a little 'off', not to himself, snappy or more quiet than usual is trying to tell something which can be used by parents. Parents usually notice and recognize few signs/ symptoms in teens but they are so occupied, that they are unable to pay attention in right time to help their wards.

Parents should not allow problems of their teens to grow and should observe teens when they seem sad, withdrawn, distant, more moody than usual, or angry. Should recognize if there seems to be greater confrontation among children, if friends stop calling or coming over, or if the teen can't seem to find his place in school. It is necessary for the parents to know all aspect of teen in right time so that situation can be handled in proper time to prevent them from anger and aggression.

45

b) Maintain relationship with teachers

Parents should visit to meet teachers before the teen land up in trouble, few parents feel that teachers are opponents of teens but they fail to understand that teachers are always there to help their teens to grow in better way; they are there to groom your teen.

If parents think that there are some issues then one should organize meeting with teacher and understand how the problem can be solved in harmony. It will be best on the part of parents to ask for the solution from teachers for the existing problem rather then accusing them.

45   Usually teachers would go for extra mile to extend their support to the teens if they find that some body in the family is sick, family going in financial crisis, family upheaval or the problems of children in family. As these all factors affect the teen's future in respect of academics and social intelligence.

c) Motivating teens for social skills

Teens to be successful in life should excel equally in academics and socially which should be encouraged by parents and teachers equally. School is a place where teens are there for maximum time of the day, where they can learn how to get with others and knowing how to develop friendships. If the teen is well adjusted and happy in school premises with his friends—teen will excel in academics or vice versa, so it is the duty of the parents and teachers to help teens in all fields of life so that they can stand with confidence in life to face any situation.

Approach!

It is best to be done by teaching life skills to teens.

a. Maintain rules and follow through with explaining consequences.

b. Fix meals time and bedtimes that establishes stability.

c. Teach him how to put oneself in shoes of others and learn their difficulty.

d. Teens should learn how to express frustration, disappointment and anger without hurting feelings of others.

e. Set basic rules of conduct: no hitting, kicking, biting, spitting, and not hurting others through words even which are always remembered.

d) Opportunity to become independent

By gaining life skills and becoming self-sufficient teens—they grow more confident in their abilities. You can watch their self-esteem take off. Every year teen should be able to point out with confidence to a new skill or additional responsibility that comes with rising age.

Approach!
- Teaching teens to pick out their clothing, dress themselves as they grow older, tie their own shoes, pack school snacks, make lunches the night before, set their own alarm clocks.
- Allow teens to complete puzzles and feed himself on his own and as he grows, to do his homework and projects by himself.
- Have your teen help around the house and gain responsibilities instead of waiting to be served.
- Teens can help with putting away laundry, setting and clearing the table, helping to serve guests, and keeping their room in order.

e) Teaching communication to teens

Teens should never be afraid of speaking with family members on any topic in any situation—may be very difficult or untoward. Parents should shower their love to them even in adverse situations—unconditional love. Teens should have faith and trust in parents that they are always available whenever they are in need.

Daily interactions with teens, sharing a smile, a good word, a laugh, a story, or a meal together. The main thing is that you put the time and energy in so that he knows that he matters in your life.
- Talk to your teen every day, may be for few minutes.
- During communication with teen do not use your gadgets, electronic appliances.
- Have an eye contact with teen which makes sure that your are interested and concern about him, it will help when teens

45

are with lower grades. It shows that you are actively listening them to solve their problems. During communication ask few questions too.

- Speak with your teen with excellent soothing tone and words.
- Express your love every day, no matter how tough the day was!

Parents should feel in their hearts that they have tried their best to help their teenagers to navigate the road of life successfully when they were standing on cross roads of life.

2. Understanding Your Teenager

45

Teenage is the age of stormy emotions in everyone's life. An age when anger and frustration takes over every form of emotion is a teenager's life. It's also the time when parents may feel that their caring teenager no longer respects them. Indeed it's not a fact.

It's just that these teenagers go through different sets on emotions in their growing years and parents need to patiently deal with them. Parenting the adolescents isn't as difficult as it appears.

a) Communicate with them

It is only when they find a good friend in their parents that they start communicating. A good way is to have open conversations with them when they are small children.

b) Develop trust

Teenagers always cherish an assurance from the parents. During their initial venture into the real world, they may never like to hide anything from their parents. The need for secrecy only arises when the begin feeling that their parents are suspicious about them.

C) Encourage teenagers

It's an age when teens have the tendency to cling to their friends more than their parents. Instead of being jealous of this development, invite your teen's friends at home. In that way you will get to know whether your teens are in a good peer group or not. If you realize that you teen have some negative company, slowly compare that particular friend with other good friends and ask your teen to judge.

d) Point out their mistakes

Occasional anger and punishment only benefits in groom your teen to be a better individual. If you notice a serious mistake, point it out to your teen without any mercy. If you have already established a good relationship with their temperaments, they will come to you and admit their mistakes.

e) Be their role model

It's age of confusion and so it's always a good idea to give them a realistic view of things and life ahead. Give them a clear idea of the vast opportunities of all academic and society at large.

45

3. Performance in Examination

Academics are given an extra amount of importance by Indian parents. They fail to understand that extra-curricular activities are essential for a teen's wholesome development. Parents need to recognize a teen's talent and help him move towards it. It's important that parents and teens work in mutual cooperation to avoid feeling of examination stress. Parents' are usually in anxiety and restlessness; the situation can be detrimental for teens.

Parents must always exhibits that they are there for their them, it's important that they stay away from doing a few things like going over the question papers again and again, as well as continuously discussing the score that they want their teens to meet.

How Teens can Help Themselves

a. Discuss not just the highs and lows of studying. Keep them in the loop about your issues and difficulties.
b. Do not create unrealistic goals. Instead, set reasonable daily targets and try to achieve them.
c. Do not allow pressure from peers. Find the difference between friendly advice and a brag that a friend might throw

at you. At the end of the day, you are your own judge and answerable to yourself.

d. Always feel proud and happy of a task well done.

It is the duty of parents to encourage teenagers to take the path of their interests so that they can excel in life academically and socially.

4. Talking About Sex

- Understand what your teen is actually asking you. It may happen that your teen wants to know something else and you're answering a completely different question before answering it is better to see in their eyes and body image.

- Today's teens have excellent grasping power and if you use language that's not proper for the age, teen might grasp it and talk in a similar language to their friends. Use a language that is extremely decent and easy to understand so that your teens are not confused or shocked knowing what you've just said.

- Teens usually convey to their friends about what they have learned from parents. So it is always necessary to tell them not to share information which they have received from parents.

- Always be careful when talking to teens—consider their psychosexual maturation.

- Teach your teens about the boundaries in physical intimacy to prevent them from sexual abuse which is rising in our country.

- Teach them about protection if they are involving in physical intimacy.

- Promote teens to develop assertiveness and self-esteem.

- Teens with religious inter-connectedness' are less involved in premature sex, it is better to promote them to be involved in religious congregations.

Parental love and affection are much needed and desired by teenagers in rearing process; parents should understand that they are making the teens overtly dependent on them. An adolescent often stops pursuing his dreams and follows his parents' dreams if in early years of his life, his creativity is restricted. Parents need to understand that after an age they need to start becoming their teen's friends than being their protectors as they can then help their teen to   grow better.

Parental interference is not just limited to deciding the career options but also includes deciding their future family life. Teen must be independent enough to make his life future decisions on his own and should be ready to face the consequences. In era of highly competitive world, an individual must be determined enough to take his own decisions and this is only possible if his parents inculcate this habit right from one's primitive years i.e. building years of the individual, things learnt at this stage help shape a person's mind and character.

45

Points to remember

1. Indian parenting is a value based system which builds respect for other people, their values and customs.

2. Conversely the authoritarian type   of Indian parenting limits individual autonomy and growth at various levels.

3. Parents should communicate effectively with the teachers. Discuss the problems so that they together find solutions to the child's problems.

4. Teach children the life skills which include effective communication, interpersonal relationship, problem solving and decision making. He should be taught to have empathy.

5. Observe, monitor, encourage, and don't be indulgent. Let him be independent. Counseling   rather than advising should be done.

FURTHER READING

1. INDIA: Parenting Styles, East vs. West
   http://www.worldmomsblog.com/2011/07/07/india-parenting-styles-east-vs-west/
2. Parent and child relationship-parenting skillshttp://timesofindia.indiatimes.com/life-style/relationships/parenting
3. Parenting and adolescent attachment in india and germany1
   Isabelle Albert, Gisela Trommsdorff & Ramesh Mishra
4. Parentinghttp://www.aish.com/f/p/5-Parenting-Goals-for-Every-Family.html?gclid=CM6BooeF_78CFZUVjgod4yEAew
5. Parenting In India: Is It Hindering For The Growth Of A Child Or More Productive When Compared To The Western Ways? #Debate 15th October, 2012 **With:** 3 Opinions-Priyanka Vaid/Nayan Bhatnagar:
6. Traditional Indian parenting practices http://www. indiatribune. com/index.php?option=com_content&id=4357:-traditional-indian-parenting-practices&Itemid=462

45

Adolescence and Defiance

Preeti Galgali

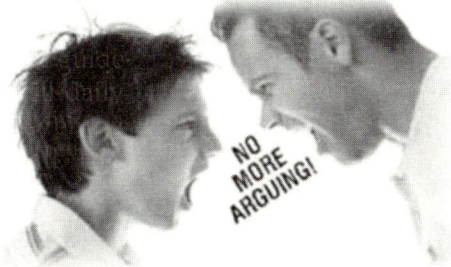

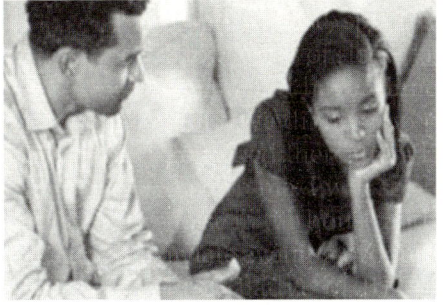

First understand, and then be understood!

—Stephen Covey

WHAT IS DEFIANCE?

For practical purposes defiance by a teen is defined as resistance to follow previously taught rules of conduct and failure to comply with an adult's request within a reasonable time. Teen defiant behavior includes use of disrespectful language, incomplete school work, failure to contribute to household chores, indulging in late night parties, sexual promiscuity, violence, aggression, drug abuse and all such behaviour that adults often term as 'risky', 'irrational', 'crazy', 'immoral' or 'Irresponsible'.

Is Defiance in Teens Normal?

One of the primary developmental tasks of adolescence is independence and formation of a unique identity. And the main task of parenting is to ensure that the adolescent grow into responsible emotionally stable independent young adult. Though most parents will love to have adolescents who are 'xerox copies' or clones of themselves, in reality this is far from truth. And rightly so, because then we would have dredging monotony and no progress in the world! So teenagers should begin to question their parents, should seek more freedom and should develop their own thinking. Infact a 'little' defiance in adolescence is desirable! Parents should not stifle such normal behaviour and thought process. Instead they should guide their teens lovingly and gently, express the family rules and expectations clearly with lucid reasoning, assist them in decision making and are there to hold their hand, even when they fail/fall sometimes!

Defiance is a problem if the teen's behaviour is much worse than those of his age or if it is interfering with his functioning at home, school or with peers or if it is causing a lot of emotional distress or harm to the teen or parent. Such defiance is nerve-wracking and creates havoc that disrupts the functioning of the entire household. In this article, the word 'defiance' will refer to the 'problematic defiance'.

What are the Causes of Defiance?

To tackle defiance appropriately, it is important to know the factors responsible for it. These interrelated factors are as follows:

1. Characteristics of teens

Some teens have a 'difficult' temperament. They are impulsive and get easily frustrated. Some are physically challenged and a few are diagnosed as attention deficit hyperactivity disorder, depression, bipolar disorder, anxiety, oppositional defiant disorder, conduct disorder, substance abuse or suffering from child abuse. All these conditions adversely affect teen thinking, emotions and behaviour leading to increased defiance.

2. Characteristics of parents

Some parents like their adolescents may be high strung and emotionally labile and manage their anger poorly leading to increased aggression and defiance in their children. A few parents may be suffering from chronic physical or mental health disease like diabetes, cancer, depression, attention deficit, substance abuse that may not leave them with much energy to deal with maturing teens and their developmental issues. Their distressed mood and poor communication may trigger defiance in the teen. Some parents may be perfectionists and fail to appreciate their teen's efforts and magnify mistakes. Their attitude sets them on the path of confrontation with their teens.

3. Family environment

Family stressors in the form of financial problems, divorce, marital conflicts and violence or professional pressures may not allow some parents to spend 'quality and quantity' time with their teenagers. They are often irritable, short tempered and inconsistent in implementing household rules. This results in defiance in the teenager.

4. Parenting style

Authoritative parents shower unconditional love on their teens and have the right balance of control and authority. They nurture compliance in their teens and have a strong bond with them. Such parents are accepting, firm and democratic. They lay down clear boundaries in terms of family rules, limits and expectations and consistently enforce positive discipline. Defiance amongst teens is common if parents follow authoritarian, permissive or neglectful styles of parenting and use abusive methods of disciplining like demeaning, calling names, hitting, slapping and kicking.

How Should Parents Tackle Defiant Teens?

The basic principals to deal with defiant teens are discussed briefly in the next few paragraphs. The interested reader can go through the suggested reading section at the end of this article for an in depth discussion of the management techniques.

1. Be knowledgeable about normal adolescent development

It is said that forewarned is forearmed. A few conflicts are normal in adolescence. Parents should be 'ready' to handle conflicts and failures in an empathetic, respectful and non abusive manner during the adolescence period. They should negotiate more and dictate less. They should avoid using the phrase—".... because I said so!" Questions asked by the teen should be answered with reasoning in a calm and reassuring manner.

2. Identify and manage factors that contribute to defiance

Parents must look into the various factors (enumerated above) that may be responsible for defiance in their teens. They may consider seeking help from health professionals and supportive family members in seeking solutions. Out of the four aforementioned factors, the parenting style is the most amenable to change. The next few points will emphasise on the authoritative parenting 'essentials' that are needed for deftly handling defiant teens.

3. Make a list of negotiable and non-negotiable rules

Parents should form a list of rules and discuss the same with their teen.

Non negotiable rules are strict rules that a family feels are needed for living in a civilised household. The list of negotiable and non negotiable rules is highly 'individualised' as it varies with each family according to its values, beliefs, expectations, culture and customs. For a particular family, 'contributing to household chores', 'no drugs or alcohols', 'no violence', 'no foul language', 'doing Pooja (prayers) everyday' may form a list of non-negotiable rules. The implementation of some of the non-

46

negotiable rules should be negotiable. For example, if doing household chores is a non negotiable rule, how much, when and what is to be done by the teen should be open to negotiation. Such a rule would be followed much more easily and happily by the adolescents than the one in which, their opinions are not sought for.

Some rules that should not be considered negotiable are usage of drugs even though the teens may insist that the other parents are allowing their children to do so. The parents should counsel the teen in a gentle but firm way about the personal risks Vis-à-vis rewards of such behavior and teach them appropriate skills to handle negative peer pressure.

46

4. Spend one-on-one time

Parents should make a habit of giving undivided attention to their teen for at least 15 minutes everyday. This 'fun time' could be spent in chatting, walking or playing. During this time, parents should refrain from criticism and concentrate on bonding with their defiant teen. Sometimes parents get caught in the cycle of negativism and dread to spend time with the teen that further aggravates defiance. The special time between the parent and teen will enhance communication and positive feelings.

5. Establish consequences for behavior

A behavior that is appreciated will be repeated is the dictum. Teens love being appreciated and more so a defiant teen who is always scolded and criticised. Any good behavior, even if it is considered 'insignificant' by the parent should be genuinely appreciated. For example, if a teen promptly gets a glass of water when asked for, the parent should respond by saying, "I like it when you help me. Thank you!" Such a reaction will go a long way in winning compliance from a defiant teen. A parent who fails to pay attention to good behaviour and is quick to reprimand bad behavior will find that his/her teen will vie for this parental attention, by repeatedly showing defiance as even 'negative' attention is preferred over 'no' attention.

For teens with severe defiance problems, tangible rewards like CDs or extra TV viewing time may have to be instituted to maintain compliance. Penalties in the form of withdrawal of privileges (restrict TV/computer usage, outings with friends, etc.) or grounding may have to be imposed in case the adolescents persist in breaking rules. The reward and the penalty system should be discussed with the teen prior to its implementation.

Defiant teens usually have problems in completing school work. Inculcating healthy study habits is the first step in dealing with this problem. Teachers should work closely with parents to ensure compliance in completing home assignments. They should form a system of daily or biweekly home–school report system in which the problem behaviors and appropriate consequences for compliance and non-compliance are listed.

6. Use effective communication and negotiation skills

The parent should use both non verbal and verbal skills effectively to communicate with adolescents. They should never humiliate or degrade the teenager. They should verbalise requests and commands, clearly and precisely. Parents should face the teenager and make appropriate eye contact while communicating with them. Defiant teens fail to comply with vague poorly worded commands. Short requests and comments have a greater impact factor than long lectures. Using the word 'I' is better than using accusatory 'you' while conversing with defiant teens. For example if a parent finds the bed of the teenager untidy, he should avoid saying words that may escalate anger, "You dirty boy! You have no sense of cleanliness!" Instead he should calmly reword it as, "When I returned after a tiring day at office, I was upset to see your bed still unmade." This may make the defiant teen to respond in a more empathetic desirable way.

Negotiation skills in the form of problem solving are useful if the defiant teen is motivated to make a desirable change in behaviour and is keen to seek solutions in collaboration with parents. Here the problem behavior is listed, various solutions are brainstormed, evaluated and the best solution that is acceptable to both parents and teen is selected and implemented. A feedback is later elicited to evaluate the success or failure of the chosen solution. If it is a failure, another back up solution is

46

picked up. Involving the adolescent in problem solving facilitates compliant behavior.

It has been proved by research that defiance amongst children increases with age and should be handled appropriately at the earliest. In case parents and teachers are not able to tackle defiance, they should not hesitate to contact a mental health professional. The old adage 'A stitch in time saves nine.' holds good here. If childhood and teen defiance is managed poorly, it can lead to antisocial and delinquent behaviour in adulthood. But more than 80% of teen defiance is known to respond to a well researched parent training program, provided it followed to the 'T"! Parenting is definitely the key in managing teen defiance.

46

Points to remember

1. Be knowledgeable about normal adolescent development.
2. Authoritarian, permissive or neglectful styles of parenting use of abusive methods of disciplining causes defiance.
3. Family stressors in form of financial problems, divorce, mental conflicts results in defiance in the teenager.
4. Spend one-on-one time.
5. Use effective communication and negotiation skills.

FURTHER READING

1. How to Talk so Teens will Listen and Listen So Teens Will Talk Adele Faber, Elaine Mazlish Harper Collins, 2006.
2. The Parenting Journey Gregory Moffat Praeger, 2004.
3. How to Talk so Kids will Listen and Listen So Kids Will Talk Adele Faber, Elaine Mazlish Harper Collins, 2000.
4. Your Defiant Teen Russell Barkley, Arthur Robin the Guilford Press, 2008.
5. A Parents Guide to Building Resilience in Children K. Ginsburg, M Jablow American Academy of Pediatrics, 2006.

Behavioral Problems in Adolescence

Shrikant Chorghade

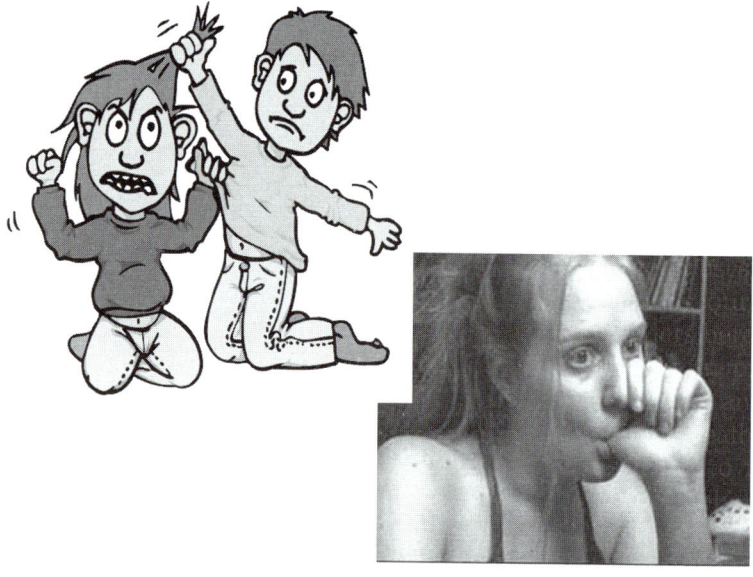

Till the end of nineteenth century in India, the family pattern used to be a joint family. Large number of children with different age groups in a family used to mix up and play with each other. The older children used to play the role of parents and teachers for the junior children and teach them the social and moral values and their roles in the society. The boys in the family usually used to take over the business of their parents and the transition from childhood to adulthood used to be a smooth affair. The term and state of adolescence never existed, so also did the behavioral problems of adolescence.

Adolescence is a gift of twentieth century where indus-trialization and urbanization started all over the world. The family pattern started changing gradually. The family size started shrinking and number of nuclear families started increasing. Formal school and college education was introduced and concept of family business started becoming obsolete. The children were required to take formal education to get an employment. All these factors were responsible for creation of stage   of adolescence between childhood and adulthood. In developing countries like India where industrialization and urbanization started later, the adolescents in these countries were described as "adolescents in adolescent countries".

47

Adolescence is name given to a period in human life when the childhood is over and adulthood has not yet arrived. It is described as a period between beginning of sexual development and end of physical development. It is roughly a phase between ages of ten years to eighteen years. Psychologists have described this period as the period of "Psychological turmoil". It has also been poetically described as "Child's mind in adult's body", viz. a period when human body has size and shape of adult but mind and thinking of a child. Erik Erikson (1902–1994), a clinical psychologist specialized in psychology of adolescents, described the period as "A period of identity crisis". The word 'Identity he meant ego identity while by 'Crisis' he meant turning point. This is the period when adolescents are in search of the answers to the questions related to own identity like "who am I"? "What is my role in life"? "what am I going to be"?.

During the period of adolescence the children feel that they are grown up but parents and seniors around treat them like children. They get a feeling that parents are always indulging, probing and asking unnecessary questions about their activities and movements. Different people around express different opinions about the same adolescent. When the parents praise them for their obedience and mannerism, their peers ridicule them for being shy and conservative. Such diverse opinions lead them to confusion about their identity.

Adolescents in same age group have different patterns of physical developments. Some boys and girls put on disproportionate weight in early adolescence and look plumpy and obese; at the same time some of their peers in the same age group increase in height faster and look skinny and bonny. Therefore, in a given adolescents' peer group of same age, there is variety of body forms. This difference in body size, shape, structure and forms in the peers confuses individual adolescents giving them a feeling of inferiority complex when they compare themselves with their peers. Sexual development also occurs during this age which has different patterns for different adolescents. Some boys may get moustaches and beard early when some others of same age group have a baby like clean shaven look. In boys the quality of voice changes. It becomes hoarse and deep. This change in voice also may appear at different ages in the same peer group.

In the same way some girls have breast development at early age while others of same age group are still flat chest. The age of beginning of menstruation also varies from one girl to another in the same peer group. These changes related to sexual development are due to hormonal changes. These hormones have psychological effects making the adolescents over anxious and emotional. Heightened emotions make the adolescents moody and unduly sensitive, which intrigues the parents.

This is the period when the children have to make choice of their career. Their academic performance may not match with their aspirations, leading to frustration. All these factors combined, lead to a state of stress and confusion. The adolescents have many unanswered questions and unsolved problems, but do not have maturity to handle them.

Developmental psychologists advice the parents to change their perception about behavioral problems in adolescents. They should perceive them as "adolescents having problems".

The common problems in adolescents with which their parents report to me are listed below.

1. Disobedience
2. Adamancy
3. Argumentative
4. Temper tantrums
5. Violent behavior
6. Restlessness

7. Neglecting studies

8. Watching television for long hours

The teachers also may have following complaints:

1. Doesn't complete homework

2. Disturbs other children

3. Truancy

Some adolescents may be having speech disorders like stammering and stuttering, while some adolescents may be having enuresis and encopresis without organic defects; the cause being unresolved stress. The list may extend longer but only common problems are enumerated above.

There are some problems which need urgent attention of the parents.

1. Progressively declining scholastic performance

2. Isolation

3. Addiction

4. Rash driving

5. Criminal activities

6. Attempt to suicide

7. Frequent expressions like "I want to die"

As has been expressed earlier adolescents having behavioral problems are to be treated as "Adolescents who are not finding solutions to their problems and they are disturbed and frustrated". Punishment is never a solution. Some solutions are with parents, while others need referral to pediatricians, psychologists and counselors.

What parents can do?

1. Parents should be able to convey love in words, facial expression, body language and action

2. Healthy parenting of an adolescent includes paying attention to the child without being indulgent.

3. Being involved in adolescent's life to the extent of creating an atmosphere of friendliness

4. Establishing positive communication which will help in satisfying the curiosity and difficulties in an adolescent.

5. Keeping a watch on tendency to material desires and addiction.

6. Parents should set examples by their behavior, which will give them value and moral education.

The adolescent who is disturbed due to identity crisis is considered as problem adolescent by the parents and they too get disturbed due to the behavior of the adolescent. The pattern of behavior of the adolescent arouses concern and discomfort among parents and caretakers. The aggressive reactions of the parents are likely to disturb the adolescents further, complicating the issue. Parents should be able to accept the adolescent whatever he or she does or behaves. They should try to create a congenial atmosphere in the house and have positive communication. This will encourage the adolescents to open up freely and express his or her concerns and anxieties which may help the parents to mellow them down.

The parents should understand that, ultimately adolescents themselves will solve their own problems. What they need is a feeling of being loved by the parents and feels secure in the family.

Summary

The number and severity of behavioral problems in adolescents go down as the adolescence progresses and as the identity crisis is resolved. Vast number of complex interacting factors which include genetically earned skills to resolve stress, the parental behavior and attitude, the family environment, the peers and friends, decide how and when the problems will be resolved. Each adolescent has his or her unique personality structure which decides the resolution of the problems? The most adolescents seem to have little trouble in coming to satisfactory resolution. The role of parents is to offer them support, health, love and a feeling of security.

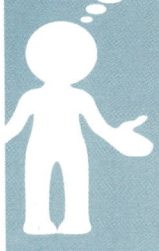

Points to remember

1. Common behavioral problems in adolescence on, disobedience, argumentative, temper tantrums, violent behavior, restlessness, neglecting studies, watching television for long hours.

2. Problems which require urgent attention are —scholastic underachievement, isolation, addiction, rash driving, criminal activities, and suicidal ideation.

3. Parent should be role model. Establish effective verbal communication and nonverbal communication in form of facial expression body language and action.

4. Be friendly—observe and monitor the adolescent's activities. Be non-indulgent.

47

The Way to Success Try, Succeed and Tell All

Hemant Joshi, Archana Joshi

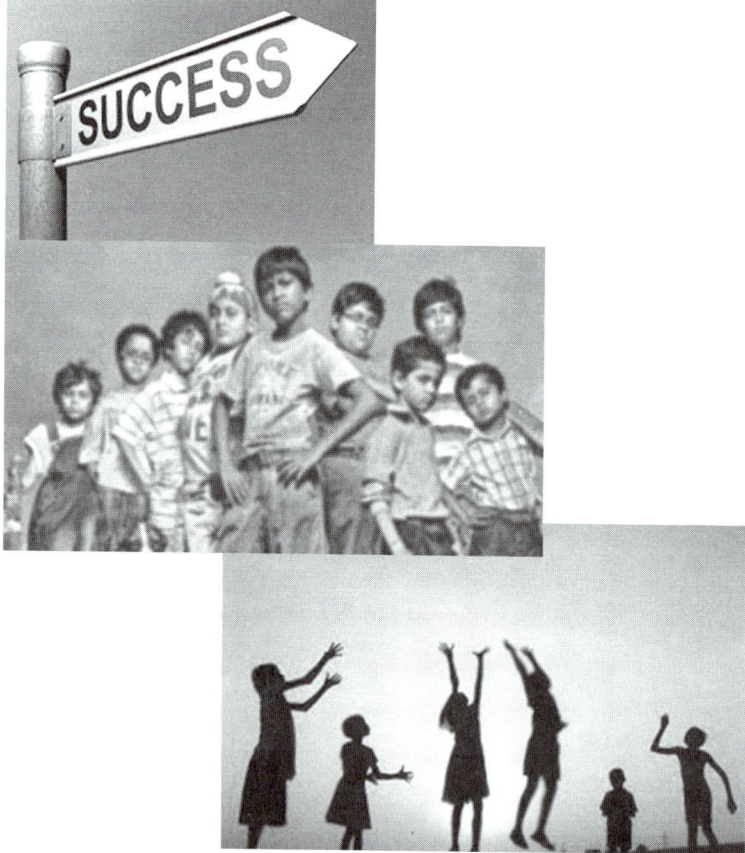

This write up is based on lessons learned from Mr. Bhishmaraj Baam's Marathi book Maarg Yashaacha. You should read all his books. He is guru of all Indian world sports champions. These ideas have created successful players. In Cricket, Snooker, Billiard, shooting Tennis, Table tennis, Badminton etc. Rahul Dravid, Om Agrawal, many shooters, and many others have benefitted. We all must learn this, succeed and tell all.

To succeed, we need sound body and sound mind. Something no one teaches. All Olympic winners use these ideas. These are mental exercises. They are derived from Indian art and science of mind control called Yoga, created by our fore fathers. Let us learn them, with a clean slate of mind. With full faith. Doubt nothing. With mental exercises we get control on our mind. With body and mind in control and focused on our aim, we succeed. Do, succeed, and tell all. Using this mind training, Russians won many Olympic medals. American weight lifter Charls Garfield did not believe this. That day he had lifted 300 pounds weight. After 2 hours of relaxation and mind training he lifted 365 pounds of weight. He was amazed. Later he taught this to all and wrote a book titled "peak performance."This is based on Yoga shastra. Do learn it. With Yogasana, Surya namaskar body becomes flexible. Do it in morning daily. With exercise body becomes strong. Do it daily. If not in the morning, do it in evening, or whenever you can or play in ground 1 hour daily. With mind exercise mind becomes strong. Napoleon lost war at Waterloo. He did not get help of his reserve forces. Similarly we fail when we do not use all our mental power. When we use a lens and focus sunrays, they burn paper. Similarly focused mind does super human jobs and give us success. Learn to do this. We look for errors, think about them and repeat them. Let us make a list of our good things. Our successes. Write them on wall of our room. Then they will grow. Larry Bashom was an American shooter. He scored 598 out of 600 marks in shooting. One asked him," "By which errors your lost 2 marks?" "He said I am focusing on how I got 598. So next time I will get 600. He actually did. There are many reasons to lose. There is only one reason to win. Look for your reason to win. Suppose 3 pieces of pipe are connected and water has to flow

Through it (see picture). If one pipe is small, the total water flowing will be less. Same is true about our result. In our case the first pipe is efforts done giving adequate time for training.

48

Second pipe is our skills, and third pipe is our self confidence, our self image, our opinion about us. This third pipe, self image usually is small. Let us make it big. If our self image is good, at the time of viva, match or interview or discussion, we are relaxed and confident and we win.

Develop a good self image as follows

1. Write diary daily. In beginning, write down all the good things you have done. List all successes. This makes the base for future successes.

2. Do mind training for success

48

Visualize your success in mind. Suppose you have to go for a viva, interview or group discussion, visualize that you are performing well in that. Once our guru Bhishmaraaj Bam was in bed for 4 months with sever back ache. Doctors asked him to severe leave sports and do operation. He daily visualized that he was improving. He rapidly recovered and became champion in shooting. All world champions use this technique. One surgeon uses this for his surgery. We do not succeed without focusing our mind fully on our aim. And our mind always wanders here and there. In past and in future. But our body is always in present. Link mind with body. For this learn Pranayam and Tratak. These are yogic kriyas. When we focus on our breathing the mind comes back to present moment. Let us learn to focus mind on breathing. Take long breathes comfortably. Imagine that as we breathe in the air rubs at tip of the nose and make noise as "SO". As we breathe our air rubs at the tip of the nose and makes a noise "HAMM". Together it becomes "SOHAM". Focus mind on that and mind comes to present moment. When a leopard relaxes on a tree branch, his 4 limbs hang down limp like dead limbs but his eyes are alert. We should be able to relax like that. This relieves our tension. A relaxed mind performs best. A tense man can make errors. One orphan tiger baby was being raised by a herd of sheep. He was behaving like sheep. One tiger took him to water and showed him his face and told him that he was a tiger. Always keep a small mirror and tell yourself that you are a winning tiger. And then go and win. Every moment. Use Yogiraj Bhagawat's following yoga system to relax and improve concentration. Yoga says, we have 27 power centres in body.

They are

1. Right foot
2. Right calf
3. Right thigh
4. Left foot
5. Left calf
6. Left thigh
7. Abdomen below naval
8. Naval
9. Heart
10. Right lung
11. Left lung
12. Right shoulder
13. Right arm
14. Right forearm
15. Right hand
16. Left shoulder
17. Left arm
18. Left forearm
19. Left hand
20. Mouth
21. Nose
22. Right ear
23. Left ear
24. Right eye
25. Left eye
26. Forehead
27. Top of head

48

The power centers are in centre of these parts. For training, go in shawasan or sit. Keep back straight. Focus mind on first centre and say a mantra 4 times or you can also say "My right foot is relaxing." 4 times. Then go to next centre and say my right calf is relaxing, 4 times. Then go to next centre. Thus, 27 × 4 = 108 times we say the mantra and our body becomes a chain of 108 counts. With this our body relaxes. The tension goes, concentration improves. We can say any mantra, like Hari om, or

Hare rama hare rama rama rama hare hare,
Hare krishna hare krishna krishna krishna hare hare.

Tratak (stare)

Tratak means staring at a steady object without blinking eyes. One can stare at a point or a leaf or om written on wall or at a flame of a lamp. Staring at a steady lamp flame is considered good. Sit in front of a lamp at a distance of about 1 meter. Keep flame at eye level. Sit comfortably with back straight. Possibly in Vajrasana or Padmasana, or cross legged, or in a chair. Now focus your mind and eyes on the flame. Do not blink eyes. They will pain and will want to blink. Blink once, in beginning. Tears will roll down. First you will be able to stare for small time. Gradually this time increases. Increase it up to 15 minutes. This is called as external tratak (staring.) Now close eyes and try to see the same flame, with closed eyes. Initially different colours and pictures will come in front of your eyes, but gradually you will see the flame. Now focus on this and see it as long as possible. This is internal tratak (staring). Tratak improves concentration. Pranayam: This is Naath panth's Amrut Pranayam. Do it as follows.

Sit on a chair with back touching back of the chair or sit with back resting on a wall or a pillow. This way we can sit for long time, keep back straight. Now first take a few deep and long breathes. Every time empty lungs fully. When you breathe out, take abdomen in. This empties lungs fully. Next, take a comfortable long breath. While breathing say Hari om 8 times. Use fingers to count. Then breathe out through mouth, making "O" of lips as we will make for whistling. Say *hari om* 16 times while breathing our. With practice fix this proportion of 8 and 16. Instead of *hari om* one may just count numbers. This is one pranayam, add 3 to your age. We should do pranayam this many times. While breathing in, imagine that all worlds' power is entering our body and staying there. While breathing out imagine that body's all bad things are going out. This pranayam improves our health, mood, eliminates doubts and makes us successful in all we do. Learn from this example. Next time while

48

worshipping god, when we offer flower, loudly say 'I am offering flowers. While saying that we cannot think of anything else. Our mind gets focused on what we are doing. Whenever you are doing one thing and thinking of something else, say loudly what you are doing. Anderson was world shooting champion. While shooting he would say to himself "the sight is correct". No other thoughts could disturb him. "All is well" is similar sentence. Make a sentence useful to you and use it and improve your concentration. Prepare for interview, group discussion, exam match, etc. as follows:

1. Why are you giving this interview? Write on a paper or your mobile, 2–4 sentences.

2. What sacrifice have you done for this? Like, left home, stayed in hostel, studied so many, etc. Write in 4–5 lines.

3. Now imagine and see that you did the best, the way you wanted in the interview, group discussion, examination, and match.

4. After the event you are telling your friend how it happened. In this you describe how skillfully confidently your mind and body responded. How all praised your performance and celebrate your success?

48

Print or make 4–5 copies on a thick paper. Keep each paper where you may see it easily. Paste it on wall in your room. Read it with full concentration, whenever you get time. Read it loud and record it on your mobile. More you read, hear this, more benefit you will have. When you read this it will create the right visual image? It will boost your self confidence. Negative thoughts will disappear. You will know for yourself, what you want and you will succeed. If we do a thing we like, and do it by our choice, we do it best. If it is forced no one succeeds. We should do the job we love or love the job we do. And do our best. After our mind and body are ready to work for the job we have undertaken the scarcest resource is time. Suppose you have a fruit tree garden. And there is scarcity of water. Then you will plan and give water only to your chosen fruit trees and not waste it. Our time is like this water. Always scares. Devote it to your aim. Always make a plan. Plan your act and act your plan. Plan your work and work your plan. How many weeks, days, you have in hand, and how will you use them? Make a plan and follow it. Make a diary and write it. Then you will improve daily. If you do not observe or write, you will not improve. Take your one hour. Write down following things.

1. What gave you happiness in past.

2. Whose opinions are important to you?

3. Your aim.

4. How much time, efforts, money, etc. you will need

5. Then plan how to do it. One week is good time span. To plan and do and assess.

48

Review progress every week

Do not work only on your aim. You should also pursue other interests of life. Keep time for relaxation, TV, etc. Keep away from bad habits like drugs, liquor. They give momentary happiness. Then they enslave, destroy and kill you young. Write this Robert Frost poem on wall. Nehru had it. "Woods are lovely dark and deep but I have many promises to keep, Miles to go before I sleep, Miles to go before I sleep." "Every moment I will do my best" if we tell our mind this only then it will do so. Laziness, lack of interest and doubts, spoil jobs and aims. At the time of examination, interview or match, we must know that blessings of our parents and best wishes of our well wishers are with us. This helps us to succeed. So while going for exams or a match, always touch feet of parents, and take their blessing. Remember those blessing at the time of match and interview and your best performance will happen.

Bunch of Ideas

Use this to put all your ideas together on any topic. This helps to make a plan to win, to write an essay, or give a speech or for group discussion or to plan your life or career. At centre of a paper write the main topic. Suppose you want to decide your future career. So in centre of page you write words future career. Make a circle or box around it. If it is a box, you get its 4 sides to write your 4 options. Like doing a job, or doing PhD, or doing MBA, or learning a dance diploma. You can write another 4 options at the 4 corner. Make a circle or box around them. Join them to the central box by a line. Near this each of boxes write all ideas related to word in that box. Put them in boxes or circles and connect them to relevant boxes. There will be some independent ideas. Keep them in separate boxes, not linking with any other boxes. Then mark important boxes. Make a separate bunch on a separate sheet for them. Also write down names of important people and important ideas. These bunches help us to organize ideas. While making a presentation or a speech, the ideas should come like flowers arranged in a garland. It should be like a story. One point flowing seamlessly into another. The most important points should come first, the less important later. We can also write each of all these words on small pieces of paper and then arrange them in a logical order this helps in planning a program, finalizing our aim, giving speech, making presentation, participating in group discussion. Use this bunch of ideas to finalize our aim and plan our steps to achieve it. Then follow them and succeed.

48

Quality Circle

This is mind training. Do this. Doubt nothing. It helps in Examination interview, group discussion, match, everywhere. It has helped many. Including all Indian shooters. Say this loudly & Record this in mobile. audio or video. Here again and again. Do this in Shavasan first. Then we can do it sitting in chair or even during travelling. First relax full body. Then take few full long breaths. Make your stomach/abdomen loose and take a long full breath. Then push stomach in while breathing air out. Empty chest fully. After few breaths, close eyes. Draw a circle in front of your eyes. Of a color you like. Then make a list of all good qualities you need to succeed like, will to win, Skill to win, self confidence, concentration, focusing on present moment and the job, etc. fill this circle with all these qualities. This is your quality circle. Continue imagining. Go and stand in that circle. Imagine that the qualities are entering inside you and have become part of you. Now imagine that your parents or teacher or well wisher is blessing you, saying that these great qualities are a part of you. Now you choose something like a pen or a ball, etc. which you will see when you go for the examination or interview or group discussion or match. Tell yourself that whenever you will see this pen/ball, all your good qualities will rise and help you. Then imagine that with all these good qualities you are performing well, and that you have won. And that all are celebrating your success. After this concentrate on your breathing and then open your eyes. Now you have completed one practice of quality circle. Do this often. Sportsmanship: Never be jealous. Do not burn out. Excel yourself. And be generous to praise success of others. Make friends with all. If they are hurt, tears should come in your eyes. You should genuinely be happy with their success. You should neglect their shortcomings. This will give you best friends for lifetime, which will always help you. Do this, succeed. Tell all. Reach this to 131 crore Indians in all Indian languages with the help of talking, phone, sms, email, face book, whats app, TV, radio, articles, media, etc. This is the best service to our people and the country and humanity.

Ten Easy Steps to Succeed

1. Have a desire to succeed. Only then, it will happen.
2. Do the job you like. Then life time you enjoy it. It is no more work.
3. Practice practice practice. That gives us perfection.
4. Focus on the job 100%. Sunrays focused by a convex lense burn the paper. Focused mind brings success.
5. Nothing comes without hard work. Work hard.
6. Push yourself whole heartedly. Become best in that. Just as our mothers pushed us to learn new
7. Things when we were small. Push away laziness, all doubts including self doubt.
8. Persist. Do not give up in when you have difficulties or you fail. Survive, criticism.
9. Do something valuable for others and others will return the favor. They will make you rich.
10. For Thesis. Research, practice, business, etc. have a new idea. Keep looking for it.

48

Student's Oath for Happy Life

After praying to God I take an oath to live happily. For this I will follow following rules made by our fore fathers. Lord Shriram was an Ideal person. He always kept his word. I too will always keep my word. Pitamah Bhishma lived as per his wish. He even chose the time of his death. We will become like him. We are students. We take an oath to become good students. Learning new things is our duty. We will do it well. Growing up as an ideal person is our aim. We will become the best. If we go in movies, we will be better than Abhishek Bachchan and Aishwarya Rai. In politics we will be better than Modiji and Indiraji. In sports, we will be better than Sachin, Milkha Singh and Mary Kom. To achieve this we will have a strong body and a strong mind. I will apply my mind fully to each job. Vani is the name of the speech by which I talk to myself. Often while doing one job our wani keeps talking to us about something else. This spoils the job. Every second my mind and wani will be focused on my job. Then every job will happen as if God did it. And every time and in everything I will be the best on the earth. For having a sound mind and a sound body I will get up very early in the morning at 4 a.m. Then after going to toilet and after bathing I will do Yogasana. I will do 12 Surya Namaskar daily. I will jump on the skipping rope and do exercise. Then I will learn some poetry, table's formulas, etc. by heart. Before that I will recollect what I had learned on the previous day. After this I will read the lessons that are to be taught in the school/ college. Then I will have breakfast. This should be around the Sunrise time. Thus I will be ahead of the world by 2 hours' work every day. In school/college I will learn sincerely. Whatever I do not understand I will immediately ask to my teachers. I will actively participate in all the activities of the school/college. Whatever good I know I will teach all. Whatever good others know we will learn from them. In the evening I will revise what I learned in the school/college. Thus, one lesson will have 3 revisions on the same day. And studies will be easy happy thing and there will be no tension at the time of examination. This daily schedule will make us excellent in studies and in physique. I will play outdoor games and do

48

physical work so that I sweat with exercise, playing for one hour every day. I will fetch water, wash clothes, utensil, make playground, do gardening and do all the works at home school and in society. They will make us strong and intelligent and better persons. I will have the guts to say no to bad things like smoking, drugs and everything that I do not approve and society does not approve. *Man is known from the company he keeps.* I will avoid bad company. This will save me from bad habits and bad company. Most India children are physically weak. Everyone has some of the other illnesses. Following tips will make me healthy and strong. Studies show that one liquid food a day makes children weak. So except water I will drink nothing. Eating outside the house gives illnesses. I will not eat outside the house. Lord Hanuman went around Lanka with a burning tail and the whole Lanka caught fire. A sick person is like him. He spreads illnesses where ever he goes. When I am sick I will stay home and not go to school/college. This will reduce sickness in the society and the school. I understand that going to school or a public place when you are sick is a social crime. Every day at sunset we will come home, have a bath, and do some exercise, spend some happy time with all. Students need 8 to 9 hours of sleep daily. To get up at 4 a.m. one has to sleep at 8 p.m. and have dinner 2 hours before that, say at 6 p.m. So I will have dinner at 6 p.m. There after I will sit for studies and go to bed thereafter. TV, Radio and bright light and noise will disturb me. I will see no TV. After sunset and reduce light and noise in the house and in the surrounding. I will not participate in late evening programmes. *Weekends are for overtaking.* Says Prof. Badve of BTCS Ruparel College, Mumbai. I will use weekends for revising what is learned over then week. This way of living will give me maximum benefit and happiness with minimum effort and will give me plenty of time for other activities. I will follow this and tell it to all. I will always tell truth. I will hurt no body. Physically or with words or by cursing. Even in mind. I will never steal anything. I will be happy with what I have. I will not crave to get everything. I will treat all as my brothers and sisters. For my improvement I will learn something new every day. We will live together, eat together, and learn together. Become bright and powerful, we will hate none. If someone does an error we will forgive him/her. I will always have good thoughts, good words and good deeds. May all be happy healthy and may all prosper. We will take this oath daily and give it to all.

Parent's Oath

Great parents raise GREAT children. Example Jijamata and Shivaji. We will become great parent and make our children great. Children learn by example. We will do what they should. We will not do what they should not. We will help our children to follow accompanying oath. We will not see TV. after sunset. We will do exercise with them. We will read the books that they should read. We will read their all school books and guide them. We will give more time to our children. We will daily come home early in the evening and avoid late evening programs. We will take this oath daily and give it to all. This will make India a better country.

48

Points to remember

1. Visualize success. Do mind training.
2. Capitalise on your success.
3. Planning and micro planning of the things that need to be done should be noted and followed.
4. Good nutrition and daily exercise to keep you physically and mentally fit.
5. Positive auto suggestive technique.
6. Finally, burning desire to succeed, dedication, devotion, hard work, perseverance, determination, focus, are some important ingredients of success.

49 Study Skills (How to Perform Better in School) and Stress in Examination

Jaydeb Ray, Chandrashekhar Dabhadkar, Santosh Nimbalkar

| Me Before Final Exams: | "Yes.. I got this." |
| After Exams: | OH GOD WHY |

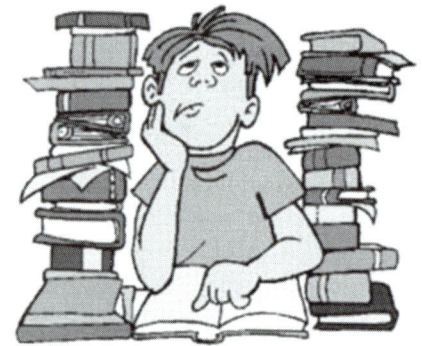

STUDY SKILLS

Learning is a tool for acquiring and developing abilities and capacities. Skill is the ability to perform a learned activity effectively and efficiently. There are many skills that can be nurtured and developed namely life skills, study skills, creative writing skills, mathematical skills, dancing skills, language skills, drawing skills, athletic skills and so on.

Definition

Study skills encompass a range of co-ordinated, cognitive skills and processes that include acquiring, recording, organizing, synthesizing, remembering and using information.

Indian Scenario

Research from India in community settings has delineated poor study habits as a major cause for poor school performance in more than 50% of the children.

Hence, it is important to inculcate good study habits in students. In hospital-based referral centre unrecognized learning disability is a major reason for poor study performance. Learning disabled children are known to benefit from remedial teaching and acquiring study skills. Latest studies from India have also demonstrated the adverse effect of low birth weight, anemia, and under nutrition, micronutrient deficiency, and poor aerobic fitness on the children's cognitive and intellectual functioning.

49

Essentials of Learning

Motivation to learn, nurturing home and school environment, balanced diet, adequate sleep and physical activity, stress management techniques and effective study skills enable children to reach their academic potential.

Motivation is the fuel that drives the engine of life. A child with high motivation to study learns study skills much more easily than a child with low motivation. To develop a high intrinsic motivation to study, the child has to love and enjoy the process of learning and imbibe the importance of education. Parents and teachers play a major role in laying a firm foundation for lifelong learning. At a very tender age, parents should nurture the feeling a "joy in learning" and teachers should further strengthen it in school.

A nurturing home environment is motivating, inspiring, encouraging, stable and supportive. Marital harmony and respect for each family member characterizes a stable home environment. In a nurturing home, the parents love unconditionally and follow authoritative parenting style with assertive communication skills. They have realistic expectations from their children. They avoid comparison with other children. They build up the self esteem of their children by acknowledging their success and help them to overcome failure. They appreciate effort and do not focus only on the end result in terms of marks scored. Parents should provide a learning atmosphere at home with plenty of interesting books and educational keys that should satisfy the child's innate hunger for knowledge. They should try to link lessons with applications in daily life. They should encourage the child to use all the three learning modalities—visual, auditory and kinesthetic.

49

The essential skills needed for schooling are the three Rs— reading, writing and arithmetic.

Concept of Multiple Intelligence

All children are not hardwired to excel in academics. Some are good in drawing while some in sports and academics. Educationists and parents should understand the concept of multiple intelligences proposed by Howard Gardner. He stated that there are different kinds of intelligence namely linguistic, logical-mathematical, musical, spatial, bodily kinesthetic, intrapersonal, interpersonal, naturalist and spiritual. Only linguistic and logical intelligence are tested by routine examination in school.

For most people, left hemisphere is associated with logical and analytical thinking and the right with creative thinking. To stimulate both hemispheres of brain, caretakers and teachers should encourage both academic pursuits and creative arts and hobbies. Parents should help children to set up SMART goals, i.e. specific, measurable, achievable, realistic and time bound goals. Career counseling for adolescents should be done on the basis of their interest and passion for a particular field.

Other Factors

A balanced diet with appropriate quantities of macro and micronutrients in form of carbohydrates, proteins, vitamins, iron, zinc, iodine, calcium and omega three fatty acids are essential for synapses, inclination and neuronal growth. Apart from ensuring fitness, physical activity also promotes neuronal growth and synaptogenesis. Sixty minutes of moderate to vigorous physical activity is recommended for all children. Sleep is the elixir for good health and memory. Each child should sleep for adequate time according to age.

Classification of Study Skills

A practical method to classify study skills is to divide then into 4 categories namely preparatory, acquisition, expression and metacognitive skills.

49

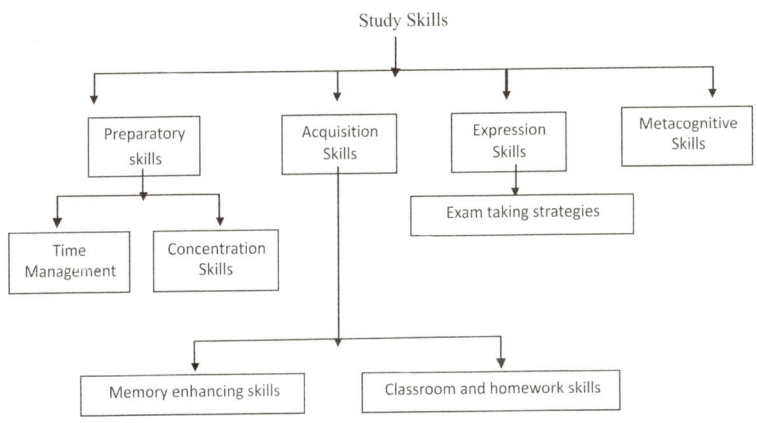

Preparatory Study Skills

Preparing skills are essential prerequisites for academic success. They enable the student to prepare for acquiring knowledge. These include the following.

Time management

Time management improves efficiency and avoids last minute anxiety. Parents and teachers can help the children to make a daily time table by asking them to list time spent everyday in sleeping, grooming, meals, school, television, meeting with friends, play and hobbies. While making a time table, it is important to leave some unscheduled time that can be used in case of an emergency. The study time can be split into time slots for revising each subject, doing home work and for extra reading. The schedule should be reviewed weekly and changes could be made according to the schedule of exams or extra-curricular or spot activities. Parents should allow children to make their 'own' time table and not dictate it to them. This will increase the likelihood of children following the time schedule.

Concentration Skills

49

Parents can help their children to concentrate better by arranging for a "Study niche" for them. It could be a separate room or even a corner of a room. It should preferably have a table and chair. Studying on a sofa or bed should be discouraged as it puts the mind in a state of relaxation and drowsiness. The study area should be free from destructions like television, computer, radio, fridge and phone. It should be well lit and ventilated. During the study time the parents should make sure that the children are not disturbed by siblings or other relatives.

It is preferable to study at the same time every day so that studying becomes an effortless enduring habit like taking a bath or brushing the teeth. Setting specific goals like planning to study one physics chapter in 40 minutes will faster concentration and focus. It has been recorded than an individual remembers best that he has read in the beginning and at the end of study period. Hence taking breaks after 40–50 minutes, helps to sustain concentration and improves memory while continuous reading causes fatigue. Parents should insist on daily revision of lessons rather than leaving the clarification to just before exams. This will help the children to be thorough with their learning.

Acquisition Study Skills

Acquisition skills develop expertise in gathering and retaining information and knowledge. These include the following.

Memory enhancing skills

There are three types of memory namely sensory, short-term and long term. Sensory memory lasts only for a few minutes and consists of what one imbibes by senses of hearing, visualizing and touch. Short-term memory lasts for one or two days. Long term memory lasts for weeks or months and even life-time.

Strategies to enhance long-term memory include the following

- Children should understand and learn the study material taught in the classroom on a daily basis. They should revise it at regular intervals preferably weekly, fortnightly and monthly to stamp it in the memory. Pre-class reading also helps in understanding the study material.
- They should use the method of association to form a mind map of the learnt material.
- Another useful technique is use of memories. For example, to remember eight planets, students can form the mnemonic - "My Very Elegant Mother Just Showed us Nine"—the pivot alphabet of each word stands for a name of the planet—Mercury, Venus, Earth, Mars, Jupiter, Saturn, Uranus and Neptune.
- SQ_3R method can be used to improve text book comprehension. SQ_3R is an acronym that stands for survey, Questions, Read, Recall and Review. First all the key points and diagrams of a particular chapter are surveyed. Then each bold heading in the chapter is converted to a question. Answers are read and then written in the student's language. Then the student recalls the answer. In the end the entire chapter is reviewed.

49

Classroom and home Work skills

Parents and teachers can teach children to actively listen in the class. They should encourage pre-class reading and ask them to correlate the newly acquired knowledge with previous knowledge to improve understanding of the subject. Teachers can guide children regarding the methodology of taking good notes in the class. Children should revise notes after the class and update the notes using text books and reference books. Children should give top priority to completion of homework. While doing homework, emphasis should be laid upon understanding and memorizing the study material.

Expression Study Skills

Expression skills enable students to demonstrate their knowledge in the tests and include exam taking strategies.

Parents should ensure that children get enough sleep and healthy nutrition especially during exam like pencils, erasers, sharpeners, rulers, pens etc. should be kept ready a day before the exam. On the day of the exam, Children should have a light nutritious breakfast. They should think and verbalize positive self-motivating statements like "I have studied regularly throughout the year and I shall do well in the exams. Last minute discussions with friends should be avoided. They should time the question paper and leave a few minutes at the end of the paper for revision. They should write legibly and neatly. They should first attempt those questions that they know the best. After the exam, the parents should refrain from discussing the answers and mistakes and should allow the children to prepare calmly for the next exam.

Students should avoid stress building beliefs like "I should always stand first" or I should always score 100%". Students believe that putting in their best effort would ensure the best results. Students should enjoy the process of learning and should not feel burdened by exams.

STRESS IN EXAMINATION

Stress is nothing but an organism's total response to environmental demands or pressures. Stress is common place in today's life. Stress can affect any one, right from a newborn baby till old age and death. But its impact varies from age to age and from underlying cause. Children are no exception to this and Stress occurs in virtually all children at some stage or other as a response to something threatening or dangerous. Stress is not bad all the time. Stress less life will stop motivation and progress of an individual (like a loose rubber band) and too much stress will be detrimental to physical and mental health (like a stretched rubber band). Therefore, we can classify stress as 'eu stress' (good stress) and 'distress' (bad stress).

People interested in well-being of children should not be only aware of physical needs of children but their psychological needs too. If psychological needs are not fulfilled properly, and then it may lead to undue stress and dire complications of stress.

WHAT HAPPENS WHEN CHILD IS STRESSED (Neuro-biological Changes in Body)

As proved, stress affects individual's mind and body also. Brain is the important organ which gets involved and affected in response to stress. How this happens is very interesting. Brain and Cardiovascular system as well as immune system have two way communications via endocrinal system. When stress is

49

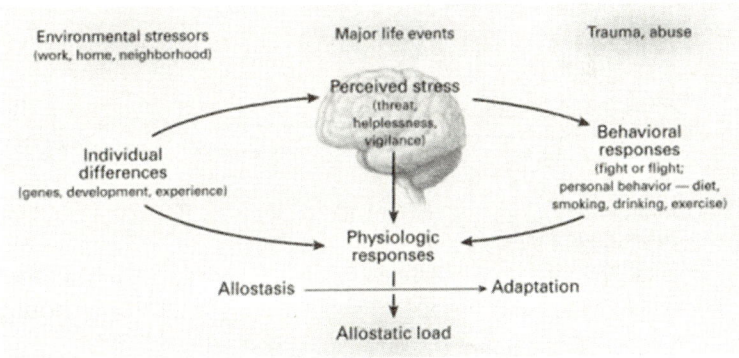

Etiopathogenesis

acute or transitional, there is "Flight or Fight" response. Various endocrinal secretions protect body and brain in short run. This is called as 'allostasis'. But when these stressful events occur daily, this produces a chronic stress ("allostatic load'). Chronic stress affects brain (particularly hippocampus, hypothalamus and other parts of brain,). Autonomous nervous system and Hypothalamo-pituitary-adrenal gland (HPA) axis is activated. This leads to adoptive as well as maladaptive effects. This alters behavior and physiological response of an individual leading to abnormal behavior and abnormal physiology (pathology/disease). Thus chronic stress affects body and mind as well.

Poor examination preparation and lack of confidence in spite of adequate preparation are two most important causes of examination stress. However, there are multiple causes leading

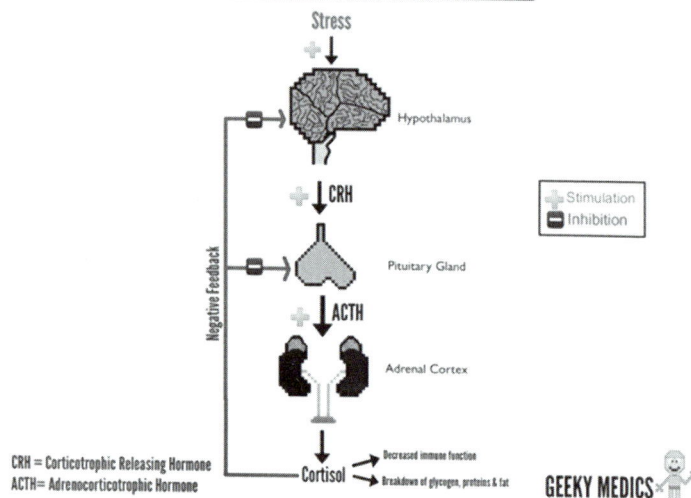

49

to examination stress.

Few of the life style issues are also important. Inadequate rest, improper nutrition, lot of temptations and stimulations, lack of physical movements and exercise are few of them. Even improper daily scheduling leading to less availability of time lead to lot of stress affecting their overall performance in examination.

Psychological background of an individual child may also lead to examination stress. Most of the children don't have control over examination situation. They all the time think of outcome (result) of examination and their thinking badly affect their performance. "If I get fewer marks, my parents will abuse me, my friends will laugh at me, I may not get a good branch for further study, and I may fail in my life too. Such negative thinking leads to more stress and less performance.

Every student has their own study style. However, children are not in position to identify which style will suit them. Studying without understanding, trying to recollect all portion of a subject, studying throughout night, binge studying will lead to lot of frustration and then depression.

Remember, problems at home or school can make children hard to concentrate—if family members are arguing or going through a tough time, it can make finding time to revise and concentrate even more difficult. Things affecting children's concentration could include: *family arguments,* problems with friends, *depression and feeling sad, having to look after people in your family, etc.* All these things will affect his study atmosphere and will lead to lot of stress during examinations.

Six Myths About Stress

1. *Stress is the same for every child*

   Wrong. What is stressful for one child may or may not be stressful for another. Each child responds to stress in an entirely different way.

2. *Stress is always bad*

   No. It's bad to assume that. Stress is to the human condition what tension is to a guitar string: too little and the music is dull and raspy; too much and the music is shrill or the string snaps.

3. *Stress is everywhere, so your child just has to cope*

   Not so. You can help your child plan her study so well that stress will not overwhelm your child or you. Effective planning involves setting priorities and working on simple problems first, solving them, and then going on to more complex difficulties. All the problems just seem to be equal and stress seems to be everywhere.

4. *The best techniques for beating stress are the popular ones*

   Not true. No universally effective stress-reduction techniques exist. We are all different and react to different things differently. Only a programmed tailored to the individual's needs can work.

5. *No sleeplessness, no extra sweating—so no symptoms*

   Wrong. Absence of symptoms does not mean an absence of stress. In fact, camouflaging symptoms might be distressful for your child and me. It is always a denial of symptoms, not the absence of them.

6. *Only the major symptoms of stress require attention*

Not in reality. Although the 'minor' symptoms, such as continuous headaches or stomach cramps, may be safely ignored, they may be the early warnings that your child needs stress management.

If you are free of these myths, you can take the next step to recognize the causes, which lead to reduce stress in your child.

Distorted thinking about exams is the major cause of distress.

Distorted thinking is the unrealistic way your child may think about herself and the exams. Some children feel inadequate and are afraid that exams will reveal their true inabilities. Several worry excessively about the grades/marks they will receive as if worrying over grades will help them prepare better. Many endlessly compare themselves with classmates or worry about how family or friends will react. You need to talk to your child about it and encourage her to share her feelings. This is the only way to get help! A problem shared is a problem halved.

HOW TO IDENTIFY EXAMINATION STRESS

There are no laboratory tests to diagnose examination stress. But keen and careful observation and meaningful verbal and nonverbal communication during examination period will give some hints in identifying a stressful child. A few of them are:

1. Change in sleeping pattern: Difficulty getting in sleep or problems for wake up

2. Change in appetite, may be increased or decreased appetite without any specific physical illness.

3. Feeling of tiredness, sad feeling, irritability, change in mood without any specific underlying illness.

4. Body ache, headache, migraine and non-specific pains without any detectable physical problem.

5. Stomach upsets, loose motions

6. Unnecessary forgetfulness

7. Loss of interest in routine activities, hobbies

8. Evidence of increased susceptibility for infections, especially common cold and flu.

9. Increased heart rate, perspiration without evidence of heart disease.

Before labeling any child as stressed child on above grounds, underlying physical illnesses should be ruled out carefully.

Tips to Avoid Examination Stress

1. General information

- *Make a plan:* Help and guide children to make a plan of a year. Planning will ease tension of study. This is the most important factor in avoiding future examination stress. Always update/change the plan as per circumstances and requirements.

- *Place and time of study:* Every child has own temperament, different body clock and his own liking. Respect his likings and plan time table accordingly.

- *Healthy life style:* There is direct link of stress and nutrition. Therefore, advise healthy, nutritious diet, in fact make it a habit. Avoid very spicy, very sweet or chunk food. Regularity in diet is most important aspect. Keeping child hydrated by giving enough water is important. Avoid strong beverages, soda, cold drinks, etc.

- *Regular and adequate* exercise is probably one of the best ways of dealing with exam stress. Enough and sound sleep for six to eight hours throughout year will help a lot.

- *Visualize success:* This one might seem a little out there, but sometimes it helps to imagine success. Think of yourself writing the exam and knowing the answers. Visualize the A+ on the paper. When you imagine yourself being successful, you're more likely to succeed. But don't just visualize studying—you actually have to do it!

- To have family at least one meal together in a day in relaxed mood, keeping away all worries and tension is great boost to every child. Do not discuss any serious problems of family matter during meal. It's important to have a change of scene and get away from the books and computer for a while.

- Teach children relaxation techniques. If child is really anxious, find a calm, quiet space and ask him to try breathing deeply in and out for a few minutes, *focusing your mind on something*

49

pleasant, like a beautiful place with happy memories. Though it seems difficult, this will help to reduce overall stress a lot.

- Communication and sharing is equally important to avoid stress. Teach him to communicate his anxieties and worries to, family member, school tutor or a student counselor. This will help him to relieve lot of stress.

Tips for the Revision Period

- See that your child prepares for proper and regular revision of the syllabus. Revision before main examination is important aspect to avoid stress in examination. Hence, leave plenty of time to revise, make detail plan and time table, keep time for relaxation and exercise in this time table, search and experiment alternative revision techniques, see that his books, notes and essays user-friendly. Ask them to use headings, highlighting and revision cards, and get tips on other revision techniques from teachers and friends with experience of exams.
- Everyone revises differently. Find out which routine suits your child the best—alone or with a friend or parent/care taker; early morning or late at night; short, sharp bursts or longer sessions; with music or without noise.
- Try not to make too many demands on your child during exam time. Arguments are counter-productive and will only add unnecessary stress and distract from revision.

Day before Examination

- Please see that your child gets get a good night's sleep before an exam, so discourage your child from staying up late to cram.
- Avoid stimulants; like tea, coffee, etc. can give you the impression that your child is somehow dealing with exam stress. But they can all leave your child craving more and, in excess, will either slow or bring you down, or over-stimulate your child. Therefore, better to avoid these things.
- *Sleep well:* Some anxiety and restlessness is common, especially if your child has low confidence level. But, relax your child by few encouraging words and be with him. If

49

you really, really can't sleep, don't panic. Some relaxation techniques will do a trick.

- *Relaxation:* Relaxation techniques are of great help during examination, especially before first day of examination. If your child is really anxious, find a calm, quiet space for him and ask him breathing deeply in and out for a few minutes
- Communicate/talk with your child if you feel he is stressed: Assure him that almost everyone finds exams stressful, so he is not alone. *Expressing his worries to a good friend,* family member, school tutor or a student counselor will help get him out of system.

Tips on Day of Examination

- Give adequate time for daily routines
- See that your child takes all the equipment he needs for exam, including extra pens and pencils, hall tickets and other needed papers.
- Also give a bottle of water, a snack and tissues.
- Give him very good and adequate breakfast. This is not only energy, but fuel to concentrate.
- Make sure he knows when the exam is being held and what time it starts. Give him plenty of time to get there.
- Ask him to go to the toilet beforehand!
- Avoid people who are stressing out.
- If he feel really anxious, ask him to undergo relaxation technique by breathing slowly and deeply while waiting for the exam to start.

Tips in Examination Hall

- A period from entering in examination hall till your child gets question paper is really crucial, which may create lot of tension and may affect his performance. Teach him following things before hand, make preparation and if possible, rehearsals too.
  - To read instructions carefully,
  - To see what is expected exactly, quickly survey each question,

- Divide time according to time required to answer each questions,
- To write answers of which he is very confident,
- To check time left for remaining questions in between and see that all questions are solved/attempted as expected,
- Reserve time for rechecking of answer paper
- Do not talk with anybody, do not look to other students, and do not hesitate to ask any technical problem to invigilators.
- If you think, question paper is difficult, do not get panic, and solve what you know first and your memory will help you to solve difficult questions too. Panic may trigger wrong buttons.

Tips after the Examination

Few things are really important in between crucial days of examination.

- Do not do postmortem of question paper of your children. Parents are always interested in knowing what examiners asked, what the/teachers taught and how their child performed. A quick review may be encouraging, but it may be discouraging too.
- Assessment at times is too harsh and may be wrong too. Don't assess.
- Assessment may harm next day's performance also. Avoid.
- Congratulate your child for the things he did right, learn from the bits where you know you could have done better, and then move on.
- Ask your child to relax, to relieve tension of today's examination, have some encouraging words, let him take some rest and prepare him for next day's performance.

Conclusion

Research has clearly proved those students who have learnt different study skills have a better academic performance compared to those who are not. Academic performance builds up a students' self-esteem and lays the foundation for future learning, career and employment opportunities. Hence, effective study skills should be taught to all students by parents, teachers and counselors.

Points to remember

1. Motivation to learn is of paramount importance.
2. Balanced diet, adequate sleep and physical activity is required to be effective in academic challenges.
3. Time management improves efficiency and avoids last minute anxiety.
4. Strategies to enhance memory and concentration skills should be learnt.
5. Expression study skills enable students to demonstrate their knowledge in the tests and include exam taking strategies.
6. Understanding of stress and examination stress is important and to avoid examination stress tips given are very important to remember.

49

50

Depression in Children

Ksh. Chourjit Singh, Chingthang Kshetrimayum, Suchit Tamboli

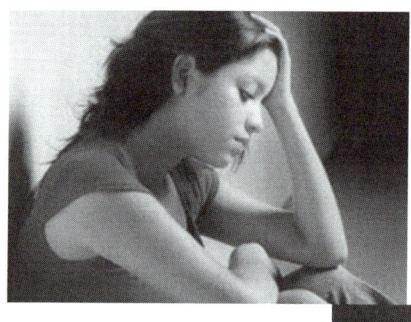

Depression in school-age children and adolescents remain long-overlooked health problems prevalent as in adults. Clinical depression is termed the common cold of mental illness. This condition, especially in childhood is a major health problem

The severity of problem in children at any given time is 5%. It affects 1% of pre-school children, 2% of school-age children and 5% of adolescents. Around 25–50% of all children and adolescents undergoing psychiatric treatment are for depression and its related problems.

It was also found that among the school going children, the problem was more common among the boys than girls (5:1) and among the adolescent, the ratio of the girls suffering from depression was more than boys (2:1).

The conclusive extent of the severity of untreated depression can be taken as important cause of suicide in adolescents, even adults.

Risk factors
- Children referred to mental health providers for school problems
- Children with medical problems
- Asthma
- Diabetes
- Epilepsy
- Many chronic childhood diseases
- Law and order problems
- Frequent bandh/strikes
- Frequent school closures
- Ethnic group clashes
- Insecure feelings
- Conflict environment
- Watching television a lot, i.e. more than 6 hours a day
- Rural versus urban children
- Sexually harassed children
- Children with family history of depression
- Genetically potential

50

Why depression runs in families?

- Genetics
  - Even if a child never contacts with depressed parents, child may also likely to be depressed
- Marital difficulties
  - Broken family/marital problems
  - Divorce plus depression in parents

- Parenting problems
  - Hard to be good parent when depressed
  - Parenting problems whether from parents or from child

At what age depression can occur?

- *Shortly after birth and very young*
  - Failure to thrive
  - Disrupted attachments to others
  - Developmental delays
  - Social withdrawal
  - Separation anxiety
  - Sleeping and eating problems
- *Between 6 and 12 years of age*
  - Fatigue
  - Sadness
  - Inability to feel pleasure
  - Irritability and Insomnia
  - Lack of self-esteem
  - Stomach ache and headache
  - Hallucinations
  - Agitation and extreme fears
  - Weight changes
  - Difficulty with school work
  - Apathy
  - Lack of motivation
  - Social withdrawal
- Adolescent
  - Over-sleeping
  - Socially isolated
  - Acting out in self destructive ways
  - Sense of hopelessness
  - Despairing thoughts
  - Weight changes

Future of Depressed School-age Children

If untreated in time—it affects the children in the following areas:
- School performance and learning

- Social interaction and development of normal peer relationships
- Self-esteem and life skill acquisition
- Parent–child relationship and sense of bonding
- Future of depressed school-age children
- Lack of trust—can lead to substance abuse
- Disruptive behavior
- Violence and aggression
- Legal troubles and even suicide

Depression thinking can become part of a child's developing personality, leaving long-term effects in place for the rest of the child's life.

50

What behavioral changes occur?

- Professional attention decreases
- Classroom disruption
- Expulsion from school
- School failure
- Injury to themselves or others
- Symptoms of ADHD
- Truancy
- Delinquency

Stress in Students Leading to Depression

- **Parental pressure to perform and to stand out among other children**
- **If not come up to their expectations, it results in**
  - Frustration
  - Physical stress
  - Aggression
  - Undesirable complexes
  - Under-performers
  - Negative traits
  - Shyness
  - Unfriendliness
  - Jealousy
  - World to loner

Results of Over-scheduling a Student's Life

- Non-availability of time for extra curricular activities after school
- No proper place for ventilation and breathing space
- Unwanted learning like music, painting or outstanding in sports
- Too many crammed schedule and unmindful of the children's choice
- Unadjusted school systems and tremendous amount of homework—spending their evenings, weekends and vacations
- Loss of interest in studies
- Under-perform due to excess academic pressure
- Students often carry enormous amount of anxiety and negative personal traits and massive attention problems
- Non-effortless learning
- Physio-psychological transition of students
- Mainly affected elementary to Junior High School

Diagnostic Points

Diagnosis: Miss world with depression crying (Dr MKC Nair)

MIS	WW	DEP C
1. Mood	↓	low or sad mood
2. Interest	↓	pleasure
3. Sleep	↓	(↑)
4. Weight	↓	Appetite

5. Worthlessness and guilt

6. Death wish or acts

7. Energy ↓ fatigue, libido

8. PMA ↓ (Psychomotor activity) slowing of movement /speech

9. Concentration C/o ↓ memory

D5/9 symptoms if present for 2 weeks one must suspect **depression**

- Transient depression or sadness
- Impairment in child's ability to function

50

- Two types:
  - Dysthymic disorder
  - Major depressions
- Dysthymic disorder—less severe but lasts longer
- Chronic depression/irritability >1 year
- Onset at about 7 years of age
- 2–6 symptoms within 5 years
- Leads to major depression/double depression
- Untreated dysthymic disorder will experience remission within 6 years
- Prevalence of depression increases with age—5 percent of all teens

50

WHAT CAN BE DONE

Psychological: Teenagers can decrease stress with the following behaviors and techniques:

1. Do daily exercise and have regular eating habits.
2. Avoid excess caffeine intake that can increase feeling of anxiety and agitation
3. Learn relaxation exercises
4. Develop assertiveness training skills.
5. Rehearse and practice situations, which cause stress
6. Learn practical coping skills
7. Decrease negative self talk; challenge negative thought about yourself with alternative neutral or positive thoughts.
8. Learn to feel good about doing a competent or 'good enough' job rather than demanding perfection from yourself and others
9. Take a break from stressful situations.
10. Build a network of friends who help you cope in a positive away.

HOW PARENTS CAN HELP

1. Monitor if stress is affecting their teen's health, behavior, thoughts, or feelings
2. Make them feel free to discuss their problems

3. Listen carefully to teens and watch for overloading
4. Learn and model stress management skills
5. Support involvement in sports and other pro-social activities.

Relaxation Training

A Class of techniques that include slow, controlled breathing; deep muscle relaxation (wherein the major muscle groups are tensed and relaxed); and guided imagery (e.g. the child is encouraged to imagine a calm, smoothing scene).

Cognitive Behavioral Therapy

50 CBT has also been used effectively in school settings. It has also been examined as bibliotherapy having children learn about the therapy components through reading, rather than interaction with a therapist.

CBT treats depression by addressing emotional, behavioral and cognitive skill deficits linked with the onset and maintenance of depression.

Core Components of CBT

1. Psycho education about the nature of depression and the treatment rationale.
2. Affective education and mood monitoring (the child learns to recognize and label his or her own feelings and the feelings of others, and to monitor and chart his or her mood).
3. Relaxation training (described previously).
4. Pleasant activity scheduling (the child learns to increases pleasant activities and decrease unpleasant and solitary activities).
5. Cognitive restructuring (the child learns to identify and challenge irrational, negative thoughts and replace them with realistic, positive thoughts).
6. Thought stopping or interruption the child learns to distract him or herself to stop ruminating, or obsessively thinking, about depressing topics).
7. Social skills and assertive communication (the child learns strategies to make friends improve his or her social support system and resolve interpersonal conflicts).

8. Problem solving (the child learns to generate and evaluate potential solutions to problems and to make plans to implement the chosen solution)
9. Reinforcement and self reinforcement (the child is awarded, and learns to reward himself or herself, for a veriety of behaviors, including increasing activity level, problem solving and social interaction).

Interpersonal Therapy for Adolescents

1. Psycho education about the nature of depression and the treatment rationale
2. Effective education and mood monitoring (described previously)
3. Attention to the primary interpersonal problems areas :
   a. Interpersonal conflicts (the adolescent develops problem solving and conflict resolution skills)
   b. Interpersonal deficits (the adolescent improves deficits in social skills and broadens his or her social support system)
   c. Grief and loss (the adolescent is assisted in mourning, in reestablishing interests and in increasing social contacts)
   d. Role transitions (the adolescent adjusts to his or her new developmental phase of life and adjusts relationships with parents and peers accordingly)
   e. Single-parent families (the adolescent accepts his or her new family situation and improves communication with parents)

Although interpersonal therapy is an adolescent focused intervention, parents and other significant individuals in the adolescent's life are sometimes brought into treatment sessions to assist the adolescents in dealing with interpersonal problems that the adolescent may be experiencing with those individuals.

- Supportive relationship with the therapist is very important: Patient and family education regarding the nature of the illness, complication, need of treatment is important.
- Relief of stress: efforts should be taken to alleviate any stressors that are identified during assessment. Presence of the stressors is known to worsen the prognosis.

- Improvement of communication of stressors through individual counseling. Improve communication between family members.

What else can be done?

- Diagnostic evaluation—success to treatment
- All disorders be discovered and addressed
- Indication for drugs:
    i. No response to psychosocial treatment
    ii. Severe symptoms
    iii. Bipolar depression
    iv. Psychotic symptoms
    v. Chronic recurrent depression
- Medication
- Mood stabilisers
    – Anti-anxiety
    – Antidepressants
    – Stimulants

Psychosocial Treatment

A. Psychotherapy
B. Supportive relationship
C. Relieve stress
D. Cognitive behavioral therapy
E. Family life education
- Individual therapy
    – Helping to cope with issues like family conflicts, low self-esteemed
    – Relaxation strategies
    – Mood and anger control
    – Better communication
- At school environment
    – Interaction with
        o School counsellor
        o Principal

  o Psychologist
  o Teachers and parents
 – Psycho-educational treatment
 – Speech and occupational therapy
 – Counselling
 – Curriculum modification
 – Resource classes
 – Behavioral modification system
 – Self-contained classrooms
- Home/parental environment
 – Family and home modification
 – Homely life environment
- Family therapy
 – Defining family members role and responsibility
 – Better communication and behavioral reward systems

50

Commonly used antidepressants

Antidepressant	Preparation	Starting dose	Usual/daily dose
Fluoxetin, e.g. Prodep Flunil	Capsule 20 mg Liquid 20 mg/5 mg 5 ml		20 mg
Sertraline, e.g. Serta Serlift	Tab. 50 mg	Children–25 mg Adolescents 50 mg	50 mg

There are three phases in the management of depression.

1. **Acute phase:** Continue the drug for 4–6 weeks.
 – Define target symptoms
 – Discuss side effects, dose schedule and delay of onset of antidepressant action.
 – Look for side effects.
 – If response is inadequate, increase the dose or change the drug.

2. **Continuation phase:** Continue the same dose for 6–12 months along with psychological methods.

3. **Maintenance**: This is to prevent recurrence of depression in the following situations:
- Multiple severe episode
- Family history of bipolar disorder or recurrent depressive disorder.
- Co morbid psychotic symptoms.
- Stressful/non-supportive environment.
- Residual symptoms.

Resistant depression: Poor treatment response may be due to the following reasons

- Inadequate dose, duration and compliance of drug treatment.
- Inadequate psychological intervention.
- Presence of co morbid condition—Psychotic/medical.
- Bipolar depression.
- Presence of chronic and severe stressors, e.g. sexual abuse.

Treatment for resistant depression
- Optimization of dose, duration
- Use a different drug
- Augmentation with and thyroid hormones, mood stabilizers (Lithium).
- Electro convulsive therapy (ECT).
- Always consider patient and family education and support.

Role of Pediatrician

Since pediatricians are the first medial persons consulted by parents for their children's problems, they have very important role in identification and treatment of depression. Diagnosis is very simple, without any costly investigation and treatment is also simple. This will definitely improve the quality of life of the child and his family and prevent morbidity and mortality. Depression a common childhood and adolescent problem can be identified and effectively managed by pediatricians. Only those children who require expert evaluation and management by a psychiatrist need be referred.

When to refer to a psychiatrist
1. No response/worsening

2. High risk of suicide
3. Relapse of symptoms
4. Atypical features
5. Psychotic features—delusion, hallucination.
6. Substance abuse.

Don't overload your child with too many after-school activities and responsibilities.

Let children learn at their pace.
Don't enrol them in every class along and don't expect them to be first in everything.

50

Points to remember

1. 25 to 50% of all children and adolescents undergoing psychiatric treatment are for depression and its related problems.
2. Family history of depression, broken families, marital problems, chronic medical problems, unrealistic expectation from self and others are some of the risk factors for depression.
3. Depressive thinking can become part of a child's developing personality, leaving long term effects in place for the rest of the child's life.
4. Behavioural modification therapy, relaxation strategies, rational emotive therapy and mood stabilisers as well as antidepressants can treat depression.

Childhood and Adolescent Suicides

Suchit Tamboli, Amol Annadate

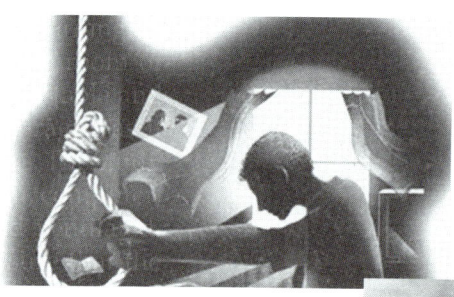

There was a time when suicide was considered as just an adult gesture and considered as adult manifestation of failure of stress management. The new era of twenty first century has come up with numerous societal changes like working parents, single parents, nuclear families, single child. All these factors has led to a new problem of increase in childhood and adolescent suicides

THE BURDEN OF SUICIDE

It is estimated that approximately one million people committed suicide in 2000; placing suicide in the top ten causes of death in many countries in the world ten to 20 times as many people attempted suicide. But, the actual figures are assumed to be higher although suicide rates vary across demographic categories, they have increased approximately by 60% in the last 50 years. Reducing the loss of life due to suicide has become a critical international mental health goal. Counselors can play a critical role in the prevention of suicide.

Suicide, Attempted Suicide and Para Suicide

Although the term suicide encompasses an intentional act of ending life, in pediatric age groups the terms Para suicides and attempted suicides are as common as suicides and also they deserve serious attention to prevent suicides. Para suicides and attempted suicides are histrionic gestures which are mostly attention seeking. But since they are most common predictors of future successful suicides they should be taken seriously and detail psycho social investigation of such child is carried out along with parents counseling.

Age

The youngest suicide recorded is of a 3-year-old child but the conceptual understanding of death starts after 7 years and hence 7 to 11 years shows the first peak age of childhood suicides the second peak being at puberty.

Protective factors that reduce the risk of suicide

They are considered insulators against suicide and include:
- Support from family, friends, and other significant relationships
- Religious, cultural and ethnic beliefs
- Community involvement
- A satisfying social life
- Social integration, e.g. through employment
- Constructive use of leisure time:
- Access to mental health care and services.

Although such protective factors do not negate the risk of suicide.

They can counterbalance the extreme stress of life events.

COMMON MYTHS ABOUT SUICIDAL BEHAVIORS

- **Myth 1:** People who talk about suicide will not harm themselves since they just want attention.
  This is *false.*

  A counselor must take every precaution when confronted with an individual talking about suicidal ideation, intent, or plan. *All* threats of self-harm should be taken seriously.
- **Myth 2**: Suicide is always impulsive and happens without warning.
  False

  Death by one's own hand might appear to be impulsive, but suicide may be pondered for some time. Many suicidal individuals give some type of verbal or behavioral message about their ideations of intention to hurt themselves.
- **Myth 3**: Suicidal individuals really want to die or are determined to kill themselves.
  False

  Most people feeling suicidal will share their thoughts with at least one other person, or call a crisis telephone which is evidence of ambivalence, not commitment to killing oneself.
- **Myth 4**: When an individual shows signs of improvement or survives a suicide attempt. They are out of danger.
  False

  Actually one of the most dangerous times is immediately after the crisis. Or when the person is in the hospital following an attempt. The week following discharge is one in which a person is particularly fragile and in danger of self-harm. Since one predictor of future behavior is past behavior, the suicidal person often continues to be at risk.
- **Myth 5:** Suicide is always hereditary.
  False

  Not every suicide can be linked to heredity and conclusive studies are limited. Family history of suicide. However. Is an important risk factor for suicidal behavior particularly in families where depression is common? Unresolved grief issues. In addition awareness of risk factors and understanding risk situations are critical counselor activities.

51

Social Factors Responsible for Childhood Suicides

1. **Low frustration tolerance:** The present day children and adolescents from all soci economic strata have a frustration tolerance for stressful situations starting from as low as wanting a toy to academic failures. Also the coping strategies are not inoculated either by parents or schools. Hence, children must be intentionally taught that ' this can happen ' and that it is ok to not have something or small failures is not the end of everything. Sports are an excellent way to inoculate these attitudes. But even failure in these sports activities also leads to frustration hence different types of games should be taught to children like purposely losing in a game against a friend and allowing him to win and see him being happy at the cost of our own loss. Such things should be appropriately rewarded by the parents but the reward should not be made the purpose of the game.

2. **Inability to accept a 'no':** Single children has lead to a trend of fulfilling all the demands of children and hence they are not used to listen a no. there have been two incidences where the cause of suicide was refusal to watch a TV program by parents and in other case it was refusal to join a dance class. These children want to revolt against slightest resistance by parents. This is a result of childhood habits and hence parents should be supportive at the same time they should teach children to accept no for few things. It is not that children should not express their likes about parental attitudes. Parents have to be patient listeners in such cases and at the same time better ways of coping with the dislikes should be taught to children.

3. **Lack of support:** In previous days grandmother and grandfather was a great support system. Uncles were proudly called ' bade papa'. But the change of family structure has left children and adolescent unsupported. All these factors supported the children and adolescents in a unbiased way. Although we have to accept the new nuclear family trend but at least a good contact should be established with modern day gadgets and children be given opportunities to interact

51

in a free environment with other family members. Instead off focusing only on ourselves as their counselors after a particular age let them select their own support systems.

4. **Academic pressure and comparisons:** Even today an academic failure stands out to be leading cause of suicides from 8th to 12th standards. Since the Indian education system follows the Chinese competitive and comparative education model students are overburdened with parental and societal academic expectations. Parents tend to compare their children with other siblings, friends, and relatives and expect them to top not just in studies but also in extra curricular activities like sports, dance, singing, etc. hence under performance and constant nagging about such failure on any front and comparison by parents leads to loss of self esteem in children leading to suicidal ideation. Hence, such things should be avoided. Children should be promoted to be what they are and they should be occasionally told that their parents love them just for being there and for no reason.

5. **Availability of easy ways and neglect of warning signals:** It is said that your eyes can lie even god but not your parents. If this is so how come we are failing to read the suicidal ideation in the eyes of our children. The reason is lack of communication and neglect of warning signals. Major depression manifesting as lack of sleep, appetite, interest in recreational activities, inability of verbalizing the problems, frequent crying, refusal to talk should be taken seriously and help by a pediatric or adolescent psychiatrist sought. In one such incidence an adolescent was brought with such complaints and the simple reason was that he had anxiety about masturbation. He had started getting suicidal ideation because of the pre occupation with masturbation and he believed it is against his cultural and religious values. He was properly counseled and the symptoms and ideation gradually settled. Family should have small meet every week where everyone talks about each ones problems and help such other for problem solving. At least one time in a day family should make it a point to have food together.

51

6. **Calf love:** Teen age break ups is a major cause of suicides in adolescents and it is associated with thrill, guilt or punishing the partner. Adolescents should be dealt in a friendly way in such situations. They should be always asking in a friendly way if they like someone. They should be taught the deep meaning of liking, love, bonding, marriage commitments and physical attraction at a particular age. Also they should be counseled about safe sex practices and explained that superficial liking and deep bonding with commitment leading to marriage are different. Also during break ups they should be supported and encouraged to speak up about suicidal ideation if any.

7. An **additional risk factor** for adolescent suicide is the suicide of prominent figures or individuals personally known by the adolescent. In particular among young people, there also exists the phenomenon of **cluster suicides**. A well-publicized attempt or completed suicide can lead to self-injurious behavior in a related peer group or similar community that mirrors the suicidal individual's lifestyle or personality attributes.

8. **Drug abuse:** Among adolescents 16 years and older. Alcohol and substance abuse significantly increase the risk of suicide during times of distress.

9. **Psychiatric disorders:** Mood and anxiety disorders, runaway behavior, and a sense of hopelessness also increase the risk for suicide attempts. A diagnosed personality disorder is associated with 10 times as many suicides as those without this diagnosis. Whereas as many as 80% of adolescents who kill themselves could be diagnosed with conduct disorder, PTSD. Or violent and aggressive symptoms. Depression is widely acknowledged as the principal factor associated with suicidal behavior.

To sum up suicide arises because of a broken bridge of communication between children, adolescents and parents, society. The rise in suicides is alarm to review our attitude of expecting the world to be our way. The best vaccine for this social epidemic is giving every child and adolescent a chance to be what he is.

51

ASSESSMENT OF SUICIDAL BEHAVIORS

A comprehensive assessment of suicidal behaviors is fundamental to effective counseling intervention and prevention. All suicide assessments should include:

- A review of relevant risk factors
- Any history of suicidal behavior
- Unchangeable biological, psychosocial, mental, situational, or medical conditions
- The extent of current suicidal symptoms including the degree of hopelessness:
- Precipitant stressors
- Level of impulsivity and personal control
- Other mitigating information, and
- Protective factors.

51

Suicide assessment requires an evaluation of the behavior and risk factors, the underlying diagnosis of mental disorders, and a determination of the risk for death.

Once an assessment is completed, it is important to rate the overall suicide risk in terms of severity. The scale below. Based on a **5-point** continuum from *nonexistent* to *extreme* suicide risk. could serve as general guidance for such a **rating**:

1. Nonexistent: Essentially. No risk of harm to self.

2. Mild: Suicidal ideation is limited, there are no resolved plans or preparations for harming oneself, and there are few known risk factors. The intent to commit suicide is not apparent. But suicidal ideation is present: the individual does not have a concrete plan and has not attempted suicide in the past.

3. Moderate: Resolved plans and preparation are evident with noticeable suicidal ideation. Possible history of previous attempts, and at least two additional risk factors, or more than one risk factor for suicide is present. Suicidal ideations as well as intent are present. But a clear plan is denied, the individual is motivated to improve his or her current emotional and psychological state if possible.

4. **Severe:** Clearly resolved plans and preparation to inflict self-harm or the person is known as a multiple attempter with two or more risk factors. Suicidal ideation and intent are verbalized along with a well-thought out plan and the means to carry it out. This individual demonstrates cognitive inflexibility and hopelessness about the future and denies available social support there have been previous suicide attempts.

5. **Extreme:** A multiple attempter with several significant multiple risk factors. Immediate attention and action is a must. Ultimately. The counselor's responsibility is to make a judgment and locate a point on the suicide lethality scale that helps identify the individual's potential for fatal self-harm.

51

It is often best to make a false positive than a false-negative error in judgment. Assessment data also can be useful in comparing an individual's pre- and post-counseling level of functioning for intervention and prevention purposes.

Adolescent and child assessment must minimally include:
- Clinical interview
- Behavioral observations:
- Collateral information from parents. Teacher's relatives and friends
- Assessment of risk and situational factors
- Assessment of ideation plan and intent and reasons for living.
- Availability and quality of family and peer support.

NEVER IGNORE A SUICIDE THREAT OR ATTEMPT!

Suicidal ideation is present in approximately 60% of children with a depressive disorder, and half of those reporting suicidal ideation will attempt suicide. Female patients are more likely to attempt suicide, but male patients have a higher success rate. Risk of suicidal behavior increases with history of previous attempts, co morbid psychiatric disorders, impulsivity and aggression, exposure to abuse or violence, and a family history of suicidal behavior.

MANAGEMENT OF SUICIDAL BEHAVIORS

Unfortunately. There are no agreed upon, set procedures for handling a suicidal or potentially suicidal individual. However counseling services must be responsive to the needs of the suicidal individual. The identification, assessment, and treatment of suicidal individuals call for the consideration of many important variables. Suicidal individuals have a range of needs from information to counseling to medication.

COUNSELING SUICIDAL CHILDREN AND ADOLESCENTS

Counseling is appropriate for all children and adolescents with suicidal behaviors and should focus on cognitive behavioral treatment with an emphasis on coping skills.

Effective counseling goals might include a better understanding of self, identifying conflicting feelings. Improving self-esteem, changing maladaptive behaviors, learning effective conflict-resolution skills, and interacting more effectively with peers.

Students are likely to turn to a friend during the initial stages of suicidal ideation. Training students to identify peers at risk for such behavior can assist with students receiving the help that they need.

Peer counseling programs have been found to increase student knowledge about suicidal risk factors. How to contact a telephone hotline or crisis centre and how to refer a friend to a counselor. Students need a forum in which they can receive information, ask questions and learn about how to help themselves and their friends with suicidal preoccupations. Unfortunately only about 25% of students will tell an adult if a friend is having suicidal ideations. Engaging parents and collaborating with other health agencies and schools also are effective prevention processes.

Parents of children in schools with suicide prevention programs should be involved in the school's efforts to educate. Identify and assist young people with suicidal intentions.

Teachers spend a lot of time with children and adolescents and also are generally good informants of student mental health issues. Moreover. When properly trained, school personnel can identify suicidal risk factors among students. When suicidal behavior occurs in a school setting it is important to contact parents.

Ensure that the student has received adequate assessment and support prior to returning to school and upon return. The student is received in a positive manner. Often students who have been confronted with the suicide of another student need to talk about the event and try to understand what has happened. Bereavement support group counseling at school can be an effective method for helping students copes.

When children have a combination of feelings of loss, hurt, anger, and frustration. Attention should focus on potential suicidal ideation and intention. Such counseling interventions should include follow-up or aftercare since some children might have difficulty for some time following the suicide of a friend or fellow student.

Management of suicide among adolescents becomes more important in the presence of substance abuse, personality disorders, and impulsivity and stressed peer relationships.

In terms of *suicide prevention*. Primary, secondary, and tertiary levels of intervention are important considerations. The primary level is concerned with groups of people who do not yet show signs of suicidal disturbance or where the disturbance is very limited. Prevention should focus on sustaining and enhancing role functioning within interpersonal and social contexts as well as significantly decrease emotional, physical, and economic risk conditions.

Education programs within the school can assist teachers in learning about identifying potentially suicidal students and train students to be aware of how they can be helpful to their troubled peers.

Community programs that focus on positive mental health also are helpful in suicide prevention. Although their effectiveness appears to be mixed. Suicide crisis centers and hot lines are central to many communities' efforts to prevent suicide.

PROVIDING HELPFUL INFORMATION TO THE COMMUNITY

- Counselors can provide community education and awareness that can help reduce the incidence of suicide. For instance , it is important for counselors to publicize the warning signs of suicidal behavior.

- Educating people about suicide may help to make communities aware of the warning signs of suicide, dispel suicide myths. as well as offer hope to those that are potentially suicidal and in need of rethinking their options.
- Community organizations, primary health care workers. Counselors can be helpful in disseminating suicide information such as specific circumstances (e.g. loss of jobs or failure in exam and subsequent family stability) and risk factors for suicide (e.g. depression mental disorders, drug and alcohol dependency family history).
- *Moreover.* It is important for counselors working in schools to assist with informing and educating teachers and parents about identifying students at risk for suicide. School counselors must train students to detect suicidal behavior and learn how to obtain help. For example, students involved in prevention programs need information and training in demonstrating empathy and active listening. As well as how to reach out to friends who may need help. Also, information that helps students weather the emotional storm of a well-publicized suicide or attempt goes far in helping to prevent "copy-cal" suicides.
- It is important for counselors to have a plan for dealing with the media in the event of a suicide. This plan should include **asking the media to not glorify glamorize or dramatize the death in order to prevent the possibility of contagion suicides.** For specific information, counselors, survivors' self-help groups are a constructive and empowering post vention method for people to use in helping themselves. Such self-help groups organized by those who are left behind can provide useful information on the grief process. Information about suicide, as well as the various roles of counseling professionals in helping survivors.
- Counselors involved with survivors' groups can be of tremendous comfort to the friends and families affected by suicide. Survivors often vacillate between feelings of guilt, anger and grief. In such cases counselors can provide an opportunity for survivors to process their feelings. Many

51

families have reported a need for counseling immediately following a suicide attempt. Such counseling helps families deal with the stress of the attempt and can clarify their role in attending to the attempter or dealing with the loss of a friend or family member to suicide.

- Where relevant, counselors also can help families and friends better understand the role of mental illness in suicidal behavior as well as reduce the risk of contagion or imitative suicides.
- Postvention group counseling includes procedures to alleviate the stress and mourning associated with a suicide and promotes a healthy recovery for the bereaved. Counselors can help people to accept the suicide. Move on with life in a positive manner, and develop a way to cope with their loss by establishing a survivors' group.

DRUG MANAGEMENT

Very important part of treatment. Only counselling is useful in mild cases but medicines plays important role in psychiatric disorder, depression, drugs like fluoxetin, sertraline should be given in proper dosage.

> **Points to remember**
>
> 1. Childhood and adolescent suicides are a failure of stress management.
> 2. Attempted suicides in childhood and adolescence are predictors of future successful suicides.
> 3. Conceptual understanding of death starts after 7 years and hence 7 to 11 years shows peak age of childhood suicides.
> 4. Low frustration tolerance, inability to accept 'no', lack of support (changing family structure), academic pressures and comparisons are major reasons of suicides in children and adolescence.

5. Major depression manifesting as lack of sleep, appetite, emotional labiality, and feeling of hopelessness should be taken seriously.

6. Effective communication with children and adolescents will strengthen his emotions and prevent suicidal tendencies.

7. Counselling and drugs with peer support group and parental awareness is important part of management.

8. Prevention of suicide should be given utmost importance to respect human life.

51

52

Substance Abuse in Children and Adolescents:
Assessment, Pattern of use, Early Detection and Treatment

N Heramani Singh, S Gojendra Singh, Ksh. Chourjit Singh,
Chingthang Kshetrimayum

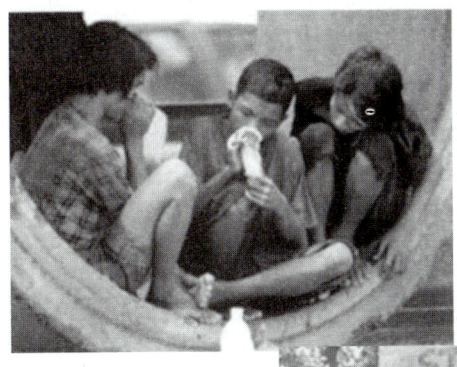

INTRODUCTION

Adolescence is a transitional stage of physical and psychological human development that generally occurs during the period from puberty to legal adulthood. The period of adolescence is most closely associated with the teenage years though its physical, psychological and cultural expressions may begin earlier and end later. It is largely a time of exploration and making choices, a gradual process of working towards an integrated concept of self. Even though for many adolescents drug use is just another form of experimentation, some of them do not spontaneously stop and continue it. Use of tobacco, alcohol, and other substances is a worldwide problem and affects many children and adolescents and early initiation of substance use is usually associated with a poor prognosis and a lifelong pattern of deceit and irresponsible behaviour.

The type of substances used has varied depending on the society and age of the adolescent. In India, an NGO survey revealed that 63.6 % of patients coming in for treatment were introduced to drugs at a young age below 15 years. According to another report 13.1% of the people involved in drug and substance abuse in India, are below 20 years. Heroin, Opium, Alcohol, Cannabis and Propoxyphene are the five most common drugs being abused by children in India. Another survey shows that of all alcohol, cannabis and opium users 21%, 3% and 0.1% are below the age of eighteen.

Recent studies also show that there has been a steady rise in inhalant addiction among the teenagers and majority of them use petrol, diesel, whiteners and nail polish removers. These inhalants contain organic solvents like toluene that could permanently damage their brain and organs, like liver and kidney.

Detailed Assessment

Once a substance use issue has been identified through screening, further assessment may be needed to determine the nature, extent, and impact of the substance use. The assessment process is longer and more detailed than screening, and it requires more experience and expertise. The objective of the assessment is to determine the meaning and significance of the (substance-using) behaviour to the adolescent and in relation to his or her family and environment. The type of intervention, its focus and its outcome depend to a large extent on the result of the assessment. The assessment also aims at identifying the deficits that need to be addressed (such as social and life skills deficits, family communication problems, educational difficulties, etc.) and the assets that could be potentiated. An important issue is matching patients with treatment. The main factor in deciding this is the degree of handicap, the level of use and the adolescent's circumstances. For example, less affected adolescents, with a relatively short period of use and less severe or absent psychopathology, respond better to cognitive behavioural approaches than those with antisocial problems, who respond better to interactional therapy, particularly group therapy. Clinical experience suggests that those using socially often need less-intensive treatment—family intervention or individual counselling may suffice. The treatment process should have a well-defined and realistic goal and should address all the therapeutic needs of the adolescent, including substance misuse problems.

52

The assessment should also determine the most suitable treatment setting for the adolescent. The possibilities include outpatient, residential and day programmes. Most cases that are not severe and chaotic can be dealt with on an outpatient or day basis, with particular attention to educational needs. However, most will need input from different professionals with different skills and the support and collaboration of a number of agencies such as social services, voluntary organisations, education and health.

Pattern of Use and its Significance

Adolescents use psychoactive substances for many different reasons. There are five different clinical contexts of adolescent involvement.

Exploratory or experimental

The primary motive in this type of substance misuse is curiosity and risk-taking. The mood-altering effects are secondary to the adventure of use. Use takes place mostly with others. The user may try more than one substance, but usually not more than a few times. The adolescent is experimenting with the 'mood swing' caused by psychoactive substances.

Social

The context here is strictly social, for example, parties, friends' houses, car parks, bicycle sheds, etc. The primary motive is social acceptance. The peer group plays a large role. Substances are shared freely or sold at cost. The aim is to fit in with the crowd and to loosen up. The adolescent is usually still experimenting with the mood swing.

Emotional or instrumental

In this context, the adolescent learns to use substances purposefully to manipulate feelings, emotions and behaviour, that is, to elicit or to inhibit certain behaviours and feelings. The adolescent is generally seeking the mood swing.

Generative/hedonistic

52

The purpose is to seek pleasure and to have fun. Use is characterised by binges motivated by the desire to 'get high' and feel good. The purpose is to elicit pleasurable feelings or to explore new feelings or emotions.

Suppressive/compensatory

The purpose is to cope with stress and uncomfortable feelings, that is, to suppress negative and distressing emotions. Mostly, use is solitary but also takes place with the peer group.

Habitual

Typically, the frequency of use begins to show a characteristic of compulsiveness and preoccupation. Lifestyle and activities begin to converge around psychoactive substances. Former relationships, activities and friends begin to be replaced by new substance-related ones. Sleep and concentration difficulties begin to appear. Withdrawal symptoms appear occasionally, especially after periods of heavy sustained use. Craving may occur, tolerance may increase and the adolescent may begin to think about use most of the time. Behavioural problems increase and school performance becomes seriously affected. The adolescent is preoccupied with the mood swing.

Dependent or addictive

This is the stage at which physical and psychological addictions become the main feature. Tolerance, craving, withdrawal symptoms and the compulsion to use become prominent. The adolescent is completely preoccupied with use and life centres around the substance and the next 'fix'. The adolescent takes substances only to feel normal.

• **Associated psychopathology (comorbidity):** Conduct problems have long been recognised as associates of substance misuse.

The strong links with emotional problems are now universally accepted. Consistently, reports indicate that affective symptoms predominate in females whereas conduct problems are more common in males.

Substance misuse is also related to increased suicidal ideation and attempted suicide. Many adolescents who 'overdose' do so while under the influence of alcohol or other drugs.

A major risk factor for completed suicide after parasuicide in adolescents is substance misuse.

Young substance misusers also show higher rates of psychosomatic complaints, anxiety, relationship problems and social dysfunction. Adolescents with poor coping skills tend to use psychoactive substances to deal with stress and as a means of emotional self-regulation.

There is also an emerging link between eating disorders (both anorexia and bulimia) and substance misuse, particularly alcohol use.

American literature consistently reports strong links between attention-deficit hyperactivity disorder and substance misuse in adolescents.

Another important point in the assessment is the need to ascertain the temporal relationship between existing psychopathology and substance misuse. Particular care should be taken when assessing adolescents with coexisting affective problems and substance misuse. Psychiatric problems may be the result of substance misuse, particularly in the case of central nervous system depressants. On the other hand, many adolescents with psychopathology may turn to psychoactive substances for psychological relief.

52

What are the highest risk periods for drug abuse among youth?

Research has shown that the key risk periods for drug abuse occur during major transitions in children's lives. These transitions include significant changes in physical development (for example, puberty) or social situations (such as moving or parents divorcing) when children experience heightened vulnerability for problem behaviours.

The first big transition for children is when they leave the security of the family and enter school. Later, when they advance from elementary school to middle or junior high school, they often experience new academic and social situations, such as learning to get along with a wider group of peers and having greater expectations for academic performance. It is at this stage—early adolescence—that children are likely to encounter drug abuse for the first time. Then, when they enter high school, young people face additional social, psychological, and educational challenges. At the same time, they may be exposed to greater availability of drugs, drug abusers, and social engagements involving drugs. These challenges can increase the risk that they will abuse alcohol, tobacco, and other drugs.

A particularly challenging situation in late adolescence is moving away from home for the first time without parental supervision, perhaps to attend college or other schooling. Substance abuse, particularly of alcohol, remains a major public health problem for college populations.

When young adults enter the workforce or marry, they again confront new challenges and stressors that may place them at risk for alcohol and other drug abuse in their adult environments. But these challenges can also be protective when they present opportunities for young people to grow and pursue future goals and interests. Research has shown that these new lifestyles can serve as protective factors as the new roles become more important than being involved with drugs.

Early Detection

The following warning signs but they do not mean that the youngster is using drugs, but they do raise suspicion.

School

- Drop in grades or achievement levels
- Skipping classes or days of school

- Dropping out of extra-curricular activities
- Defiance of teachers
- Breaking rules and regulations
- Excessive sleepiness
- Frequent suspensions

Family

- Change in attitude towards parents and siblings
- Isolating in one's room
- Lying
- Breaking curfew
- Blaming other for irresponsible behavior
- Selling possessions
- Stealing
- Strange, secret telephone calls
- Has money but no job
- Physically or verbally violent
- A variety of excuses for improper behavior

Changes in behavior

- Withdrawn, overly quiet
- Confused, disoriented
- Odor of alcohol
- Erratic eating and sleeping patterns
- Poor hygiene
- Overly defensive
- Easily upset
- Mood changes
- Started using street language
- Dilate pupils
- Reddened eyes
- Nervous, agitated, trouble sitting still

Religious behavior

- Decreased *davening, shul* attendance
- Ignores *Shabbos* rules and *kashrus*
- Cynical, skeptical

52

Legal

- Driving while under the influence
- Accidents
- Careless driving
- Possession of drugs
- Selling drugs
- Thefts

Prevention

Preventing or delaying use of psychoactive drugs, alcohol, and tobacco among adolescents is a critical and the simplest and most cost-effective way to lower the human and societal costs of drug abuse is to prevent it in the first place. Prevention is most promising when it is directed at impressionable youngsters. Adolescents are most susceptible to the allure of illicit drugs. Delaying or preventing the first use of illegal drugs, alcohol, and tobacco is essential. Not only does hazardous drug use put young people at risk of negative short-term experiences but those who do not use illegal drugs, alcohol, or tobacco during adolescence are less likely to develop a chemical-dependency problem. Like education in general, drug prevention is demonstrably most effective among the young. In addition to deterring some initiations completely, drug prevention programs help people who use drugs to use smaller quantities. Successful substance-abuse prevention leads to reductions in traffic fatalities, violence, unwanted pregnancy, child abuse, sexually transmitted diseases, HIV/AIDS, injuries, cancer, heart disease, and lost productivity.

The Central Role of Parents

While all parents are critical influencers of children, parents of children aged eight to twelve are especially influential. Children in this age group normally condemn drug use. Such attitudes and attendant behavior are easily reinforced by involved parents. Parents, who wait to guide their children away from drugs until older ages when youngsters are more readily influenced by peers or may have started using alcohol, tobacco, and other drugs, decrease their ability to positively influence children.

Parental example is a determinant of adolescent drug use. Children whose parents abuse alcohol or other drugs face heightened risks of developing substance-abuse problems themselves. There are an estimated eleven million such children under age eighteen in the United States. Everyday, these youngsters receive conflicting and confusing messages about substance abuse. Nevertheless, specially crafted prevention messages can break through the levels of denial inherent in these families. SAMHSA's Children of Substance Abusing Parents program is developing community-based interventions services to reduce those risks.

52

Teachers, coaches, youth workers in all areas of life from faith communities to scouts, and extended family members also provide youth with important protection from drug abuse and support for positive parental training by modelling, teaching, and reinforcing positive behavior. Such "occasional preventionists" are vital in touching the lives of children from chemically dependent families. Adult addiction can have a devastating impact on children. By taking small steps, adult mentors can make a permanent difference in the course of a child's life.

Treatment Options

The need for treatment and the type and intensity of treatment depend on the stage of involvement and the degree of impairment or handicap caused by substance use. However, the treatment plan should involve addressing the complex of the personal and environmental needs of the adolescent, including any concurrent psychiatric illness, social skills and educational deficits, physical health and family problems.

Detoxification

A process where an individual who is physically dependent on a drug is taken off the drug either abruptly or gradually. The purpose of detoxification is to minimize subjective and objective discomfort.

Individual Counseling

A recent development in individual counseling is the use of brief intervention techniques. This began with the use of simple advice in primary care settings leading to significant reduction in use, particularly in relation to alcohol use.

The cycle of change identifies 5–6 stages—intervention begins with identifying where in this cycle the person is. The objective is to help the young person move along from one stage to another through increasing motivation to change behavioural patterns, including substance use. This approach is particularly useful with resistant clients (such as adolescents). Different stages require different techniques. The stages and main objectives of the therapist at each stage are:

Stage I: Pre-contemplation

User is not thinking about stopping drinking—raise doubt; increase perception of risks and problems with substance use.

Stage II: Contemplation

User is thinking about change: "May be I should stop drinking"—tip the balance; evoke reasons for change; strengthen self-efficacy for change.

Stage III: Determination

User is determined to change: "I must stop drinking"—help to determine the best course of action for change.

Stage IV: Action

User actually changes: "I stopped drinking"—help client to take steps towards maintaining change.

Stage V: Maintenance

User continues not to drink—help client to identify and use strategies to prevent relapse.

Stage VI: Relapse

User goes back to drinking—help to renew contemplation.

Family Work and Therapy

Families can be helpful in the process of therapy. Families and family dynamics have been shown to be influential as risk factors for initiation and progression. On the other hand, most recovered addicts report family systems as being very helpful in their recovery. In particular, the family can help improve compliance with treatment that involves medication.

A recent approach in family therapy is multi-dimensional family therapy (MDFT). This is an outpatient, family-based, behaviorally–strategically oriented approach. It views adolescent drug use in terms of a matrix of influences (i.e. individual, family, peer and community). Behavioural changes occur via multiple pathways, in differing contexts and through different mechanisms.

During individual sessions, the teenager is helped to acquire communication skills and problem-solving skills to deal better with life stressors. Job skills and vocational training are also part of treatment. At the same time, sessions with the parents address parenting styles and belief systems. The parents are helped to examine their particular parenting style, to distinguish influence from control, and to develop parenting approaches that lead to positive influence on their child.

Group Work (Therapy)

Group therapy which involves peer confrontation seems to be effective for adolescents, at least in the short term. However, most substance misuse-oriented work has really been based on the Alcoholics Anonymous (12-step) model. The basic objective is self-help and relapse prevention. However, although this model of work can be beneficial for adults, there are some problems with adolescents.

External Support Network, Education and Employment

For adolescents in treatment, abstinence is a major change in lifestyle, and needs support to be maintained. Once treatment is completed, it is important for the adolescent, in order to function satisfactorily and 'stay off' drugs, to be able to return to an environment that will support this. The nature and degree of support must be explored as part of the continued review and assessment process. Such support will inevitably involve opportunities for adequate accommodation, education, training and employment. Often, it is also useful to provide psychological support either on a regular or an *ad hoc* basis.

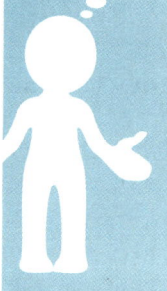

Points to remember

52

1. Curiosity and risk taking is the primary motive of substance misuse. (Exploratory or Experimental.)

2. To be accepted socially and peer group, to manipulate feelings, emotions and behaviours and inhibit certain behaviors and feelings is another reason.

3. Substance abuse is done to cope with stress and also to have pleasure and fun.

4. Abuse occurs during major transitions in children lives vis-à-vis puberty, divorced parents, separation from home to hostel where there is no parental supervision.

5. Early detection in school, family can be easily done when there are changes in behavior and personality as well as non-social behavior.

6. Multidimensional family therapy and group therapy is effective for adolescents.

FURTHER READING

1. en.wikipedia.org/wiki/Adolescence
2. www.childlineindia.org.in › Vulnerable Children › Children's Issues
3. Inhalant abuse on the rise.TNN | Jun 28, 2014.
4. Brogen Singh Akoijam, M. Nukshisangla Jamir, Ebenezer Phesao, Gojendra Singh Senjam. Inhalant Use among Schoolchildren in Northeast India: A Preliminary Study. Substance Abuse: Research and Treatment. Substance Abuse: Research and Treatment 2013:7 1–7.

5. National Institute of Drug use among children and adolescents: a research based guide for parents, educators and community leaders. 2nd Edition.
6. Harish Swadi. Substance Misuse in adolescents. Advances in Psychiatric treatment(2000), 6:201–210.
7. http://www.nida.nih.gov/prevention/principles.html
8. Preventing drug abuse. National Drug Control Strategy, 1999.
9. Nageotte CA, Murphy KM. Child-adolescent substance use disorders. Program and abstracts from the 153rd Annual American Psychiatric Association Meeting; May 13–18, 2000; Chicago, Illinois. Issue workshop 79.
10. Nageotte CD, Amato J. *Treatment of Addiction in Adolescent Populations.* Philadelphia, Pa: WB Saunders; 1997.
11. Chatlos JC. Adolescent drug and alcohol addiction: diagnosis and assessment. In: Miller NS, ed. *Comprehensive Handbook of Drug and Alcohol Addiction.* New York, NY: Marcel Dekker Inc.; 1991:211–233.

52

53

Value Education and Life Skill Training

Shailaja Mane

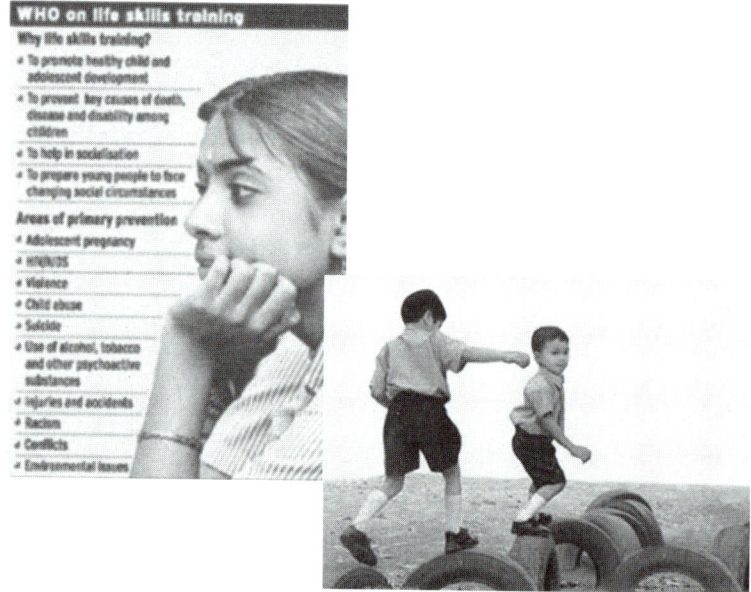

WHO on life skills training

Why life skills training?
- To promote healthy child and adolescent development
- To prevent key causes of death, disease and disability among children
- To help in socialisation
- To prepare young people to face changing social circumstances

Areas of primary prevention
- Adolescent pregnancy
- HIV/AIDS
- Violence
- Child abuse
- Suicide
- Use of alcohol, tobacco and other psychoactive substances
- Injuries and accidents
- Racism
- Conflicts
- Environmental Issues

"Children are the wealth of a nation and it is duty of the society to take good care of them."

—Jawaharlal Nehru

India is youngest country in the world at present. Adolescents form about 22% of India's population (approximately 331 million). Childhood and adolescence is a vital stage of growth and development. Adolescence is a period of transition from childhood to adulthood. It is characterized by rapid physiological changes and psychosocial maturation. These are the years when teens are most vulnerable to negative peer pressure, risk-taking, experimentation and misinformed decisions on crucial issues, especially relating to their carrier, behavior, bodies and sexuality. These decisions affect self development of the individual, family and society also. Adolescence is thus a turning point in one's life, a period of increased potential but also one of greater vulnerability.

Need for Life Skills Education

Current education practices are mostly knowledge based, least highlighting on life skills and attitude. Education system does not fulfill need of complete health education (mental, physical, emotional and spiritual). Education system does not prepare students for real life challenges. High level of stress, expectations along with changed lifestyle is leading to increased incidence of lifestyle diseases.

53

The host factors that promote high risk behavior are alcoholism, drug abuse, casual relationships, boredom, rebellion, disorientation, peer pressure and curiosity. The psychological push factors such as the inability to tackle emotional pain, conflicts, frustrations and anxieties about the future are often the driving force for high risk behavior.

Life skills training is an efficacious tool for empowering the youth to act responsibly, take initiative and control. It is based on the assumption that when young people are able to rise above emotional impasses arising from daily conflicts, entangled relationships and peer pressure, they are less likely to resort to anti social or high risk behaviors and suicides. Life skills include psychosocial competencies and interpersonal skills that help people make informed decisions, solve problems, think critically and creatively, communicate, effectively, build healthy relationships, empathize with others, and cope with managing their lives in a healthy and productive manner.

INTRODUCTION TO LIFE SKILL EDUCATION

A skill is a learned ability. Life skills are competencies that assist people for functioning well in the environments in which they live. Life skills enable individual to transforms knowledge, attitudes and values into actual abilities, positive and healthy behavior.

Acordina to Delors, learning life skills is to find "The Treasure Within". It is learning to know, learning to be, learning to do and learning to live together.

It is the need of the hour to shift concept of skills from survival and income generation skills (i.e. livelihood skills) to individual's capacity to fully function and participate in daily life (i.e. life skills).

53 Definition

World Health Organization (WHO) has defined life skills as "the abilities for adaptive and positive behavior that enable individuals to deal effectively with the demands and challenges of everyday life".

'Adaptive' means that a person is flexible in approach and able to adjust in different circumstances. *'Positive behavior' means* that a person is forward looking, even in difficult situations, can find a ray of hope and opportunities to find solutions.

UNICEF defines life skills as "a behavior change or behavior development approach designed to address a balance of three areas: knowledge, attitude and skills".

Life skills include psychosocial abilities and interpersonal skills that help people take decisions, solve problems, think critically, communicate effectively, build healthy relationships, empathize with others, and cope with the stress and strain of life in a healthy and productive manner.

Key Life Skills

The goal of life skills approach is to promote healthy, sociable behavior and to prevent or reduce risk behaviors, as well as make an impact on knowledge and attitudinal components. *There are two kinds of life skills*

1. *Thinking skills* are regarding thinking and relate to reflection at a personal level. It includes decision making, problem solving, creative thinking, critical thinking, etc.

2. *Social skills are* related to dealing with others, include interpersonal skills and do not necessarily depend on logical

thinking. It includes communication skills, empathy, interpersonal relationship skill along with self management skills like self esteem, self awareness, coping with stress and coping with emotions, etc.

The combination of these two types of skills is needed for achieving assertive behavior and negotiating effectively.

GENERIC LIFE SKILLS

1. **Cognitive skills:** Including search, selection, analysis of information; critical thinking; problem-solving; understanding consequences; decision-making; adaptability; creativity.

2. **Emotional coping skills:** Including motivation; sense of responsibility; commitment; managing stress; managing feelings; self-management, self-monitoring and self-adjustment.

3. **Social or interpersonal skills:** Including communication; assertiveness.

WHO has identified ten core life skills as vital, essential for everyday life. These skills are at the heart of skills based initiative for the promotion of health and well being of children and adolescents.

1. Self-esteem and self-awareness
2. Empathy
3. Critical thinking
4. Creative thinking
5. Decision making
6. Problem solving
7. Effective communication
8. Interpersonal relationship
9. Coping with stress
10. Coping with emotion

Self-Esteem and Self-Awareness

Self-esteem is how we value ourselves; perceive our value to the world and how valuable we think we are to others. Self-esteem affects our trust in others, our relationships; our work means every part of our lives. Positive self-esteem gives us the strength and flexibility to take charge of our lives and grow from our mistakes without the fear of rejection.

Self-awareness is the capacity for introspection and ability to recognize oneself as an individual separate from the environment and other individuals. As a form of intelligence, self awareness means understanding one's own knowledge, attitudes, opinions, our character, our strengths and weaknesses, desires and dislikes. Self awareness means recognition of 'self. It helps to recognize when we are stressed or feel under pressure. It is often a prerequisite to effective communication and interpersonal relations, as well as for developing empathy.

53 Self-control is the ability to control one's emotions, behavior, and desires in order to obtain some reward, or avoid some punishment.

Empathy

It is the ability to imagine what life is like for another person. It helps to have a successful relationship with our loved ones, society and to understand needs, desires, and feelings of other people. Empathy can help us to understand and accept others, to elicit support from others, to improve social interactions

Critical Thinking

It is an ability to analyze information and experiences in an objective manner by recognizing, assessing the factors that influence attitudes and behavior like values, peer pressure, media influence, values, social norms, beliefs, etc.

Creative Thinking

It is a novel way of seeing or doing things that is characteristic of four components—fluency (generating new ideas), flexibility (shifting perspective easily), originality (conceiving of something new), and elaboration (building on other ideas).

Decision Making

This skill helps us to make appropriate decisions about our lives. It helps to take active decisions about actions in relation to healthy assessment of different options and their effects.

Making decision after examining the choices and consequences in view of one's values and goals is **"Responsible Decision Making "**.

Problem Solving

It helps to deal constructively with problems in our lives by gathering information, evaluating future consequences and influence of values. Unresolved problems can cause mental stress and physical strain.

Interpersonal Relationship Skills

It helps to establish a rapport with the people interact and relate in a positive ways. It helps to make and keep friendly relationships for mental and social well-being. It may also mean being able to end relationships constructively.

Effective Communication

It is ability to express ourselves, both verbally and non-verbally, in ways that are appropriate to our cultures and situations. So that our ideas are effectively transmitted to others. Verbal communication means using language can be oral or written and nonverbal means communicating through body language, sign language, eye contact, through media, i.e. pictures, graphics and sound, etc. and writing. It also includes active listening, expressing and receiving feedback. It helps to express opinions, desires, needs and fears. It prepares ability to ask for advice and help in a time of need.

Coping with Stress

It is recognizing the sources of stress in our lives, its effects on us and ways to control levels of stress, by changing our environment, lifestyle and learning how to relax.

Coping with Emotions

It means recognizing emotions within us and others, being aware of how emotions influence behavior and being able to respond to emotions appropriately. Intense emotions like anger or sadness can have negative effects on our health if we do not respond appropriately. It includes assertive skills, negotiation skills, listening and saying NO, accepting refusal, etc.

Emotional Quotient and Social Quotient

Emotional quotient (EQ) is a measurement of a person's ability to monitor his or her emotions, to cope with pressures, demands and to control own thoughts and actions. It is very popular in the corporate world, where many businesses use EQ tests to help their employees determine and measure their emotional responses to various situations.

Social intelligence is the capacity to effectively negotiate complex social relationships and environments. Social intelligence is defined as "the ability to deal efficiently and thoughtfully, keeping one's own identity, employing apposite social inputs with a wider understanding of social environment; considering empathetic co-operation as a base of social acquaintance."

Advantages of Life Skills Education

Life skill education for adolescent is the need of today's world. It makes a person "a balanced adult" who contributes meaningfully to society. Life skills are applied in various aspects of life, in human relationships, learning about rights and responsibilities, in health issues like mental health, stresses, prevention of HIV-AIDS, sexually transmitted diseases, drug abuse, sexual violence, teenage pregnancy, suicide prevention, *social cultural issues*, etc.

Life skills are also very important for personal safety in prevention and management of child marriage, sexual abuse, physical abuse, child labor, dowry, child trafficking, child injury, puberty and reproductive health issues, etc,

Adolescents must learn about *'Life skills' because it empowers them to take positive actions to protect themselves, to promote health and positive social relationships.*

Life Skills-based Education (LSBE) has a long history of supporting child development and health promotion. In 1986, the *Ottawa Charter for Health Promotion* recognized life skills in terms of making better health choices. The 1989 *Convention on the Rights of the Child* (CRC) linked life skills to education by stating that education should be directed towards the development of the child's fullest potential. The 2000 Dakar World Education Conference included life skills in two out of the six EFA Goals. Life skills-based education is now recognized as a methodology to address a variety of issues of child and youth development.

Life Skills Education Program

The life skills program is a school based program where life skills are imparted in a supportive learning environment. They are applicable for all ages of children and adolescents in school. However, the age group targeted is mainly 10–18, adolescent years, since young people of this age group seem to be most vulnerable to behavior related health problems. The program is for the promotion of health and well being and targeted group is all children.

Life skills education involves a dynamic teaching process. The methods used to facilitate this active involvement includes working in small groups, pairs, brainstorming, role plays, games debates, etc.

Effective acquisition and application of life skills can influence the way one feels about others, ourselves and will equally influence the way we are perceived by others.

We all use Life Skills in different situations in daily life. The appropriate combination of life skills in a given moment is an art. Children learn their life skills from parents, teachers and significant others who act as their role model. They gradually learn to use a particular skill effectively in diverse situation to cope with challenges of life.

Life skills program empowers the youth to choose the appropriate values and behavior which are ingredients of positive health.

Various evidences shows that preschool enrichment and social development programs, which target children early in life, can prevent aggression, improve social skills, boost educational achievement and improve job prospects.

Interventions that Support Children in the Development

Of life skills can have positive impacts on young people's opportunities through improving pro-social abilities, educational attainment and employment prospects and can help prevent violence.

Schools need to be recognized as the single most important recognized forum to reach out to the young population. Any program to reach the adolescents and youth has to be incorporated into the educational system to be feasible, effective, and cost-effective. The teachers are the personnel who interact with the adolescents closely. They could be trained to transfer these skills to the adolescents.

53

Life skills based education is a Coordinated School Health Program can be implemented by using various components like comprehensive school health education, physical education, school health services, school nutrition services, school counseling, psychological, social health services, etc.

LSBE teachers training for all secondary teachers must be organized. Comprehensive social mobilization and advocacy materials covering all beneficiaries of the Country should be developed. Pediatricians, Adolescent pediatricians, Life Skills trainers, Teachers, Parents along with various NGOs and Government should work together for betterment of children and adolescents.

Children's Health is Nation's Wealth!
Our Future is in Our Hands!

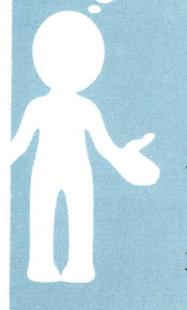

Points to remember

1. Life skills is defined as "the abilities for adaptive and positive behavior that enable individuals to deal effectively with the demands and challenges of everyday life".
2. Life skills training is an efficacious tool for empowering the youth to act responsibly, take initiative and control.
3. WHO has identified 10 core skills as follows
    i. Self-esteem and self-awareness.

ii. Empathy

iii. Critical thinking

iv. Creative thinking

v. Decision making

vi. Problem solving

vii. Effective communication

viii. Interpersonal relationship

ix. Coping with stress

x. Coping with emotion

4. Life skills program empowers the youth to choose the appropriate values and behavior which are ingredients of positive health.

53

FURTHER READING

1. WHO (1999), *Partners in Life Skills Training: Conclusions from a United Nations Inter-Agency Meeting*, Geneva.

2. WHO (2004), *Skills for health: An important entry-point for health promoting/child-friendly schools*, Geneva.

3. World Health Organization. *Life skills education for*
   a. Children and adolescents in schools: introduction
   b. Guidelines to facilitate the development
   c. *Implementation of life skills programs.* Geneva
   d. World Health Organization, 1997.

4. www.unesco .org

5. Life Skills Education and CCE- CBSE

6. CCE-CBSE Presentation

7. NAEP Teacher's Workbook for student Activities

8. Indian J Psychiatry. 2010 Oct-Dec; 52(4): 344–349.

9. "http://en.wikipedia.org/w/index.php?title=Life_skills-based_education&oldid=622227345"

10. http://www.who.int/violenceprevention/publications/en/index.html

11. *World Vision's Way of Contributing to Child Well-being-* August 2009

12. Life skills education for children and adolescent in schools. Division of Mental Health, World Health Organization, 1211, Geneva 27, Switzerland.

13. Knowledge and Resources for Adolescents- Kalinga institute of social sciences.

Reproductive Health Counseling in Adolescents

Sushma Desai

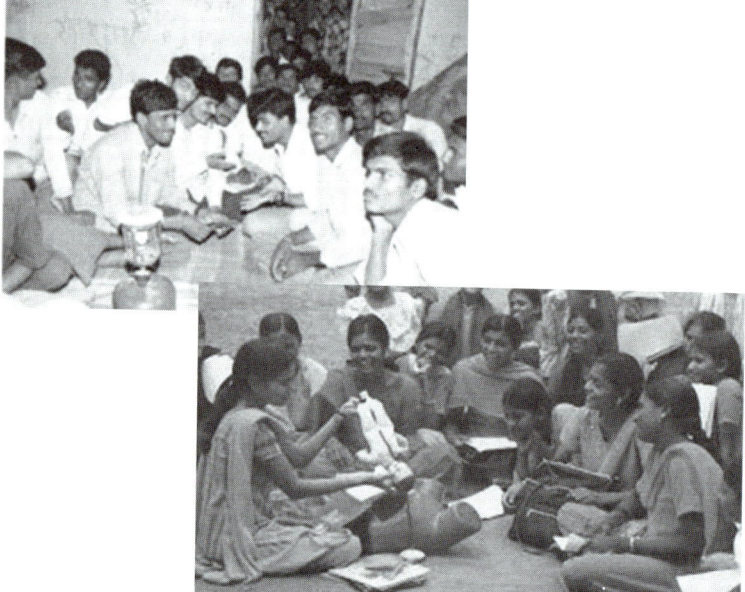

INTRODUCTION

Adolescents are those aged 10–19 years. Characteristic 'risk taking behavioral pattern, peer pressure, media influence, all contribute to sexual experimentation. Depending on their age and development, they are not always able to foresee the consequences of their behavior and to make safe decisions for themselves.

Children and adolescents need accurate and comprehensive education about sexuality to practice healthy sexual behavior as adults. Early, exploitative, or risky sexual activity may lead to health and social problems, such as unintended pregnancy and sexually transmitted diseases, including human immuno-deficiency virus infection and acquired immunodeficiency syndrome.

There is substantial increase in STD and HIV in the past decade. Children most likely to engage in early sexual activity will have learning problem or low academic attainment. Children will also have other problems like social, behavioral, emotional, substance abuse and mental health problems.

Counseling which contributes to their overall development will help them to clarify their feelings and thinking, and make more advantageous decisions. A style of counseling which is "non-directive ", that is it .helps young people to make their own decisions, is greater value to them in long run.

54

The International Conference on Population and Development recognized that "Full attention should be given to

1. The promotion of mutually respectful and equitable gender relations
2. Particularly to meeting the educational and service needs of adolescents
3. To enable them to deal in a positive and responsible way with their sexuality
4. Taking into account the rights of the child to access to information, privacy, confidentiality, respect and informed consent, as well as the responsibilities, rights and duties of parents and legal guardians to provide, in a manner consistent with the evolving capacities of the child, appropriate direction and guidance.

In 2007, GOI introduced HIV and AIDS chapter in the school curriculum for Xth std students. However, the content of discussion does not provide full details.

Adolescent Health Objectives

Identified by the Healthy People 2010, are as follows

1. Reduce the pregnancy rate
2. Reduce the incidence of HIV, Chlamydia, and other sexually transmitted diseases.
3. Increase the number of adolescents who practice abstinence.

Strategies to successful communication with adolescents
1. Address the patient directly and ask open ended questions.
2. Listen attentively without interrupting.
3. Observe non-verbal communication, posture and eye movements.
4. Avoid making judgment based on patient's appearance
5. Ask an explanation for unfamiliar slang terms the patient raises.

Recommendations for counseling
1. Put sexuality education into a lifelong perspective.
2. Actively encourage parents to discuss sexuality and contraception consistent with the family's attitudes, values, beliefs, and circumstances beginning early in the child's life.
3. Do not impose values on the family. Be aware of the diversity of family circumstances, such as families with samisen parents. Guide these families or refer them to agencies or clinicians that can help them if they report difficulties or if you are not comfortable assisting them.
4. Encourage parents to offer sexual education and discuss sex-related issues that are appropriate for the child's or adolescent developmental level.
5. Use proper terms for anatomic parts. Discuss masturbation and other sexual behaviors of all children, even those as young as preschool age, openly with parents.
6. Initiate discussions about sexuality with children at relevant opportunities, such as the birth of a sibling or pet.
7. Encourage parents to answer children's questions fully and accurately. Offer parents resources to assist their communication efforts at home.
8. Provide sexuality education that respects confidentiality and acknowledges the individual patient's and family's issues and values.
9. Promote communication and safety within social relationships between partners.
10. Ask about special friendships and relationships and explore their character.

54

11. Complement school based sexuality education, which typically emphasizes unintended pregnancy, STDs, and other potential risks of sex. When appropriate, acknowledge that sexual activity may be pleasurable but also must be engaged in responsibly.

12. Address knowledge, questions, worries, or misunderstandings of children and adolescents regarding anatomy, masturbation, menstruation, erections, nocturnal emissions ("wet dreams"), sexual fantasies, sexual orientation, and orgasms.

13. Information regarding availability and access to confidential reproductive health services and emergency contraception should also be discussed with early adolescents and with parents.

14. During these discussions, also be open and non-judgmental toward those with homosexual or bisexual experiences or orientation.

15. Acknowledge the influence of media imagery on sexuality as it is portrayed in music and music videos, movies, television, print, and Internet content.

16. Obtain a comprehensive sexual history from all adolescents, including knowledge about sexuality, sexual practices, partners and relationships, sexual feelings and identity, and contraceptive practices and plans. In discussing reasons to delay sexual activity or use contraception, frame the suggestions in terms of the individual's development, language, motivation, and history.

17. Be sensitive to cultural and family norms, values, beliefs, and attitudes, and integrate these factors into health promotion or behavior change counseling. Think of the potential of ask about, abuse or coercion in relationships or sexual activity.

18. Counsel parents about sexuality. Suggest opportunities for them to provide guidance about abstinence and responsible sexual behavior to their children.

19. Encourage reciprocal and honest dialogue between parents and children.

20. Counsel parents and adolescents about circumstances that are associated with earlier sexual activity, including early

dating, excessive unsupervised time, truancy, and alcohol use.

21. Ensure that adolescents have opportunities to practice social skills, assertiveness, control, and rejection of unwanted sexual advances. Provide specific, confidential, culturally sensitive, and **nonjudgmental counseling** about key issues of sexuality.

General Counseling

54

Counsel children and parents about normal sexual development before the onset of sexual activity, and encourage parent–child communication about sexuality. Parents should be encouraged to discuss explicit expectations for abstinence, for delaying sexual activity, and for responsible expression of one's sexuality.

Advise children and adolescents to discontinue high-risk sexual behavior and avoid or discontinue coercive relationships.

Discourage alcohol and other drug use and abuse not only for the direct benefits to the adolescent's health but also to prevent unwanted sexual activity or adverse consequences of sexual activity.

Handouts to reinforce safe sex practices and responsible decision making should be made available in the office or clinic.

Pediatricians may directly provide this counseling, and other members of the office staff, such as nurses, social workers, or health educators, may also provide counseling and health education.

   i. **Preventing unintended pregnancy.** Discuss methods of birth control with male and female adolescents ideally before the onset of sexual intercourse. Barrier methods should always be used during intercourse in combination with spermicide or with hormonal contraceptives. Providing access to contraception for adolescents who are sexually active is an important method of reducing pregnancy rates.

  ii. **Strategies to avoid STDs, including HIV infection and AIDS.** Abstinence should be promoted as the most effective strategy for preventing HIV infection and other STDs as well as for prevention of pregnancy. Adolescents who become sexually active need additional advice and health care services. Adolescents should be counseled regarding the importance of consistent use of safer sex precautions.

Pediatricians should assist adolescents in practicing communication and negotiation skills regarding use of condoms in every sexual encounter and should consider providing adolescents with information and demonstrations about how condoms should be used. Provide appropriate counseling or referrals for children and adolescents with **special issues and concerns.**

   i. **Gay, lesbian, and bisexual** youth. Maintain nonjudgmental attitudes and avoid a heterosexual bias in history taking to encourage adolescents to be open about their behaviors and feelings. If adolescents are certain of homosexual or bisexual orientation, discuss advantages and potential risks of disclosure to family and peers, and support families in accepting children who identify themselves as gay, lesbian, or bisexual.

   ii. Children and adolescents **with disabilities**. Rates of sexual activity for adolescents with disabilities are the same as those for adolescents without disabilities. Children in special education may not receive sexual education in school. Children and youth with disabilities should be provided developmentally appropriate sexual education. Parents may need reassurance and support in getting sexual education for children and adolescents with disabilities. Discussions should be initiated with parents or guardians of children with disabilities at a young age to encourage self protection and acceptable forms of sexual behavior. Community resources and support groups may also be of assistance

   Adolescents who are homosexual should be screened carefully for depression, risk of suicide, and adjustment related mental health problems. Similar issues are important to children unsure of their sexual orientation.

   iii. Other children at risk. Identify children at risk for early or coercive and unintended sexual behaviors at an early age. Children at increased risk include: a) Victims of physical or sexual abuse b) Those who have witnessed sexual violence

54

or physical abuse; c) Children with precocious puberty; and d) Children with social risk factors, such as learning problems, drug or alcohol use, and antisocial behavior.

Provide or arrange for counseling about sexuality for these children or adolescents. Refer to mental health services if appropriate.

Routine gynecologic services should be provided to female adolescents who have become sexually active. Screening for cervical cancer and STDs should be performed for sexually active females,

Become knowledgeable about sexuality education offered in schools, religious institutions, and other community agencies. Encourage schools to begin sexual education in the fifth or sixth grade as a component of comprehensive school health education and to use curricula that provide effective and balanced approaches to puberty, abstinence, decision making, contraception, and STD and HIV prevention strategies and information about access to services.

As many schools do not provide any information about contraception regardless of whether students are sexually active or at risk, pediatricians should consider presenting material at the school. The American College of Obstetricians and Gynecologists publishes the Adolescent Sexuality Kit: Guides for Professional Involvement. This series addresses AIDS, date rape, contraceptive options, and other topics that may be useful to pediatricians who plan to provide sexuality education.

Work with local public planners to develop a comprehensive strategy to decrease the rates of unsafe adolescent sexual behavior and adverse outcomes.

ADOLESCENT INTERVIEW QUESTIONS BASED ON THE HEADDSS MODEL

1. Home/health
Where and with whom do you live?
Are your parents your legal guardians?
How well do you get along with the people you live with?
How is your health in general?
Do you have any health problems?

54

2. Education/employment
Do you go to school?
What grade are you in and what school do you attend?
Are you in a specialized education program?
Do you have a job?

3. Activities
What do you do for fun?
Do you have friends to socialize with?

4. Drugs
Do you smoke?
Do you drink? If so, how much and how often?
Do you use drugs?

5. Depression (including suicidal feelings)
Do you ever feel depressed?
What do you do to cheer yourself up?
Do you ever want to hurt yourself?
Do you have anyone to discuss your problems with?

6. Safety
Do you feel safe at school?
Do you feel safe at home?

7. Sexuality
Have you ever had sex?
Are you using birth control?
Do you use condoms every time you have sex?
Have you ever been pregnant?
Did anyone ever make you do something that you didn't want to do?

The Transactional Analysis (TA) Model

Simple way to get across to the client the type of behavior he/she is practicing and why and how he/she can change.

This model is helpful for better understanding of emotional behavior.

Rational Emotive Therapy

Helps client to realize that his/her problem is not catastrophic, awful but has been made so by irrational views held.

Simple A-B-C therapy.

A= Activating event.

B= Beliefs which helps the client to identify his/her irrational behavior.

C= Concluding event.

P-LI-SS-IT Model

P= Permission giving.

LI= Limited Information.

SS= Specific suggestion

IT=Intensive therapy.

54

Points to remember

1. Children and adolescents need accurate and comprehensive education about sexuality to practice healthy sexual behavior as adults.

2. Early, exploitative, or risky sexual activity may lead to health and social problems, such as unintended pregnancy and sexually transmitted diseases; they also have behavioral, academic, emotional, and mental health problems.

3. Effective communication can be achieved by addressing the patient directly and asking open ended questions.

4. Listening attentively without interrupting, observing nonverbal communication, posture and eye movements, and being non-judgmental helps in counseling.

5. Adolescent Interview Questions Based on the HEADDSS Model and Rational Emotive Therapy: P-LI-SS-IT Model helps in giving therapy.

FURTHER READING

1. W.H.O. counseling skills training in Adolescent Sexuality and reproductive health.
2. Sexual counseling in Adolescents by Dr. Manjunath Hulliyappa, Wikipeadia.
3. Sexual and Reproductive Health of Young People: Dr. M.K.C. Nair.

54